European
School
of
Oncology

Monographs

Series Editor: U. Veronesi

E.J Freireich (Ed.)

New Approaches to the Treatment of Leukemia

A.M. Marmont, E.A. McCulloch, J.K.H. Rees
P. Reizenstein, P.H. Wiernik

With 37 Figures and 36 Tables

Springer-Verlag Berlin Heidelberg New York
London Paris Tokyo Hong Kong Barcelona

Emil J Freireich, M.D., D.Sc. (Hon.)

Ruth Harriet Ainsworth Professor
The University of Texas
M.D. Anderson Cancer Center
1515 Holcombe Boulevard, Box 55
Houston, TX 77030, USA

The European School of Oncology gratefully acknowledges sponsorship for the Task Force received from Farmitalia Carlo Erba.

ISBN-13: 978-3-642-75486-9 e-ISBN-13: 978-3-642-75484-5
DOI: 10.1007/978-3-642-75484-5

Library of Congress Cataloging-in-Publication Data
New approaches to the treatment of leukaemia / E.J. Freireich (ed.) ; A.M. Marmont . . . [et al.]. p. cm.–(Monographs / European School of Oncology) ISBN 3-540-52261-1 (alk. paper).–ISBN 0-387-52261-1 (alk. paper) 1. Leukemia–Treatment. I. Freireich, Emil J., 1927– . II. Marmont, A.M. (Alberto M.) III. Series: Monographs (European School of Oncology) [DNLM: 1. Leukemia–therapy. WH 250 N532] RC643.N48 1990 616.99'41906–dc20 DNLM/DLC for Library of Congress 90-10316 CIP

Softcover reprint of the hardcover 1st edition 1990

Bookbinding: J. Schäffer GmbH & Co. KG, Grünstadt
2123/3145-543210 – Printed on acid-free paper

Foreword

The European School of Oncology came into existence to respond to a need for information, education and training in the field of the diagnosis and treatment of cancer. There are two main reasons why such an initiative was considered necessary. Firstly, the teaching of oncology requires a rigorously multidisciplinary approach which is difficult for the Universities to put into practice since their system is mainly disciplinary orientated. Secondly, the rate of technological development that impinges on the diagnosis and treatment of cancer has been so rapid that it is not an easy task for medical faculties to adapt their curricula flexibly.
With its residential courses for organ pathologies and the seminars on new techniques (laser, monoclonal antibodies, imaging techniques etc.) or on the principal therapeutic controversies (conservative or mutilating surgery, primary or adjuvant chemotherapy, radiotherapy alone or integrated), it is the ambition of the European School of Oncology to fill a cultural and scientific gap and, thereby, create a bridge between the University and Industry and between these two and daily medical practice.
One of the more recent initiatives of ESO has been the institution of permanent study groups, also called task forces, where a limited number of leading experts are invited to meet once a year with the aim of defining the state of the art and possibly reaching a consensus on future developments in specific fields of oncology. The ESO Monograph series was designed with the specific purpose of disseminating the results of these study group meetings, and providing concise and updated reviews of the topic discussed.
It was decided to keep the layout relatively simple, in order to restrict the costs and make the monographs available in the shortest possible time, thus overcoming a common problem in medical literature: that of the material being outdated even before publication.

Umberto Veronesi
Chairman, Scientific Committee
European School of Oncology

Contents

Introduction

The spectrum of disseminated malignancies that are grouped under the heading of Leukaemia have played a signal role in the development of therapy for systemic cancer of all sites. A few milestones in treatment include the first complete remissions, the first anti-metabolites, the effectiveness of oral alkylating agents, the first combination chemotherapy regimens, the first immunotherapy and the first biological anti-tumour agent interferon, the first major supportive therapy modalities including platelet replacement, infection therapy, and both allogeneic and autologous bone marrow transplantation.

The primary reason that leukaemia is such an important diagnosis is the unique clinical characteristics of this disease which render it highly susceptible to systematic study in the clinic and in the laboratory. Firstly because the disease is systemic from the outset in virtually all of these patients. Localised treatment modalities thus play only a minor role and the need for systemically effective therapeutic strategies is evident. Perhaps more important is the fact that, because in leukaemia the organs of origin are the myeloid bone marrow, the lymphatic tissue and the blood, repeated sampling is technically simple and the samples are both liquid and relatively pure suspensions of tumour cells.

The fact that the last 40 years have seen major improvements in both the palliative and curative strategies of treating this group of diseases, has revealed enormous heterogeneity. This heterogeneity allows basic clinical investigations into the biology of the disease. In acute leukaemia, for example, patients who achieve a complete haematological remission provide the investigator with an opportunity to compare tumour cells collected at diagnosis to normal organ cells collected during periods of complete remission and to recurrent cells, if a relapse occurs.

Over the last 40 years there has been a wealth of clinical research productivity in this area. There are excellent animal models. The leukaemic cells and the normal cells can be grown *in vitro* and manipulated both in short-term and long-term culture. Particularly important is the fact that molecular genetics has been pioneered in the leukaemias, giving a major increment in our understanding of the biology of the malignant transformation.

It is for these reasons that the authors of this monograph were assembled as a Task Force. The task was to identify areas of basic clinical research which provide the most promising opportunities for the understanding of the biology of leukaemia and for developing new treatment and prevention approaches to this disease. We identified five major areas. The first is historically the senior strategy, chemotherapy. It is clear that the chemical agents have been responsible for a major change in the natural history of the leukaemic disorders. This has been associated with both an increase in the quantity of life and, even more importantly, a dramatic improvement in the quality of life for patients with these disorders. Certainly, a field that has been so prolific and productive over the last 40 years represents an area where continuing innovation and progress have occurred in the past and will most certainly occur in the future.

A second exciting area is the area of immunotherapy and host defense against the malignancy. This field was born with the observations of the non-specific immunostimulation associated with BCG scarification, but has now led to a broad spectrum of chemical and biological immunological stimulants which have definite anti-tumour activity. The observations of the effectiveness of allogeneic bone marrow transplantation has established the presence of "graft-versus-leukaemia" effects which are in a major way responsible for the curative activity of the allogeneic transplant. The exciting new information about natural killer cells (NK cells), and lymphokine-activated killer cells (LAK cells) has greatly stimulated the field of host defense against malignancy.

The third area that we chose was the new biologicals manufactured by recombinant technology. These human proteins have now begun to be studied in clinical trials. It is clear that a wealth of agents is available and an understanding of the stimulation and inhibition of proliferation and differentiation is now being systematically investigated both *in vitro* and *in vivo*. This area will certainly profoundly affect future developments in leukaemia therapy.

The fourth area we identified was bone marrow transplantation. Allogeneic transplantation has an established role in the treatment of acute leukaemias, but the recent important observations that allogeneic transplants can effectively cure chronic granulocytic leukaemia has provided an enormous impetus to our understanding of the treatment and biology of these diseases. In addition, the gradual amelioration of one of the most menacing complications of allogeneic BMT, graft-versus-host disease, by means of sophisticated depletion procedures of the offending immune-competent cells, will most probably afford relevant progress. On the other hand, the exciting developments in the area of autologous transplantation will almost certainly prosper in the immediate future. The introduction of the new growth factors in both types of marrow transplantation has also the potential of substantial progress. Finally, the observation that normal diploid cells have growth advantages *in vitro* in a number of culture situations and the possibility of chemotherapy directed at bone marrow *ex vivo* are areas of innovation which will certainly lead to new insights and to new therapeutic strategies for these diseases.

Finally, cytogenetics and molecular genetics have already had a major impact on the treatment strategies that are used for controlling leukaemic disorders. The most important aspect of the molecular genetics is the profound insight that it has provided for understanding the genetic basis of malignancy. The unique genes that have been discovered in a number of malignancies now offer the clinical scientist the long sought after specific target for a fundamental difference between the tumour cells and normal cells of the host. The observations relating to anti-oncogenes or suppressor genes, loss of heterozygosity, and point mutations in specific genes such as the RAS gene, have provided exciting new leads for developing new strategies for the treatment of these disorders.

Our Task Force met for three full days and reviewed our choices of therapeutic strategies. We decided to assign the six chapters in the book to the individual authors. It is our hope that this volume represents the productivity of the authors, because we found an enormously positive interaction during the deliberations of the Task Force.

Emil J Freireich, Chairman
A.M. Marmont
E.A. McCulloch
J.K.H. Rees
P. Reizenstein

Chemotherapy of the Leukaemias

John Kempton Harold Rees

University of Cambridge, Department of Haematology, Clinical Trials Unit, Addenbrooke's Hospital, Cambridge CB2 2QQ, United Kingdom

This review attempts to discuss the most recent developments in the treatment of the leukaemias, but in one chapter it cannot hope to be exhaustive. Some of the well established views and policies have been given less emphasis than the areas where debate remains, or where there have been interesting new ideas on the pathogenesis of the diseases and the therapeutic opportunities that these may provide. They are discussed in order: Myelodysplastic syndromes, acute myeloid leukaemia, acute lymphoblastic leukaemia, chronic myeloid leukaemia, chronic lymphatic leukaemia and hairy cell leukaemia. The section begins with a short history which may help to put our ideas today into perspective.

History

The first accurate clinical descriptions of leukaemia were reported simultaneously in 1845 by Craigie and Bennett [1,2] in Edinburgh and by Virchow [3] in Berlin. Craigie had seen a case in 1841 but had not recognised its significance until he watched the autopsy on Bennett's first patient in 1845. The interpretation of the findings are to some extent given in the titles of the papers. Bennett referred to "enlargement of the spleen in which death took place from the presence of purulent matter in the blood" whereas Virchow's paper was simply entitled "Weisses Blut" (white blood).

Barth [4] in Paris had, meanwhile, seen a similar case with massive splenomegaly. The microscopic appearances of the blood were examined by Donne [5] and reported in a publication on microscopy in 1844; the clinical features were described a little later in 1856.

At a meeting of the Royal Medical and Chirurgical Society of London on June 23rd, 1846, Fuller described a further case in which there was "enormous enlargement of the spleen and liver (...) coincident with a peculiarly altered condition of the blood" [6]. The blood had been examined on 3 occasions during the 8 days the patient had been in hospital before his death. On each occasion, he found "in addition to the natural corpuscles, a very large proportion of abnormal, granular, colourless globules".

Further cases were soon reported and in 1852 Bennett [7] published a monograph on "Leucocythaemia" in which 37 cases were described. Four years later Virchow [8], who had introduced the term leukaemia in 1847, published a very scholarly review entitled "Die Leukämie".

However, the condition was not uniformly recognised. In a discussion on Leukocythaemia in Paris on 9th January 1856, Barthez [9] is quoted as saying "There are enough diseases without inventing any new ones".

The predominating theory for 20 years following the initial description of the disease was that the principal organ involved was the spleen. This changed following the publication in 1868 of 2 papers drawing attention to the role of the bone marrow.

Neumann's paper [10], published on October 10th, 1868, associated the appearance of the "dirty yellowish-green" material in the bone marrow with an aetiological role in a patient who had died from "splenic" leukaemia. He therefore proposed an alternative "myelogenous" leukaemia in addition to the splenic and lymphatic forms. He subsequently developed his ideas in a review published in 1878 [11] and was the first to recognise that the production of cells by the bone marrow was a continuing process following birth.

The second classic paper appeared one month after Neumann's on November 10th, 1868. Bizzozero [12], its author, was at the time only 22 years old and faced considerable opposition within his own town. Referring to his earlier work in frogs and chickens, his paper concluded "In summary, the marrow probably contains an active site of production of white and red blood cells". Bizzozero later turned his studies to the coagulation system and introduced the term "platelet" [13].

A very interesting historical review of bone marrow function has been included in Tavassoli and Yoffey's monograph on bone marrow structure and function [14].

Lissauer, meanwhile, had not waited for the finer points of the pathogenesis of leukaemia to be established. He reported the treatment of 2 patients with Fowler's solution - liquid potassium arsenite [15]. He relates, in his graphic account of 1865, that his patient, "on bleeding from a small cut on the finger said, 'mein Blut ist ja ganz weiss' - 'my blood is completely white' - not realising this self-diagnosis condemned her to death".

The patient was treated with arsenic because the head of the hospital, Dr. Rosenkranz, had noticed that horses treated with arsenic for a long time had sleek shiny coats and improved digestion. A second patient with, what appears to be from the account, the first case of priapism associated with leukaemia, also received arsenic with a good short-term response. Unhappy love affairs were thought to be aetiological factors in both cases.

Arsenic remained a popular drug for the treatment of chronic myeloid leukaemia for the next 65 years, enabling Forkner and Scott [16] in 1931 to state that the "use of potassium arsenite in chronic myelogenous leukemia can be well supported by scientific data".

Other potential therapeutic agents were being investigated. Foremost among these were dichloroethyl sulphide (mustard gas) and the related B chlorethylamines and sulphides.

A detailed review of the history of the development of chemotherapeutic agents is outside the scope of this chapter, but the reader wishing to gain some perspective on the subsequent development of leukaemia treatment would find the effort very worthwhile. In general, original articles contain an authenticity and impact which cannot be fully reproduced in historical reviews, although excellent accounts have been published [17].

Only 2 examples of the early work will be taken here; the studies on nitrogen mustard and the discovery of the properties of 11 dehydro-17 hydroxycorticosterone (Compound E).

The toxic effect of dichloroethylsulphide in animals and man were first reported at the end of the first world war [18-21] and later by Pappenheimer and Vance [22]. Their experiments studied the effect on rabbits of intravenous injection of dichloroethylsulphide which had been distilled from a German Yellow Cross shell. Rabbits which survived more than 24 hours showed a marked decrease in the leucocyte count, the granular series being most severely affected.

Following the war, research declined but was resumed with increased energy again with the advent of World War II. The first clinical results were reported by Gilman [23,24], then a major in the army, and Goodman in 1944 [25,26]. The physical properties of Sulphur mustards had made them unsuitable, but nitrogen mustards in the form of their hydrochloride salts were stable and water soluble. The response of patients with Hodgkin's disease was good but disappointing in the leukaemias.

The first report of the action of steroids on a malignant tumour appeared in 1944 [27], although the manuscript had been received by the editor nearly 2 years earlier, on June 1st, 1942. The reason given for the delay was that the authors wished to repeat the studies before raising the hopes of patients and physicians, particularly as the quantity of steroid available was very limited. The tumour, a transplantable lymphoma in mice, was very sensitive to 11 dehydro-17 hydroxycorticosterone when the steroid was included in the drinking water of 7 of 14 mice which had been injected with the tumour: the female mice responded better than the male.

Myelodysplastic Syndromes

The myelodysplastic syndromes (MDS) are a heterogeneous group of clonal disorders of the bone marrow haemopoietic stem cells, characterised by normal or hypercellular bone marrows and peripheral cytopenias of varying degree.
Patients who would satisfy the criteria for this disease have been described for the last 90 years. Rhoads and Halsey Barker [28] reported 100 cases of refractory anaemia, which included cases of tuberculosis, in 1938, but it is to Hamilton Paterson [29] that the credit is given for coining the term "preleukaemic anaemia". It was subsequently known as preleukaemic leukaemia, smouldering leukaemia [30], low-percentage leukaemia [31], the preleukaemic syndrome [32,33] and subacute myeloid leukaemia [34].
In 1956, Bjorkman [35] described "refractory anaemia with sideroblastic bone marrow" in 4 elderly patients in Malmo, Sweden, using the technique and terminology originally described by Gruneberg in the flex-tailed mouse [36]. Nearly 15 years later, "refractory anaemia with an excess of myeloblasts" was reported from France by Dreyfus [37] and Linman [38] described the features of "haemopoietic dysplasia" as a precursor of myelomonocytic leukaemia.
In 1976, the FAB group provisionally classified these individual sets of reports into 2 groups: Refractory Anaemia with Excess of Blasts (RAEB) and CMML [39]. Subsequently, a more definitive classification was developed by the same group [40] (Table 1).

Incidence

The early reports on the incidence of MDS relied on retrospective analysis and suggested a low incidence. The true value is probably higher but it is strongly influenced by the age of the population being studied. The largest analysis of the frequency of MDS comes from the Groupe Française de Morphologie Hématologique, which established a registry of 4,496 cases of acute leukaemia and myelodysplastic syndromes in 1982-83 [41]. There were 820 cases of MDS from 37 large university hospitals, but this represents an underestimate because of optional reporting during the first year and the decreased probability that all cases would have been referred to major centres compared with the acute leukaemias. More than half the patients were >50 years of age; 23% had Refractory Anaemia; 13% had Refractory

Table 1. Classification of Myelodysplastic Syndromes

Type	Peripheral blood	Bone marrow
Refractory anaemia (RA)	<1% blasts	Dyshaemopoiesis in 1, 2 or 3 lineages <5% blasts
RA with ring sideroblasts (RAS)	<1% blasts	As RA with ring sideroblasts representing at least 15% of erythroblasts
RA with excess of blasts (RAEB)	<5% blasts	As RA with 5-20% blasts
RAEB in transformation (RAEBt)	As RAEB or <5% blasts with Auer rods	As RA with 20-30% blasts or as RAEB with Auer rods
Chronic myelomonocytic leukaemia (CMML)	As any of the above with >1 x 10^9/l monocytes	As any of the above with promonocytes

Table 2. Incidence of MDS by age and sex (data provided by Dr. R.A. Cartwright)

	Subgroup of MDS									
	RAEB *		CMML		RAS		Total		RA **	
Age Group	M	F	M	F	M	F	M	F	M	F
20-29	1	-	-	-	-	-	1		1	-
30-39	1	1	-	-	-	-	1	1	1	3
40-49	4	1	-	-	-	-	4	1	-	7
50-59	8	4	1	5	8	5	17	14	9	9
60-69	22	14	18	10	12	14	52	38	30	30
70-79	48	33	36	27	33	30	119	93	68	57
80-89	30	25	24	39	27	28	83	83	41	52

* RAEB includes RAEB-t ** RA - considerable regional variation produced less reliable incidence values

Anaemia with Sideroblasts (RAS); 40% had Refractory Anaemia with Excess of Blasts (RAEB); 8% had evidence of transformation (RAEB-t) and 16% had Chronic Myelomonocytic Leukaemia (CMML). There is considerable variation in the percentage of sub-groups of MDS in the series reported which may reflect inconsistency in the use of the FAB classification or differences in the referral pattern from one area to another [42-46].

A recent review of haematological malignancies in England and Wales (1984-88) gives an overall incidence of 3.6/100,000 population, but it was more common in males (4.69/100,000 compared with 2.51/100,000 for females) [47].

The median age at the time of diagnosis is 65 years, but the incidence increases sharply with age (Table 2).

Primary and Secondary MDS

The majority of patients who develop MDS have no apparent cause and, in the absence of any evidence, are arbitrarily assigned the status of primary MDS. However, exposure to ionising radiation and cytotoxic drugs are known to increase the risk of MDS and AML. The capacity for producing malignant change varies between the cytotoxic agents, but the alkylating agents have been implicated more often than any other group [48,49]. Cuzick [50] has estimated the risk of developing MDS to be 3% for each year of treatment with melphalan for myelomatosis.

Secondary myelodysplasias are associated with a much higher incidence of karyotypic abnormalities [51], which may be related to the nature of the original disease and the treatment given.

Pathogenesis

The preleukaemic nature of MDS suggests that the same processes involved in leukaemogenesis are also involved in MDS.

Some of the most convincing evidence that the disease is clonal and that the target cell in MDS is the pluri-potent stem cell comes from the analysis of the glucose-6-phosphate dehydrogenase (G6PD) isoenzymes in women who are heterozygous for the enzyme.

Following the demonstration by Prchal [52] of the presence of a single G6PD iso-enzyme in the erythroid, granulocytic, B and T lymphocyte lineages, but not in the fibroblasts, from a woman with RAS, a single G6PD isoenzyme was found in the myeloid cells and B cells but not in the T cells of another patient with RAS [53].

Evidence from work on the heterozygous offspring of the domestic cat and the Geoffroy Wildcat has shown that clonal growth may be more common than previously suspected. After recovery from the myelosuppression induced by dimethylbusulphan, the Geoffroy-type G6PD emerged as the single dominant form in 50% of the cats treated [54]. Therefore, stem cell depletion alone can result in clonal evolution without malignancy being evident.

The theory of the pathogenesis of MDS is based on the proposal that there are at least two events involved: one causing the proliferation of a clone of genetically unstable pluripotent stem cells, and another inducing chromosomal abnormalities in its progeny.

The recent development of techniques which can identify point mutations in oncogenes in very small quantities of DNA, has provided further opportunities to examine the theories in a wider group of patients.

Hirai [55] and his co-workers in 1987 demonstrated that a point mutation at codon 13 of the N-ras oncogene was present in 3 of 8 patients with MDS, and they suggested that this might be related to conversion to a leukaemic phase of the disease [55].

The frequency of mutational activation of the N-ras oncogene has been well established in AML [56-58], but the rate of such events and their significance in MDS awaited the prospective study on patients with MDS carried out in London and Ulm [59]. Mutations were found in the K-ras and N-ras genes but there was no correlation with a conversion to AML. It was argued that this is compatible with the multistep theory of leukaemogenesis, if one assumes that the order in which the steps occur may vary. There is no clear agreement on whether ras activation is an early or late event in MDS [59], but other malignancies have recognisable patterns; human lung adenocarcinoma and colonic carcinoma show an early expression of K-ras [60,61], whereas ras mutation has been associated with tumour progression in malignant melanoma [62].

One of the striking findings in this large collaborative study on MDS was that the point mutations were heterogeneous. This may provide important information on the role of a variety of carcinogens in producing specific mutations [63].

In another large study in Wales [64], point mutations were found in 20 of 50 patients with MDS. There was, again, no correlation between the presence of mutations and the morphological and clinical stage of the disease, nor was there any evidence of preferential activation of a particular ras gene. In general, there is a higher frequency of activated N-ras and a lower frequency of activated K-ras in haematological malignancies [65], which again contrasts with the findings in other tumours such as urinary tract cancer, in which H-ras is preferentially expressed, and colon and lung adenocarcinoma, in which the K-ras is commonly activated [66]. The increased expression of N-ras and K-ras compared with H-ras reflects the degree of expression in normal haemopoiesis [65].

A second report from Cardiff established the incidence of mutations in the fms [67] gene which encodes for the cell surface receptor for the macrophage and monocyte-specific growth factor. 12.7% of 115 patients (67 with MDS and 48 with AML) had mutations at codon 969 and 1.8% had mutations at codon 301. The fms mutations were most common in patients with CMML (20%) and in patients with AML M4 (23%). In 2 patients the mutations appeared as the condition progressed from MDS to AML, but in one other case the mutation disappeared. They concluded that the expression of a fms mutation was not an initiating event in the development of MDS.

The role of autocrine growth factors in the leukaemic transformation of MDS may also be important and offers clear opportunities for therapeutic intervention, which have been reviewed by Russell and Reilly [68].

The evidence that MDS is a multistep disorder is also supported by identification of chromosome abnormalities. The report of the 6th International Workshop on Chromosomes in Leukaemia [69] included a correlation between the clinical and cytogenetic features in MDS. Forty-three percent of 247 had chromosomal abnormalities and 55 patients (22%) showed evidence of clinical progression during the period of observation. This was more common among patients with abnormal karyotypes than for those with normal chromosomes (29% vs 17%). The more complex the chromosomal changes, the shorter the survival. A greater proportion of patients with RAEB and RAEB-t had chromosomal abnormalities and the changes carried prognostic significance which was independent of morphology. The findings of the workshop provided an important follow-up on a group of patients reported earlier [70].

Similar conclusions came from the Third Morphologic, Immunologic and Cytogenetics (MIC) Workshop [71]. There was general agreement that the appearance of a chromosomally abnormal clone in a patient with MDS, who had previously been found to have a normal karyotype, was usually associated with accelerated disease.

The most common karyotypic abnormality is a deletion of a part or the whole of the long arm of chromosomes 5, 7 or 20, and the acquisition of additional genetic material such as chromosome 8. There is no correlation between a particular chromosomal abnormality and a specific FAB subtype [70-72], but some abnormalities have clinical and morphological features in common; patients with an interstitial deletion of the long arm of chromosome 5 (5q-) as the only abnormality, are often females with RA or RAEB [73]. Monosomy 7 is associated with a hypocellular bone marrow, pancytopenia and abnormal neutrophil function [74].

The type of chromosome abnormality carries prognostic significance [70-77]. The 12 patients with normal karyotypes reported by Yunis [77] were all alive at 49 months, whereas the median survival of patients with an abnormal chromosome 7 was 12 months and that of patients with a complex karyotype was 4 months; the prognostic significance of the karyotype was independent of the FAB type.

Patients who develop MDS following exposure to mutagens usually have complete or partial loss of chromosomes 5 and/or 7. Other structural abnormalities associated with secondary MDS include t(1;3) (p36;q21); t(1;7) (p11;p11) and t(2;11) (p21;q23) [75,78,79].

It is intriguing that the genes which code for granulocyte-macrophage colony stimulating factor (GM-CSF), macrophage colony stimulating factor (M-CSF) and the c-fms oncogene, are all found on the part of the long arm of chromosome 5, which is deleted in patients with 5q- [80,81].

Clinical Features

The clinical features of MDS are associated with the pancytopenias which are a hallmark of the syndromes. The causes of death are usually evenly divided between progression to acute leukaemia and the consequences of the cytopenias in the more indolent stage. The morphological features of peripheral blood and bone marrow are shown in Table 3.

Table 3. Morphological features of peripheral blood and bone marrow in MDS

Lineage	Peripheral Blood	Bone Marrow
Erythroid	Oval macrocytosis Anisopoikilocytosis Hypochromic fragments Basophilic stippling	Erythroid hyperplasia Dyserythropoietic features Ring sideroblasts
Granulocytic	Hypogranular neutrophils	Small agranular or sparsely granular blasts
	Pelger neutrophils with round or bilobed nuclei	Hypogranularity of promyelocytes, myelocytes and metamyelocytes
Monocytic	Monocytes agranular or with abnormal nuclear lobation Presence of promonocytes	
Megakaryocytic	Agranular or giant platelets	Micromegakaryocytes Large mononuclear megakaryocytes Large polyploid megakaryocytes with dispersed nuclei

Table 4. Prognosis of MDS

	% Progressing to Acute Leukaemia				Median Survival (Months)				
Ref No	84	85	86	43	84	85	86	87	43
RA	11	12.5	15	15	32	18.5	65	52	40
RA-S	5	11.5	10	20	76	21	70	29	52
RAEB	28	42	40	44	10.5	11	10	12	10.6
RAEB-T	55	59	60	-	5	4.5	5	11	-
CMML	13	9.5	30	40	22	9.5	10	2	11.1

RA=Refractory anaemia; RA-S=Refractory anaemia with sideroblasts; RAEB=Refractory anaemia with excess of blasts; RAEB-T=Refractory anaemia with excess of blasts in transformation; CMML=Chronic myelomonocytic leukaemia

The FAB classification does not consider bone marrow histology, although distortion of haemopoiesis and variability of bone marrow density can occur.

Abnormal localisation of immature myeloid precursors (ALIP) in a trephine biopsy is always present when the bone marrow blast count exceeds 5%, and can be used to divide RA and RA-S into good and bad prognostic groups, depending on whether ALIP is present or not [82,82].

The FAB subtype can predict survival and evolution to leukaemia as shown in Table 4, but the results are inconsistent.

The 5 subgroups devolve into 2 major groups, those with a high or low risk of transformation into acute leukaemia. Unfavourable prognostic factors include increased numbers of bone marrow myeloblasts, advanced age and neutropenia.

Patients with RAEB or RAEB-t have a much poorer prognosis than the remaining groups because there is a much higher incidence of progression to AML (56% in one series) [87]. Patients with RA or RA-S have a low rate of transformation to AML, but a high mortality due to infection or bleeding.

CMML has been studied in some detail, because it has rather unusual features which take it outside the pattern seen in the other subtypes of the FAB classification system [88-91]. The marrow demonstrates ineffective erythropoiesis and haematopoiesis, but granulopoiesis is usually effective and often associated with extreme leucocytosis.

In addition, the increased numbers of granulocyte-macrophage colony forming units (CFU-GM) and splenomegaly resemble the myeloproliferative disorders [92] and there are differences in the clinical course within the CMML group [88,89]. The varied prognoses in what appears to be the same disease has led to the term subacute myelomonocytic leukaemia being applied to the rapidly progressive form [93].

Various prognostic factors have been sought, but the system which has gained widest acceptance is the modified "Bournemouth" score [84]. One point each is allocated for Hb <10G/dl, neutrophils <2.5 x 10^9/l or > 16 x 10^9/l, platelets <100 x 10^9/l and bone marrow blasts >5%. A score of 2 or more predicts a median survivial of 9 months compared with 32 months for those with a score below 2. The latter group do not require treatment, whereas the high-score group have a pattern of disease which, in terms of its clinical course, is very similar to RAEB. A similar system has been used by Varela [94] and Kerhofs [95].

Treatment

The treatment of MDS has raised some of the most fundamental questions in the treatment of haematological malignancies and has formed the basis for extensive studies of its cell biology, pharmacokinetics and pathogenesis. It has also provided an opportunity for the development of more experimental forms of treatment, particularly the differentiating agents, because in many cases there is time to study the effects of drugs which do not have rapid cytoreduction as their main aim, and because many physicians feel that aggressive chemotherapy is not justified in these conditions unless an accelerated phase of the disease has been reached.

Cytosine Arabinoside

One of the most popular drugs in the management of the condition has been low-dose cytosine arabinoside (LD-Ara-C) given at doses of 5-30 $mg/m^2/day$ [96-107]. Ara-C is the arabinoside analogue of deoxcycitidine. After passage into the cell, it is rapidly phosphorylated to the active metabolite Ara-CTP. Ara-C is incorporated into the DNA but not into the RNA of myeloblasts [96]. *In-vitro* studies of the human myeloid leukaemia cell have shown that Ara-C slows DNA synthesis and induces terminal differentiation [97]. In man, Ara-C is rapidly eliminated by conversion to Ara-U, with a plasma half-life of 90-150 minutes. The treatment schedule and the rate of drug administration have, therefore, an important bearing on the drug concentration. The interpretation of this information and the means by which it may be applied clinically has led to a wide variety of therapeutic regimens.
The efficacy of low-dose Ara-C in the treatment of MDS has been explored in a number of uncontrolled trials [97-106]. The results are variable because of the differences in the schedules and the population of patients being treated.
Clinical trials with low-dose Ara-C alone or in combination with cis-retinoic acid have been developed by the MRC in Britain and the potential role of the retinoids have been considered elsewhere in this chapter. A recent review of the interaction between retinoic acid and cytosine arabinoside has been encouraging in acute myeloblastic leukaemia and may well be of value in MDS [108].
The naturally occurring 13-trans-retinoic acid appears to hold more hope for clinical use than its geometric isomer 13-cis-retinoic acid, at least in APL [109], but the response may not be predicted by the level of retinoic acid receptor mRNA expression [110], if the evidence derived from human leukaemia cell lines holds good for MDS.

Interferon

Interferon has recently gained acceptance as a potentially useful agent in the treatment of MDS, although one of the original studies using interferon-alpha was rather disappointing [111]. The mechanism of action of the interferons in this condition is not known, but the regulatory effect of interferons on natural killer (NK) cells may be one of the major factors in human tumour immunosurveillance [112,113].
One example of the clinical expression of depressed NK activity is the Chediak-Higashi [114] syndrome, in which there is a high incidence of malignant deaths. Alpha interferon production is low in most patients with MDS and NK activity is seriously reduced [115-117].
The association of a deletion of the long arm of chromosome 5 in approximately 15-20% of patients with MDS is particularly interesting if interferon normally plays an important part in promoting NK activity, because the gene related to interferon production has been located in the 5q (15-30) band-region and patients with monosomy 5 on 5q- abnormalities have been found to be deficient in alpha interferon production [118].
The response of the NK cells depends on the route of administration of the interferon. It is also possible to exceed an optimal dose and achieve a negative effect on NK activity [119,120].
Apart from the cytopenias normally found in MDS, the clinical picture is made worse by diminished function of the mature cells which are present. Alpha interferon enhances macrophage phagocytosis, occasionally affects antibody production by B lymphocytes, and enhances the cytotoxicity of sensitised lymphocytes [120]. It has very little effect on neutrophil function but has a beneficial effect on platelet activation [121].
Galvani [122] found a very good response to alpha interferon in patients with RAEB with improvement in anaemia and increase in NK activity. This study used leucocyte interferon, which may in part explain the results when compared with the modest responses obtained with the recombinant product in early trials. It has not been possible, however, to reproduce these results in a larger study [119,123].

Long-term therapy with interferon alpha 2c has been used in good risk MDS. The doses were 9, 6 and 4 mega units/wk for the first, second and third years of the trial [124]. The main benefit was a decrease in the infection rate and in 3 of the 10 cases a good but slow response in the blood counts was obtained. After treatment was discontinued, the haematological indices deteriorated and the incidence of infection increased in some of the patients.

While the long-term results of these and other randomised studies comparing alpha interferon with supportive care alone are awaited, other opportunities have been explored with the arrival of recombinant growth factors.

Growth Factors

The first reports of the response to GM-CSF came from the MD Anderson Hospital, Houston [125]. The 8 patients with various forms of MDS all responded with increased numbers of monocytes, eosinophils and lymphocytes. Three of the 8 patients had a 2 to 10-fold increase in platelet counts and 5 patients became independent of blood transfusions. Treatment was also associated with increased marrow cellularity and a decreased percentage of blasts in the bone marrow of patients originally having an excess.

A phase I/II trial in Frankfurt [126] used doses of GM-CSF ranging from 15-150 $\mu g/m^2$ by intravenous infusion for 7-14 days. Nearly all the 11 patients in the study were transfusion dependent and the median age was 64 years. The blood leucocyte counts rose in a dose-dependent fashion to values 130% - 1800% above pretreatment levels in 10/11 patients, but no sustained increase in reticulocytes or platelets was observed. Both CD4+ and CD8+ cells were increased in number, but there was no evidence of activation judging by the interleukin-2 receptor expression. The percentage of blast cells in the bone marrow increased in those patients having >14% before treatment began. The conclusion was that patients with moderately high percentages of blast cells may require other differentiation-inducing or cytotoxic agents in addition to the growth factor. The lack of reticulocyte response is in keeping with the findings of at least one group who have used GM-CSF for the treatment of patients with AIDS [128].

The general experience with recombinant GM-CSF in MDS points towards a dose-dependent increase in the number of leucocytes, neutrophils and eosinophils. The main side effects were fever, phlebitis at the infusion site and bone pain in a small number of patients and similar results have been reported by other workers [129].

Granulocyte colony stimulating factor (G-CSF) has not been available for use in many centres, but in one study [130] there was a useful decrease in the frequency of blood transfusions in nearly one-third of the patients. There was no evidence of conversion to leukaemia in any of the cases.

Several randomised trials have now begun in Europe and the U.S. in which GM-CSF is compared with a policy of providing supportive care alone. The use of the growth factors is clearly not without risks, but a better understanding of their role in the management of MDS will come from properly designed studies. The biology and clinical applications of growth factors in MDS and other conditions has recently been reviewed by Groopman et al. [131].

Other agents have also been used as differentiation agents, including the most active form of Vitamin D, 1,25-dihydroxy-vitaminD3 [132]. The results hitherto have been modest and further studies are being conducted.

The treatment of CMML with etoposide has recently been reported [133]. Seven of 10 patients responded well to a dose of 100 mg daily for 3 days. A particularly valuable aspect of the response was the striking disappearance of pericardial and pleural effusions in 2 patients.

An oral preparation of 4-demethoxydaunorubicin (Idarubicin) has been used in 6 patients with RAEB/RAEBt by Johnson et al. [134]. The outpatient treatment produced complete remission in 3/4 patients with RAEB and partial responses in the remaining case with RAEB and the 2 patients with RAEBt.

Bone Marrow Transplantation (BMT)

The place of bone marrow transplantation in MDS is rather limited because of the average age of the patients. However, the results from several groups show that allogeneic BMT is feasible for young patients with MDS [135,136]. The success rate is highest when the transplant is performed during the "preleukaemic" phases, such as RA or RAEB, and is considered the treatment of choice for this group of patients. This aspect of the treatment of MDS will be discussed in another chapter of this monograph.

Acute Myeloid Leukaemia

Acute myeloid leukaemia (AML) presents the most formidable clinicial challenge of all the leukaemias, with the exception of the myeloid blast crisis of chronic myeloid leukaemia.
The clinical features of AML are sufficiently well known and do not need to be discussed in a review such as this. The principal exception to the features which are common to all, viz. symptoms of anaemia, neutropenia and thrombocytopenia, is the profound coagulopathy which is found in most cases of acute promyelocytic leukaemia.
There is no universal agreement on the title which should be assigned to this group of diseases. In Europe, the general term acute myeloid (myeloblastic) leukaemia is used, whereas in the Americas the term acute non-lymphocytic leukaemia (ANLL) has become popular. Although the term AML has limitations, it has the merits of historical roots, and will perhaps regain the support of most haematologists. It is encouraging to read the Footnote to the report of the second meeting of the MIC Cooperative Study Group which states "AML as used here is equivalent to the term ANLL (acute non-lymphocytic leukaemia)."

Classification

Marcel Bessis [137] in his scholarly work "Blood Smears Reinterpreted" describes nomenclature as "one of the plagues of haematologic exposition" and draws attention to the separate European and American Schools which have developed. "Some terms are simply ill chosen and carry implications other than those intended. Some are ungrammatical or consist of a mixture of Latin and Greek roots, thereby offending scholars of the language". He concludes, in his discussion of the "classification" (his quotation marks) of leukaemia that "one day the present classification of leukaemias, though useful at the moment, will probably appear as bizarre as an ancient Chinese classification of animals into 13 categories including:

1) Those belonging to the emperor
2) Tame animals
3) Four-footed animals
4) Those resembling flies
5) Embalmed animals
6) Mythologic animals
7) Those not included in the foregoing classes.

"As illogical as this classification appears to us, it was very useful: it would have been deadly not to recognise an animal belonging to the emperor". It is interesting to see that the idea of a "misfit" group (group 7) had been developed many years ago.
These passages from the writings of an expert in this field are included, not to devalue the major contributions of more contemporary workers, but to underline the need to avoid a petrified view of the classification method.
The classification of AML has been reviewed from time to time by the FAB group. The system which has been proposed most recently is shown in Table 5 [138].

Table 5. FAB classification of acute myeloid leukaemia

Subtype	Features
M 0	Undifferentiated myeloblasts
M 1	Myeloblastic without maturation
M 2	Myeloblastic with maturation
M 2 baso	M2 with basophil blasts
M 3	Hypergranular promyelocytic
M 3 variant	Micro or hypogranular bilobed promyelocytes
M 4	Myelomacrocytic with both granulocytic and monocytic differentiation
M 5	Monocytic: monoblastic (M 5a) and promonocytic-monocytic (M 5b)
M 6	Erythroleukaemia, with >50% erythroblasts and ≤30% or >30% blasts
M 7	Megakaryoblastic

Table 6. Simple classification of acute myeloid leukaemia - Hayhoe

Type I

Granulocyte (G) and for monocyte (M) lineage only:
A: Well differentiated (>50% SB or BE positivity; includes t(8;21), t(15;17), (inv 16))
B: Poorly differentiated (<50% SB or BE positivity; includes most t(v;11))

Type II

Multiple lineage involvement G and/or M + E (dysplastic/PAS-positive erythroblasts) and/or ME (dysplastic megakaryocyte/precursors) includes most 5 or 7 monosomies or 5q-, 7q-, t(1;7) and trisomy 8, whether in secondary or apparently *de novo* cases and most 9q-, t(6;9) and 3q arrangements.
A: Well differentiated (>50% SB or BE positivity)
B: Poorly differentiated (<50% SB or BE positivity)

The FAB system has undoubtedly made a major contribution to the morphological organisation of this group of diseases; it has raised the general standards of morphology and it has made comparison between clinical trials of the treatment of AML more reliable.
The main drawback of the FAB classification is that it does not take into account the fact that, in the majority of cases, AML does not involve a single cell line but often 2 or 3; the multilineage expression of AML is not accommodated. The criteria for maturation can also be misleading, based as it is on the need for later members of the granulocyte or monocyte series. No weight is given to the degree of sudanophilia, butyrate esterase positivity or presence or absence of Auer rods. In a review of 621 bone marrow slides from patients entered into the 8th MRC AML trial, the remission rate was 67.5% for 480 patients with convincing features of differentiation described, compared with 54.6% from patients lacking the features of maturation [139].
Hayhoe has proposed an alternative classification (Table 6), which has shown very close correlation with the response to cytotoxic therapy [140].
A further classification has been prepared by the members of an expanded FAB group to take into account the increasing weight of evidence presented by the pattern of cell surface antigens and karyotype analysis.
The combination of morphology, immunophenotyping and cytogenetics has led to the MIC working classification of the acute myeloid leukaemias which was put forward following the second meeting of the MIC Cooperative Study Group in 1988 [141].
The classification established 10 subtypes of AML which are characterised by unique cytogenetic, morphologic and immunological criteria. These are:

M2/t(8;21)	M1/inv(3)
M3/t(15;17)	M2/t(6;9)
M5a/t(9;11)	M5b/t(8;16)
M4EO/inv(16)	M2Baso/t(12p)
M1/t(9;22)	M4/+4

At the present stage in the development of this approach, the system is limited by the fact that in about one-third of the cases of AML, no chromosomal abnormality has been identified and in others with well recognised non-random changes, such as trisomy 8, monosomy 7, 7q- or 5q-, there is no reliable allegiance to a single morphological subtype. The suggested MIC nomenclature for a case with trisomy 8 is therefore M?/+8. The committee concluded that it is, at present, impossible to use the system as a prognostic factor because of the small numbers of patients in some subgroups, lack of uniformity in the treatment and missing information in many reported series. A strong recommendation was made, however, that cytogenetic analysis and immunophenotyping should be carried out on every case of AML. This body of information will make it possible for a useful prognostic system to be devised. The role of the

Table 7. Mortality rate per 100,000

Age Group	Male	Female
0-4	0.4	0.41
5-9	0.33	0.27
10-14	0.41	0.36
15-24	0.69	0.55
25-34	0.87	0.77
35-44	1.27	1.14
45-54	2.22	1.74
55-64	4.66	2.98
65-74	9.98	5.59
75-84	16.47	9.94
85+	18.39	10.29
TOTAL	2.29	1.82

Adapted from Selvin S et al. 1983 [142]

classification system will be discussed later in the section on prognostic factors.
Acute myeloid leukaemia is a condition which predominantly affects patients in the older age groups [142,143]. The mortality rate according to age is shown in Table 7, for white persons only.

Management of AML

There are several issues in the management of AML which have produced controversy and some on which views are generally in agreement.
There can be little doubt that the principal reason for the improvement in the care of patients with the condition has been the better development of supportive care. Many of the drugs which form the framework for the design of treatment protocols have been available for 20 years but the remission rate has improved substantially during that time.

Prognostic Factors

When a patient presents with the clinical picture of acute leukaemia, the diagnosis requires careful morphological examination of the blood and bone marrow, immunophenotyping studies and cytogenetics. Although the latter 2 factors are extremely important in the process leading to a diagnosis, the situation remains that cytochemical staining of peripheral blood and bone marrow smears is the main diagnostic method. This will allow, in the majority of patients, a decision to be made on whether the features are of acute lymphoblastic or acute myeloid leukaemia and will make it possible to allocate the patient to one of the morphological subgroups.
The list of prognostic factors which have been claimed to have an effect on the prognosis in AML is awesome. There have been many reviews of univariate and multivariate analysis which have attempted to rationalise the treatment of AML [144-154].
Many of the features which have been said to be correlated with successful induction therapy appear to be epiphenomena. Some of the prognostic factors are listed in Table 8.
The results of these have consistently shown that age, performance status, cytogenetic pattern and a preceding haematological abnormality are the most important. Even the role of the last factor may be spurious because it is frequently associated with cytogenetic abnormalities and is more common in older patients.
The reliability of the FAB classification has been disputed with advocates of its value, counterbalanced by those who have found that it does not predict outcome. The M5 subtype, which is more common in children, appears to have a poorer prognosis in this age group [149-152]. This was not the case, how-

Table 8. Factors associated with the prognosis of AML (for remission induction)

Age	Presence of Auer rods
Sex	FAB classification
Performance status	Fibrinogen levels
Cytogenetics	Lactate dehydrogenase levels
Liver/spleen size	Peripheral blood counts
Labelling index	CNS Leukaemia
Day 6 marrow appearance	Drug sensitivity *in vitro*
Clonogeneic assay	Time to complete remission
Preceding haematological disorder	No. of cycles to complete remission

ever, in the most recent POG study (8498) [153], which was an unexpected finding. Their interpretation of the results made 2 points: 1) prognostic factors can be influenced by therapy and are not static factors; 2) there is some evidence that monocytic subtypes of AML appear to respond to regimens which include an epipodophyllotoxin [154].

Table 9. Induction Therapy for AML: response rates

Drugs	No. of patients	Age Group	C/R(%)	C/R(%) patients <60 yrs	Reference
Ara-C, DNR (3+7 DA)	226	Adults*	58	72	Yates [155]
Ara-C, DNR (3+7 DA)	508	Adults*	66	--	Vogler [156]
6-TG (1+5 DAT or 3+10)	846	Adults*	65	77	Rees [157]
Ara-C, DNR (3+7 DA)	450	Adults <55	68	--	Petti [158]
Ara-C, DNR, Etop (ADE 8+3+5)	132	Adults <50	67	--	Kurrle [159]
Ara-C, DNR, 6-TG (TAD 9)	272	Adults <60	69	69	Buchner [160]
HD, Ara-C, Mit (TAD 9) (HAM)			77	77	
Ara-C, DNR, 6-TG (DAT 3+5)	439	Adults <65	67	--	Cassileth [161]
Ara-C, DNR (3+7 DA)	228	Adults <45	60	--	Hayat [162]
Ara-C, ACR (6+7 AA)	19	Adults <60	68		Labar [163]
Ara-C DNR, 6TG/Etop	350	Adults <55	81		MRC10 Data
Ara-C, DNR, VCR (DOA 3+1+17)	515	Children <11 Adults <65	67.4		Jehn [164]
Ara-C, DNR (3+7 DA)	171	Children	82		Amadori [165]
Ara-C, DNR, 6-TG (3+10 DAT)	40	Children	91		MRC10 Data
Ara-C, DNR, Etop (8+3+5) Ara-C, DNR (3+7)	40 64	Children	70		Grier [166]
Ara-C, DNR, 6-TG (3+7 POG 8498)	254	Children	85		Steuber [167]
Ara-C, DNR (7+3)	194	Children	70		Lampkin [168]
Ara-C, DNR (7+3)	182	Children	80		Ritter [169]

Ara-C = Cytosine Arabinoside; DNR = Daunorubicin; 6TG = 6Thioguanine; Mit = Mitozantrone; ACR = Aclarubicin; VCR = Vincristine; Etop = Etoposide

* less than 5% children in this population

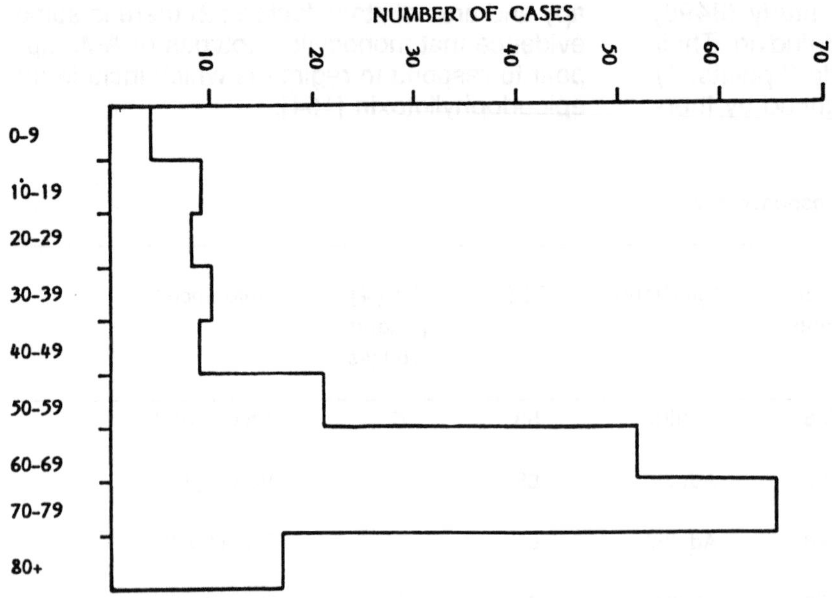

Fig. 1. Age distribution of patients not entered into MRC 9th AML trial

The complete remission rates reported from many large groups are usually about 65%. Some are summarised in Table 9. The reasons for the similarity is that the treatment regimens are often similar but a more important explanation - one that is not often acknowledged - is that the degree of selection of the patients is similar. Some idea of the degree of selection which was occurring in the U.K. during the running of the 9th AML trial was obtained by asking collaborating physicians to report all the patients treated at the centre who were not entered into the trial and to give a short explanation of the reasons. The distribution of the age groups is shown in Figure 1, from which it can be seen that the majority of patients were elderly (median age 65 years compared with a median of 55 years for the patients who entered the trial). The principal reason given for excluding the patients was the reluctance of the physician to give aggressive chemotherapy to the elderly and frail patients. The small number of younger patients who were not included reflected a personal preference on the part of the haematologist for one or other of the induction treatments being randomised. As a result of this simple questionnaire, it became clear that 1 in 3 patients arriving at collaborating centres were selected out of the study and that this was almost certainly an underestimate. The question of selection is a very important one as it can produce a misleading impression of the success rate in the treatment of AML. Another aspect of the problem was underlined by the Toronto Leukaemia Study Group [170], who showed that the remission rate varied between 44%, for all 272 patients registered with the group in a 4-year period, to 85% if patients were excluded who had received no treatment or partial treatment, were over the age of 70, or had evidence of a preleukaemic phase or other disease. The same issues have been raised by Copplestone [171].

Reasons for Failing to Achieve Remission

Although it is now recognised that certain characteristics carry a poor prognosis for achieving remission, relatively little attention was paid to the exact reasons for failure until Preisler's analysis in 1978 [172]. Similar studies have been carried out since [173,174]. Estey found that two-thirds of the patients who died after the third week of induction therapy, during which time very few patients have achieved remission, had bone marrow hypoplasia and might have entered complete remission had they survived; infection accounted for three-quarters of the patients who died during the first course of treatment.
The original categories of failure of Preisler have been modified in the analysis of the U.K.

Table 10. Reasons for failure to achieve remission in AML

% All cases	% Failures only	Types of failure	
9	23	A	Inadequate trial. Patient dies during or less than 7 days after completing the first course of therapy
2	5	B	Marrow hypocellularity attained but regenerating population consists predominantly of blast cells
8	21	C	Marrow hypocellularity with no peripheral blood blasts attained but patient dies during the hypoplastic period from haemorrhage
7	20	D	Decrease in bone marrow blast cell population to 10-15% (partial remission)
7	19	E	Failure of therapy to achieve any or significant effects on the marrow blast cell population
4	11	F	Any other course of events not covered by A-E

results in Table 10, which is based on 900 patients entered into the study over a 5-year period [174].

The important conclusion from this and other studies is that the majority of patients fail to achieve complete remission because they die of haemorrhage or infection soon after presentation or during the hypoplastic phase which follows treatment. This highlights deficiencies in supportive care rather than the inability of the therapy to clear the disease from the bone marrow. A minority of patients regenerate with blasts having passed through a period of hypoplasia, suggesting that the leukaemia population of cells has retained its advantage in growth rate or the pool of normal stem cells is inadequate. It seems rather inappropriate to place too much emphasis on subtle or radical changes in the induction therapy while infection and haemorrhage retain such a major role in the cause of death. Continued reappraisal of the toxicity and efficacy of first-line treatment is, however, important, not least because of the possible effect on long-term survival.

Supportive Care

There is a vast literature on the management of febrile episodes in neutropenic patients [175-188].

The principal papers are based around a knowledge of the spectrum of antibiotics available, their toxicity and the type of organisms which are likely to be involved. Although gram-positive and gram-negative bacteria make up the majority of causative organisms, the increase in the numbers of unsuspected fungal infections has been spectacular in the last 5 years. Traditionally, combinations of 2 or 3 antibiotics are given intravenously until the patient has been apyrexial for 48 or 72 hours and antifungal agents may be added if no response has been obtained with first-line therapy. The plethora of new antibiotics becoming available with conflicting claims of efficacy combined with a lack of toxicity, makes it difficult to make recommendations which would be appropriate for general adoption. However, aminoglycosides have become one of the most consistent components in an antibiotic cocktail - usually with one of the B-lactam antibiotics or second- or third-generation cephalasporins. More important, perhaps, than the combination which is selected, is a sound clinical approach with appropriate investigations to identify abscesses or obtain adequate material for culture being a prerequisite of good treatment. Adequate volumes of blood are required for microbiological studies to improve the success rate.

Prophylactic oral antibiotic therapy has been criticised because of the theoretical risk of developing resistant organisms. These views have generally been set aside and many larger units have now established collaborative trials on the use of prophylactic antibiotics for patients whose white counts fall below 1.0 x 10^9/l.

The period of neutropenia is the most dangerous phase of patients' treatment and attempts to shorten this by the use of growth factors therefore have a great deal of appeal. GM-CSF has mainly been used after bone marrow transplantation and chemotherapy for solid tumours [187-191].

The preliminary studies are very encouraging but there has been some natural reluctance to move on rapidly to clinical trials in AML because of the risk of stimulating the leukaemic population and conferring autonomy [192-195]. However, this does not appear to be the case from the evidence provided by a study at the University of Munster [190] in which 23 elderly or relapsed patients were treated with intensive chemotherapy followed by GM-CSF 250 μg/m^2 daily by continuous infusion if bone marrow hypocellularity had been achieved; treatment continued at this dose until the neutrophil count reached 2.0 x 10^9/l and the dose of GM-CSF was gradually decreased over the next week. The median period to recovery of neutrophils was decreased by 6 days for the relapsed patients and by 10 days for the elderly. The early death rate in patients over 65 years of age was 20% compared with 39% for the same group of patients who did not receive GM-CSF. In one patient, the peripheral blood contained a high percentage of monoblasts, which disappeared after GM-CSF was discontinued; the patient remains in remission over a year later.

In a similar study by Estey [196], patients with AML with a poor prognosis were treated with high-dose Ara-C and non-glycosated recombinant GM-CSF at a dose of 120 μg/m^2 per day by continuous infusion starting 2 days after completing the 6-day course of Ara-C.

Half the patients achieving remission attained a neutrophil count of 1.0 x10^9/l within 19 days of starting treatment. Previous experience at the same institute predicted that only 10% of patients achieved these white counts without GM-CSF.

In only one patient there was evidence of growth of leukaemia following GM-CSF, which contrasts with the frequency with which GM-CSF stimulates the *in-vitro* proliferation of blast cells from patients with AML.

These preliminary studies, which indicate no serious toxicity, raise the very exciting prospects that the use of growth factors may in future play a very important part in shortening the period of exposure to serious infection.

Moreover, there is equally interesting evidence that GM-CSF can enhance the cytotoxicity of Ara-C by increasing the recruitment of myeloid blast cells into S phase [192].

Clinical studies on the use of GM-CSF, in combination with cytotoxic therapy in its role as a cell cycle inducer and as a rescue agent, are now being conducted in Europe.

The use of platelet transfusions during phases of thrombocytopenia has varied a great deal, depending on the distance from the regional supply or the availability of HLA-matched donors. There is little doubt that the latter situation is the ideal and some units are fortunate enough to have a large group of donors who are prepared to spend the extra time required for a platelet phoresis. Most European hospitals do not enjoy such facilities and a more pragmatic approach is required.

Platelet concentrates are preferable to platelet-rich plasma and should be hepatitis B negative and, if possible, CMV negative, particularly if bone marrow transplantation is being considered as an option for post-remission treatment. The general policy on when to give platelet transfusions has changed to a more clear-cut decision based on the peripheral platelet count rather than wait for evidence of bleeding. The guidelines for platelet counts adopted in a large number of British centres lie between 10-20 x 10^9/l, with the proviso that platelet transfusions are given more frequently when patients are pyrexial. Support with platelet transfusion is also particularly important in older patients and in association with APL (vide infra). The principal difficulty following regular platelet transfusions is the development of non-haematological febrile reactions, refractoriness and virus transmission [197-200].

There is evidence that lymphocyte-contaminated blood products are the major cause of alloimmunisation and refractoriness. The incidence is probably as high as 40% in multiply transfused patients. While white-cell depleted red cells and platelets for transfusion can be prepared by a filtration procedure [201] in the transfusion centre, this practice has been largely replaced by filtration in the patients' transfusion lines. Red cell filters have been in use for some time but a new

Table 11. AML 9: Supportive care - remitters only

	No. courses to C/R	Days in hospital	Units blood	Platelets	Antibiotics	(N=)
1+5	1/2	40	14	62	18	155
	3/4	57	21	96	28	93
3+10	1	32	13	62	18	195
	2	56	17	85	24	68
All remitters						
	1+5	47	16	75	22	249
	3+10	39	14	68	20	264
p=		0.01	0.002	0.16	0.13	

range of platelet filters are currently being tested.

One other advantage of more intensive treatment has recently been apparent from the MRC trials. The more aggressive 3+10 DAT regimen achieved remission more quickly and required less supportive care (Table 11). The effect was seen in all ages and was almost equally convincing for patients who achieved remission as it was for the group as a whole.

Consolidation Therapy

The interpretation of consolidation is traditionally held to be intensive post-remission therapy incorporating a combination of drugs which were successful in achieving remission plus a novel combination designed to abrogate the growth of a totally or partially resistant minor clone [202-206]. Consolidation therapy has to be interpreted in the light of the induction treatment as the tolerance of this post-remission treatment is to some extent dependent on the speed of response to the induction therapy. High-dose Ara-C has been used extensively in post-remission treatment and in induction therapy. In the mid 1980s, there was an extraordinary range of regimens incorporating intermediate or high-doses. The clinical response to Ara-C depends on the pharmacodynamics of Ara-CTP; the area under the curve being more important than the peak values [212].

The principal problems encountered at a dose of 2-3 g/m^2 2 hourly has been cerebellar toxicity. Thus, the German Collaborative Group [159] were unable to complete the post-remission therapy as planned, in approximately 15% of the patients entering remission because of the toxicity of the previous treatment, refusal, death in remission or relapse. However, the theoretical arguments are attractive and prolonged remissions have been described by some groups using this form of post-remission therapy.

The data of Ara-C have gradually been reduced to 0.5-1 g/m^2 for each dose, thereby coming closer to the theoretical maximal capacity of Ara-CTP production [211-213].

Maintenance Therapy

Orthodox maintenance chemotherapy has usually been designed to produce relatively little toxicity, minimal dependence on inpatient care and a high degree of patient tolerance. However, it has been interpreted differently by the inclusion of blocks of more intensive treatment. It is difficult, therefore, to assess the value of maintenance treatment, particularly when the induction and consolidation phases of treatment also vary a great deal. The most important factor in long-term survival may be the degree of success of the induction and consolidation therapy in decreasing the tumour load.

The BFM (Berlin, Munster, Frankfurt) group in Germany have examined the relative success of maintenance therapy for 3 years, incorporating 3 recycling monthly courses which included daunorubicin + Ara-C (2+5); 6-thioguanine 200 mg/m^2 orally for 5 days; and a third course of cyclophosphamide 1 g/m^2 i.v. daily x 3.

There was a significant difference between the group receiving maintenance therapy and those who did not, although this is partly explained by the poor survival of the non-treated group [2]. Buchner [160] reviewed the evidence from 10 multicentre studies, comparing maintenance therapy with no therapy. The maintenance group appeared to do better, but as all the papers were published in the first half of the last decade - and most had started in the 1970s - the early treatment was almost always less intensive than it would be at the present time.

The present MRC 9th AML Trial found no difference at 2 years between a group of patients receiving maintenance therapy with Ara-C and 6-thioguanine (100 mg bd of each for 5 days/month) and no treatment, although there was a slight early advantage for the group receiving maintenance. In summary, the role of maintenance therapy is probably changing. Protocols which include this phase of treatment will not rely on the low toxicity outpatient schedules alone but include phases of more intensive treatment.

Acute Promyelocytic Leukaemia

Acute promyelocytic leukaemia (APL) is a distinct subtype of AML comprising about 10% of the cases [214]. The classical chromosomal abnormality is the t(15;17) translocation and 2 morphological subtypes are recognised. The classic FAB M3 form is characterised by the presence of promyelocytes which are packed with prominent purple or pink-staining granules. The M3 variant [215], in contrast, has fine granules and a complex folded nucleus. The ratio of M3 to M3V is approximately 3:1.

The principal clinical problem in the treatment of APL is the management of disseminated intravascular coagulation (DIC) and the consequent high risk of massive haemorrhage [216-218]. Although the long-term prospects for patients with APL are generally held to be better than other forms of leukaemia, the prognosis only holds good for patients who have entered remission and have survived the initial bleeding problems. The bleeding is precipitated by the release of a procoagulant, which is antigenically related to brain tissue factor [219], from the azurophilic granules in the promyelocytes [220].

The chemotherapy regimens used in the treatment of APL have generally been the same as for other forms of AML but some groups, particularly French centres, have relied on single-agent therapy in the form of an anthracycline - usually daunorubicin with impressive results [221-223].

The principal laboratory findings in DIC include a prolonged prothrombin time, a prolonged partial thromboplasbin time, thrombocytopenia and a reduction in plasma fibrinogen level [216].

Depending on the severity of DIC, there is a variable risk of developing renal and respiratory failure probably caused by the deposition of small thrombi in the kidney and lungs. The more serious cases can result in acute respiratory distress syndrome, characterised by pulmonary platelet sequestration leading to haemorrhage and thrombosis. Although it is uncommon at the time of diagnosis, all the coagulation problems associated with this form of AML may be exacerbated by treatment [224].

The role of heparin in the control of DIC has been debated for some years [225,226], but a recent report analysing the results of the treatment of patients with APL in the British MRC trials strongly supports its use [227]. The analysis was a retrospective look at the remission rates among 115 patients with APL, depending on whether the collaborating physician used heparin or not. Eighty-six percent of patients who received heparin achieved a complete remission, compared with 49% among those who did not receive it. The dose of heparin varied between 12,000 and 24,000 units daily, usually given as an infusion at a rate of 500-1000 i.v. per hour. The optimal dose is usually between 15,000 and 20,000 i.v. per day.

In addition to heparin, platelet transfusions will be necessary in the majority of patients and some have recommended that the platelet count should be maintained above 60 x 10^9/l by intensive platelet transfusions [223], while heparin treatment continued; in many cases this may not be necessary beyond 5 or 6 days. The replacement of coagulation factors must be maintained by transfusion of fresh frozen plasma and transexamic acid has been found valuable in reducing the number of platelet and red cell transfusions in a small randomised trial in Rome and Amsterdam [228]. Treatment was continued for only 6 days and there were no thromboembolic complications.

Transexamic acid acts by replacing fibrin on the binding sites in the plasminogen molecule and thereby preventing the conversion of plasminogen to plasmin [229,230].

Treatment Following Relapse

In spite of the more intensive treatment programmes, a high percentage of patients will relapse. The prospects of achieving a second remission are closely related to the duration of the first remission (Table 12).

It was also closely related to the patient's age (Table 13).

The treatment of relapses has introduced a range of experimental therapy which may later be adopted in first-line treatment of the disease. The problems set by an early relapse or refractory case provide a very informative proving ground for new drugs.

One of the main problems in interpreting the results of these studies has been the lack of detail which has been provided about the duration of the first remission and the varied definition of refractoriness. There is an understandable but misleading tendency to allow enthusiasm for a new drug to influence the objective assessment of what has been achieved.

Valuable information on the biology of relapsed and refractory disease could include further insight into the mechanism of drug resistance. This may develop as a result of an increased expression of the P-glycoprotein as part of the activity of the multidrug resistance gene 231- or the levels of glutathione or topoisomerase II.

While some tumours are inherently resistant, this is uncommon in AML. Resistance can, however, be acquired by a variety or mechanisms which may in the future be circumvented.

Pharmacological studies have shown that MDR cells usually have a reduced accumulation of drugs with the MDR phenotype; these include daunorubicin, adriamycin and vincristine.

An increased expression of P-glycoprotein has been demonstrated in leukaemia cells from patients at relapse [236] and the MDR gene has been located to chromosome 7q36 [238]. Similar genes have been found to be amplified in drug-resistant Plasmodium falciparum [239] and the product of the STE6 gene in the yeast S cerevisiae can produce sterility by enhanced loss of α-factor pheremone [240].

Attempts to alter the structure of the anthracycline molecule have started to produce encouraging results. An alternative approach is

Table 12. Second remission rate by duration of 1st C/R (MRC AML9 trial)

Duration of 1st remission	2nd C/R rate
<6 months	12 %
6-12 months	37.5 %
1-2 years	42 %
2+ years	69 %

Table 13. Second remission rate (by age group)

Age	C/R rate
0-39	42 %
40-59	25 %
60+	19 %

the use of "resistance modifiers" (RMs) which, when administered with cytotoxic drugs, lead to a partial or complete restoration of sensitivity in resistant cells. The prototype compound is the calcium transport blocker verapamil, first shown to be a resistance modifier by Tsuruo in 1981 [241]. Since that time, many other compounds, particularly calcium transport blockers and calmodulin inhibitors, have been used. The majority of studies have found that, as far as Verapamil is concerned, the action is through an interference with the efflux process [242]. It is of clinical interest that Twentyman et al. [243,244] have found that aclacinomycin A does not share the characteristics of the drugs with the MDR phenotype. *In-vitro* testing of fresh leukaemia cells can help in predicting response to treatment [245].

Another mechanism of multi-agent (pleiotropic) drug resistance involves the tripeptide glutathione [246,247], which is the principal cellular non-protein thiol and is able to react with and detoxify many of the reactive alkylating agents used in chemotherapy. This interaction is catalysed by the family of enzymes known as glutathione-S-transferase (GST) [248].

Methods of lowering intracellular GSH - and thereby increasing drug sensitivity - include the use of ethacrynic acid, which was formerly used as a diuretic. This has now entered clinical trials as a resistance modifier in the U.S. [250].

A further target for chemotherapy is the topoisomerases, which may also be involved in drug resistance in human malignancies [251]. The DNA topoisomerases are ubiquitous enzymes which alter the configuration of DNA. They assist in relaxing and supercoiling DNA and prevent the double helix of DNA from tying itself into impossible tangles when it divides into 2 separate strands. The topoisomerases can create a break in either one strand (topoisomerase I) or in both strands (topoisomerase II).

Many active drugs such as daunorubicin, amsacrine and etoposide achieve their effect by binding to topoisomerase II and preventing DNA strand separation and resistance is achieved either by the presence of low concentrations of topoisomerase II or by modifying uptake of the drug and the catabolism of the topoisomerase cleavable complex [252].

A prospective study is being conducted in patients with myeloid leukaemia to try and predict the response to amsacrine by screening for low concentrations of topoisomerase or mutant enzymes [251].

The Use of Differentiating Agents in Acute Myeloid Leukaemia

The Theory

Two hundred billion erythrocytes and 70 billion granulocytes are produced and destroyed in a human weighing 70 Kg each day [253] and the process continues throughout life [254]. Because of the hierarchical and complex structure of myelopoiesis, a subtle abnormality in an early stem cell (such as an imbalance between self-renewal and differentiation) could profoundly affect myelopoiesis, e.g., if a transformed cell remained in the replicative pool for 2 additional generations, there would be a 4-fold multiplicative impact on the number of mature end-cells produced.

The fine balance between proliferation and differentiation is essential for normal myelopoiesis to be maintained [255]. In a tissue where cells tend to undergo 10 cell divisions in the time taken for all the necessary differentiation steps between stem cell and mature cells, a 10% increase or decrease in proliferation rate will double or halve the number of mature cells produced by each stem cell [255].

Normal human myelopoietic tissues have an extraordinary ability to produce a large but tightly regulated number of cells in the steady state, yet they respond to environmental stimuli by increasing the production and activity of the relevant mature cells without affecting the others [256]. Myelopoiesis is a dynamic process controlled by a group of specific stimulatory and inhibitory regulatory factors [257,258] which are secreted by T-lymphocytes [259-261], monocytes/macrophages [262] and fibroblasts and endothelial cells [263]. Macrophages can also produce both a stimulator [264] and an inhibitor [265] of the stem cell proliferation, and another inhibitor of the pluripotent stem cell, named the tetrapeptide AcSDKP with a molecular weight of 497 kD, has been isolated from foetal calf bone marrow [266].

Table 14. The human myelopoietic growth factors

Haemopoietic factor	Chromosomal localisation
1 - STIMULATORY FACTORS:	
IL-1	2q14
IL-2	4q
IL-3	5q23-31
IL-4	5q
IL-5	5q31-q33
IL-6	7q15
GM-CSF	5q23-31
G-CSF	17q11-q23
M-CSF	5q33
2 - INHIBITORY FACTORS:	
AIF	11q13
LF	3q21-23
PGE	
INF-gamma	12q24.1
TNF-a	6q21.3

IL-1 = interleukin-1; IL-2 = interleukin-2; IL-3 = interleukin-3; IL-4 = interleukin-4; IL-5 = interleukin-5; IL-6 = interleukin-6; GM-CSF = Granulocyte-macrophage colony stimulating factor; G-CSF = Granulocyte colony stimulating factor; M-CSF = Macrophage colony stimulating factor; AIF = Acidic isoferritins; LF = Lactoferrin; PGE = prostaglandins E; INF-gamma interferon; TNF-a = Tumour necrosis factor-alpha

Human bone marrow stromal cells, and the extracellular matrix produced by them, provide anchorage sites for myeloid progenitor cells [267], and binding sites for myelopoietic growth factors [268] to facilitate adhesive interactions between these growth factors and their respective immobilised target cells [269].

Several factors which inhibit normal human myelopoiesis have been identified in the past 10-15 years [270]. They include acidic isoferritin (AIF) [271]; lactoferrin (LF) [272]; prostaglandin E (PGE) [273]; gamma interferon [274]; tumour necrosis factor [275]; adenosine diphosphate - ribosylation inhibitors [276] and inhibin [277].

The human myelopoietic regulator factors are shown in Table 14.

The suppression of normal myelopoiesis in AML is one of the most spectacular phenomena in cellular haematology [278]. By suppressing normal myelopoiesis, AML cells set up conditions that favour their own expansion. The infiltration of the marrow stroma could limit the capacity of stromal cells to produce/release myelopoietic growth factors which may impair normal myelopoiesis in AML [279]. The suppression of normal myelopoiesis in AML has been reproduced *in vivo* in Shay Chloroleukaemia (an AML in the long-Evans rat), which was abrogated when the leukaemic influence was removed [279]. Whereas undifferentiated K562 and HL-60 cells exerted an inhibitory effect on normal bone marrow colony formation, prior induction of differentiation by butyrate, or hemin and retinoic acid, respectively, resulted in loss of their ability to suppress normal human myeloid progenitor cells [279,280]. Reversal of the suppression could be due to the more differentiated state of the leukaemic cells and their apparently "less malignant" nature after chemical induction of *in-vitro* differentiation and not due to changes in the numbers of cocultured leukaemic cells [279,280]. Also, HL-60 cells treated with DMSO showed a significant decrease in the production of acidic isoferritins [281]. The induction of monocytic differentiation of HL-60 cells also led to a cessation of the release of a fibroblast growth inhibitory factor which was constitutively produced by HL-60 cells [282]. More significantly, the induction of granulocytic differentiation of AML blast cells in primary culture by retinoic acid was associated with the reversal of their suppression of normal human bone marrow myeloid colony formation [283]. Therefore, the loss in the ability of butyrate or hemin-treated K562 cells and retinoic acid-treated HL-60 cells to suppress normal myelopoiesis could be related to a decrease in the production of the inhibitory factors [279].

Evidence of the inhibitory role of protein kinase C on retinoic acid-induced differentiation has been provided by the inclusion of sphinganine, an inhibitor of protein kinase C in *in-vitro* studies with HL-60. Sphinganine enhanced differentiation, raising the question of the clinical value of modulators [284] of protein kinase C.

Various combinations of drugs have been used in an attempt to induce differentiation in acute myeloid leukaemia, rather than rely on cytotoxic agents [285].

Hassan et al. [286] have shown that combinations of all-trans retinoic acid (all-trans RA), low dose concentrations of cytosine arabinoside (LD Ara-C) and hexamethylene bisacetamide induce differentiation in human blasts in primary culture. These studies were carried out *in vitro* on fresh AML cells over a 6-day period.

Although some degree of differentiation was obtained with one of the drugs used alone in some cases of AML (notably acute promyelocytic leukaemia and acute myelomonocytic leukaemia), the combination of the 3 agents was generally more potent in achieving differentiation than any of the individual agents.

The biological activity of Vitamin A (retinol) has been known for nearly 80 years, but initial emphasis was placed on the consequences of its deficiency [287]. More recently, it has been shown that it plays an important part in cell differentiation and embryo morphogenesis [287]. *In-vitro* studies showed that derivatives of Vitamin A - particularly retinoic acid - were capable of reversing the malignant phenotype of many cell lines [288].

13-cis-retinoic acid has been shown to be effective in inducing differentiation *in vitro*, either alone [289-292], or in combination with other drugs [291], and has been fairly extensively used in myelodysplastic syndromes [293]. The role of retinoic acid receptors may be the critical factor in the response, but this has not yet been resolved [294]

Three retinoic acid receptors (RARs) have been identified, alpha, beta and gamma [295-297]. The alpha and beta receptors map to different chromosomes (17q21 and 3p24, respectively) [297] and have different affinities for all-trans retinoic acid (beta>alpha). Moreover, the RARB gene has been shown to be autoregulated by retinoic acid, as RARB mRNA is increased up to 50-fold in retinoic acid-treated hepatoma lines. As the alpha gene is not effected, the evidence strongly suggests that the first target gene for retinoic acid is the RAR beta gene.

A fascinating parallel in the relationship between retinoic acid receptor expression and a dose response to retinoic acid has been demonstrated in the progenitor cells (blastema), which regenerate amputated limbs in the newt. Multiple retinoic acid receptors are exposed during limb regeneration in amphibians, suggesting that receptor heterogeneity may underlie the different effects of retinoids on limb development [298].

All-trans RA has been spectacularly successful in acute promyelocytic leukaemia with recent reports from France confirming the original work in China [299-302]. Thirteen patients with APL and 1 patient with a variant of APL were treated with oral 45 mg/m^2/day all-trans RA for 3 months. Eleven of the 13 patients achieved complete remission with this outpatient schedule after an interval of 30-90 days. The remission duration was of the order of 6 months; future policy may include oral all-trans retinoic acid as induction therapy followed by consolidation with an anthracycline such as daunorubicin.

6-thioguanine has been substituted for Ara-C in combination with all-trans RA and HMBA without any discernible difference in the response of fresh acute myeloid leukaemia cells *in vitro* [303].

Synergistic effects on differentiation have also been shown when all-trans RA is combined with hydroxyurea, DMSO, interferons, verapamil and human recombinant GM-CSF [304-307].

High-dose retinoids in the form of retinyl palmitate at a dose of 50,000 IU/m^2 orally daily have been given as maintenance therapy for children with AML. This non-randomised phase I Norwegian study on a small group of children has found little toxicity, although the drug has been given for up to 3 years; only one relapse has occurred at 37 months [308].

Vitamin D (1,25 dihydroxycholecalciferol-1,25 (OH) 2-D3) has also shown a capacity to induce differentiation [309]. Its potential role in the management of AML has been reviewed by Kelsey et al. [310].

The use of a selection of differentiating agents to treat at least some forms of acute myeloid leukaemia seems a great deal closer, particularly with the development of analogues of HMBA, retinoic acid and Vitamin D. They would be of particular value for the treatment of elderly patients who cannot tolerate aggressive cytotoxic therapy.

Central Nervous Disease

The incidence of CNS disease in AML is substantially lower than in ALL, but children are more frequently affected than adults.
Estimates of the incidence of initially overt CNS disease at diagnosis has varied from 5-10% [311-313], but occult involvement of the CNS may be a little higher. It is an uncommon site of isolated relapse, occurring in less than 3% of cases [314,315]. In a large collaborative study in Britain, patients under the age of 55 were randomised to receive no CNS prophylaxis or 6 alternating intrathecal injections of Ara-C and methotrexate. The relapse rate in the CNS in the group as a whole was so small (<0.5%) that the value of prophylaxis could not be assessed.
CNS prophylaxis has therefore been excluded from subsequent MRC trials on AML in adults, but it has been retained for children as the incidence of monocytic and myelomonocytic leukaemia is higher in this age group and carries a higher risk of CNS disease [316].
An unusual form of CNS disease is associated with specific chromosome abnormalities INV 16 and t(8;21) rearrangements have been associated with isolated tumour masses (chloromas). The explanation for these associations is not yet clear [317,318].

Treatment of AML in the Elderly

The remission rate among patients with AML over the age of 60 is less than 50% and the success rate falls sharply after 70 years of age. The reasons for this are complex but include a number of factors which include changes in the biology of the disease - a higher percentage of secondary leukaemias following a pre-existing haematological disorder on chemotherapy and both are more commonly associated with chromosome abnormality - and in the patient's capacity to cope with the side effects of intensive therapy.
Obvious mitotic inadequacies in the maintenance of the bone marrow population are not a generally recognised feature of advancing age, but there is probably a progressive depletion of the stem cell compartments, both numerically and functionally.
Studies with cultured human fibroblasts from donors of different ages show that the replicative lifespan of the cultures is inversely proportional to the age of the tissue donor [319-320].
There is also a great deal of evidence to suggest that the process of aging alters the pharmacokinetics of some drugs and more care is needed in prescribing antibiotics, analgesics, hypnotics, digoxin and Beta-blockers as well as cytotoxic drugs, in order to avoid clinical disasters which may have no intrinsic relationship to the disease being treated. The modifications to drug availability and metabolism may include the rate of absorption, metabolism by the liver, renal excretion and plasma binding [321-323].
In a very comprehensive review, Brinker [324] has examined the results of treating several thousands of patients with AML. He notes that 55-59% of the patients are over the age of 60 and that the remission rate is 35%-49%.
Low-dose Ara-C has been used in many combinations and doses, with varying results. These have been reviewed by Cheson [325], who found a remission rate of 32% in patients with primary AML, but the toxicity was fairly high. A recent study on the treatment of patients with low-dose Ara-C (10mg/m^2 bd s.c.) over the age of 60 obtained a complete remission rate of 23%, lasting a median period of 10 months. The median survival of all the 44 patients was only 3 months but was 19.5 months for the remitters. The conclusion from the study was that the response rate was similar to that obtained by other treatments, but the toxicity was lower.
One of the difficulties in assessing the value of low-dose Ara-C is that it is usually reserved for the patients with a low performance score [326,327]. In a report by Sebban, patients receiving low-dose Ara-C had a poor prognostic index and a median survival of 17 days, while aggressive therapy for another group with a higher performance status achieved a remission rate of 48%. They concluded that the diagnostic characteristics were not helpful in directing the therapeutic plan; the decision to treat patients actively should be based on the patients' general condition and socio-economic criteria rather than on age.
A trial of more aggressive therapy for patients over 70 years of age at the MD Anderson

achieved a C/R rate of 35%, but the median duration of remission was only 33 weeks and the median overall survival for all the patients was only 6 weeks [328].
A potentially very useful addition to the range of cytotoxic drugs in the elderly has been the oral preparation of Idarubicin (4-demethoxy-daunorubicin). It combines the potency of the newer anthracyclines with the convenience of an oral preparation.
Studies at the Memorial Sloan Kettering Hospital in New York [329] have demonstrated efficacy in phase I and II studies and these have been confirmed by the Italian GIMEMA Group [330].
A combination of cytotoxic agents plus growth factors or a range of differentiating agents may prove potentially very valuable in the management of this large group of patients with AML.

Acute Lymphoblastic Leukaemia

During the last 10 years, there has been a remarkable increase in our knowledge of the biology of acute lymphoblastic leukaemia (ALL) and the management has improved to the point where over half the patients developing the condition will be cured. The outlook remains less optimistic for adults than for children and the problems which remain to be resolved differ to some extent in the two groups. In summarising the current state of the management of ALL, an attempt will be made to highlight the differences.

Incidence

Acute lymphoblastic leukaemia is the second most common cause of death in children under the age of 16 after accidents [331]. The incidence in children is approximately 1-2 per 100,000 and accounts for over one-third of all childhood cancer mortality [332].
In adults, the condition is distributed fairly evenly throughout the age groups, with a median age of about 40 years [331]. ALL accounts for approximately 15% of the acute leukaemias in adults and approximately 85% in children.

Symptoms and Signs

These are well documented with symptoms of anaemia - often a late feature in children - combined with bleeding and infection to a greater or lesser degree, depending on the severity of marrow failure. Hepatosplenomegaly, lymphadenopathy, sternal tenderness, evidence of infection, fever unrelated to obvious infection and haemorrhage are the cardinal signs.
X-rays of the chest show mediastinal or hilar lymph-node enlargement in approximately 10% of patients with ALL. Other radiological findings which are more common in children include discrete osteolytic lesions, cortical destruction, periostial elevations, osteoporosis or increased bone density.

Classification of ALL

The combination of morphological and cytochemical features of ALL have been arranged into 3 groups by the French, American and British (FAB) Group [333]: a small microlymphoblastic cell (L1), a larger more undifferentiated cell (L2) and a large cell cytologically of the Burkitt cell type (L3).
The classification system has proved very valuable in coordinating the analysis of clinical studies in many countries and has important prognostic significance discussed below.
The immunological and biochemical classification of ALL is shown in Table 15.
The main current issues in the management of ALL in both children and adults are:

- What are the risk groups
- The induction therapy: How intensive can it be ?
- Consolidation therapy: Early or late intensive chemotherapy ?
- The role of other post-remission therapy such as bone marrow transplantation
- Maintenance therapy: How long and what should we give ?
- CNS treatment: Is there a preferable form of treatment to cranio/spinal irradiation?
- Testicular disease: incidence and prevention
- Treatment of relapsed patients: early and late, i.e., <1-3 years and >3 years.

Table 15. Immunological and biochemical classification of Acute Lymphocytic Leukaemia

	Non-T, non-B ALL			
	cALL- (null cell)	cALL+ (common)	T-ALL	B-ALL
Membrane markers				
Anti-Ia	-	+	-	+
Anti-cALL	-	+	-	-
Anti-T	-	-	+	-
Sheep E-rosettes	-	-	+	-
SmIg	-	-	-	+
Enzymes				
TdT	+	+	+	-
Hex I	+	+	-	-
	-			
Adenosine deaminase	+	+	+	-
	-	-		
Acid phosphatase	-	-	+	-
Incidence				
Childhood ALL (701 patients) (%)	12	75	12	1
Adult ALL (103 patients) (%)	50	38	10	2

abbreviations: anti-cALL = antisera to the common acute lymphocytic leukaemia (ALL) antigen; anti-Ia = anti-p28, 33/Oa-like antigen antisera; anti-T = xennoantisera to T-cell antigens; Hex-I = intermediate (I) isoenzyme of hexosaminidase; SmIg = intrinsic surface membrane immunoglobulin; TdT = terminal deoxynucleotidyl transferase; + designates reactivity with membrane markers or increased quantities of enzyme; - designates the opposite, and ± indicates intermediate or variable results

Data from Greaves MF: Analysis of the clinical and biological significance of lymphoid phenotypes in acute leukemia. Cancer Res 1981 (41):4752

Induction Therapy

The history of the early development of treatment of acute lymphoblastic leukemia has been well reviewed [334].

These studies and others which followed allowed paediatric and adult patients to be allocated to different risk groups [335-342].

The features which have been found to be relatively reliable include age, white blood count, cytogenetic characteristics and morphological and immunophenotypic features [337,339,343,344].

Having established these guidelines, treatment regimens have been developed to stratify therapy for children with ALL [335,339,345]. Adults are accepted as being in a bad prognostic group because of their age alone, but within this, other prognostic features come into play, including haemorrharge at the time of diagnosis [344] and T-cell subtype although, in the BFM adult study, these patients had a remission rate of over 80% [340,344,346-349]. The general improvement in adult patients with T-ALL is remarkable in view of the fact that, as in childhood T-ALL, there is a male predominance and a high proportion of patients with mediastinal mass, CNS involvement or a high WBC count. The POG study [345] defined 3 risk groups within their large series of 253 children with T-cell ALL. The best prognosis was found in patients with WBC <50 x 10^9/l without significant splenomegaly and blasts expressing CD5 antigen (65% event-free survival at 4 years). An intermediate group included 2 subsets of patients with either WBC<50 x 10^9/l with massive splenomegaly and blasts lacking CD5 expression or WBC>50 x 10^9/l with expression of the THY antigen (39% EFS at 4 years). The worst prognosis was associated with WBC>50 x 10^9/l with blasts lacking THY antigen (19% at 4 years).

Several structural chromosome abnormalities have been shown to be strong predictors of short survival including t(8:l4), t(4:11), t(9:22) and hypodiploidy. These are reviewed by Dr Freireich in another section and in other recent publications [350-353]. The incidence of the Philadelphia chromosome in children with ALL is about 2-3%, but it is considerably higher in adults (15-20%). Hyperdiploidy, the most common cytogenetic abnormality in children, carries a good prognosis [351], but it is rare in adults [350].

As therapy gradually improves the response rate, it has become increasingly difficult to define the groups with "high risk" ALL in children. There is a consensus, however, that infants with ALL do rather poorly and a high white blood count carries a poor prognosis [335,340,344-346].

The main object of the initial treatment in ALL is clearly to achieve a complete remission - unless this stage is reached the outlook is very poor.

High remission rates in children have been achieved since the introduction of the combination of vincristine and prednisone in combinations in the mid 1960s and Frei et al. achieved over 80% C/R in 166 children, using a combination of prednisone and 6MP [354].

In all the early reviews, it became clear that it was the introduction of prednisone which was the major factor in the improved remission rate. Freireich et al. had achieved remission rates of 57% in 72 patients using this drug alone [355]. What is not clear, even after the long interval which has elapsed, is exactly why lymphoblasts are so spectacularly sensitive to steroids and radiation - a feature which they share with germ cells.

The subsequent development of more intensive induction programmes has served not so much to improve the remission rate as to prolong the duration of remission [356] - an extension of Pinkel's "Total Therapy" which he and his colleagues introduced to St Jude's Hospital, Memphis, in 1962. An excellent review of the early years of effective treatment of ALL in children has been written by Pinkel in 1986 [357].

The designation of patients into high-risk and low-risk groups raises the question of whether the good-risk groups are being undertreated. However, several collaborative groups have adopted the guidelines and drawn up treatment regimens accordingly.

The most recent MRC trial (UKALL X and XA) for the treatment of acute lymphoblastic leukaemia in children and adults attempts to assess the effect of adding intensive chemotherapy after induction therapy has been completed. It is further hoping to establish whether the intensification block should be given "early"- from the end of the 4th week of treatment; "late" - from the end of the 19th week - or both "early" and "late".

The intensive block consists of vincristine, daunorubicin, VP16 (etoposide), cytosine arabinoside and 6-thioguanine. The design of the regimen for "early" intensification is shown in Figure 2.

All patients will be randomised except those with a WBC >50 x 10^9/l, who will receive early and late intensification treatment.

Before discussing the success of current regimens in achieving long-term survival in ALL, it is worthwhile noting that one of the reasons for relapse is for patients to be undertreated by falling short of the doses of drugs recommended in the protocol. Lennard [359,360] has discussed this in respect to 6-mercaptopurine doses in paediatric patients and quotes De Vita who, in a slightly different context, said "The most toxic manoeuvre a physician can make when administering chemotherapy is to arbitrarily and unnecessarily reduce the dose" [360]. Possibly as a result of a policy of enforcing sustained maximally tolerated doses of oral 6-mercaptopurine and methotrexate in the MRC 8th ALL trial (UKALL VIII), there was a 20% in-

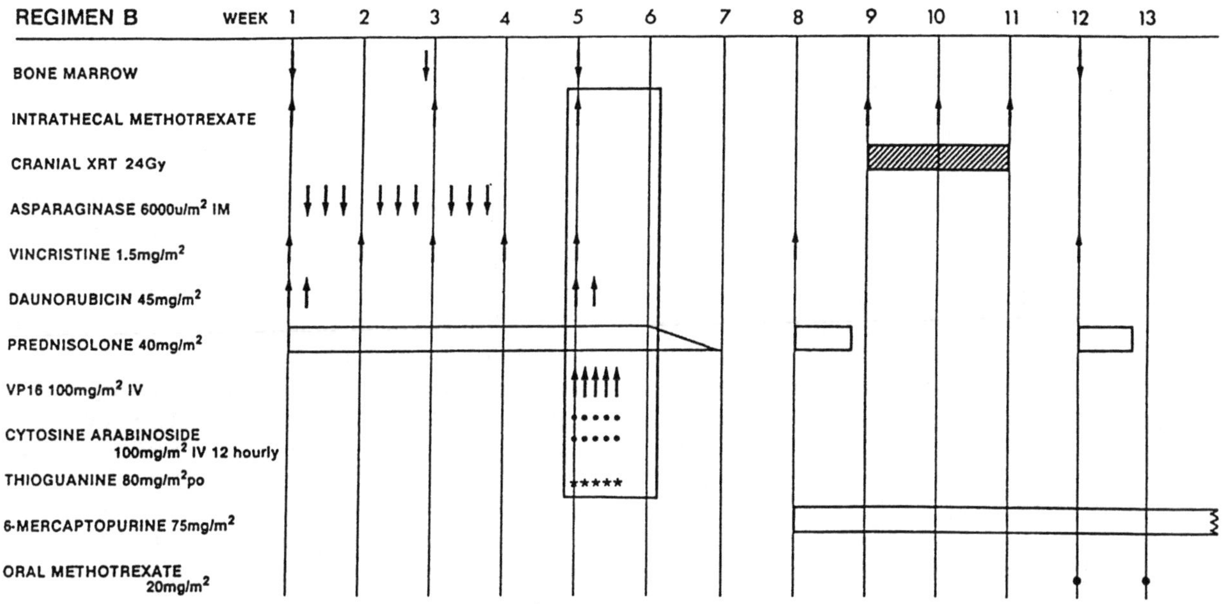

Fig. 2. Early intensification arm of MRC X trial in ALL (UKALL X)

crease in the 3-year survival in children compared with earlier studies.

The consolidation regimen employed in Britain has to some extent been modelled on the very successful West German protocol which is based on a calculation of risk factors.

$$RF = 0.2.\log(B1+1)+0.06.L+0.04.S$$

RF = risk factor, B1 = absolute number of leukaemic cells in the blood/mm^3

L = enlargement of the liver (centimetres below the costal margin)

S = enlargement of the spleen (centimetres below the costal margin).

Low-risk patients were those with a RF <0.8.

All patients received induction therapy with prednisolone, vincristine, daunorubicin and L-asparaginase followed by cyclophosphamide, cytosine arabinoside, methotrexate and IT methotrexate. No cranial irradiation was given to the CNS in this study. This intensive treatment, given over 10 weeks, was referred to as "Protocol I". The remission rate was 100%. Randomisation between a very intensive consolidation programme - "Protocol III" was compared with oral daily 6-MP and weekly oral methotrexate. The relapse rate in the intensive arm (15.8%) was half the rate seen with the oral treatment with an 82% probability of an event-free interval of 5 years compared with 61% in the oral therapy group [361].

In the German studies the standard risk score is 1.2 and comprises 60% of the patients in their population. They were not able to protect this group from an unacceptable CNS relapse rate (11%) when CNS irradiation was omitted in comparison with a 4% isolated CNS relapse rate with cranial irradiation [362].

The debate about the role of cranial irradiation; its dose and which group should receive it, has not been resolved. Randomised studies by the American CCSG group have shown that a dose of 18 Gy to the cranium is as effective as 24 Gy, except for patients with a high initial white count [363].

There is a general move towards the replacement of cranial irradiation with intrathecal therapy combined with intermediate dose methotrexate for "low-risk" and "standard-risk" patients. This has already been adopted by the Italian collaborative GIMEMA group who have analysed the results of treating 358 adults in their ALL 0183 study. The complete remission rate was 80% but only 25% of patients maintained the remission at 4 years.

The relapse rate in the CNS alone was 15% and in 7% the relapse was a combined CNS/bone marrow. Nevertheless, they conclude that CNS radiation may now be replaced by intrathecal and intermediate-dose methotrexate [364].

Testicular Relapse

Isolated testicular relapse occurs in about 5% of boys in remission [365], but may be decreasing as therapy becomes more intensive. However, a wide variation in the incidence of isolated testicular relapse has been reported, ranging from 1.5% to 41% [366-369]. The majority present with partial swelling of one or both testes within the first 2 years of completing treatment [368-370]. The bone marrow is usually still in remission but Baum et al. [358] found evidence of involvement of para-aortic lymph nodes in some patients.

The treatment recommended is radiotherapy to about 24 Gy to both testes [371,372]. Systemic chemotherapy is also necessary because of the high risk of bone marrow relapse but the prospects are good if retreatment is comprehensive and includes consolidation and maintenance therapy combined with CNS treatment, preferably with high-dose intravenous and standard-dose intrathecal methotrexate [372,373].

The policy of performing testicular biopsies to detect early infiltration has not been found to be of value [374]. Miller et al. [369] have recently reported that the percentage of boys having occult testicular disease in CCSG 141 was 11% (26/237), but a high percentage of false negative results in other studies has provided a major source of confusion [373,375].

The reliability of the technique is clearly crucial in the interpretation of the findings; in the CCSG 141 trial the disease-free survival at 5 years for boys with occult testicular disease was 62% compared with the biopsy-negative group (86%).

Testicular biopsies have now been abandoned as routine procedures, principally because of the false-negative rate but also because there is little evidence that prophylactic testicular irradiation, as used in the MRC VI and VII paediatric ALL trials, provides any safeguard against local relapse; furthermore, intensive chemotherapy has reduced the incidence of testicular relapse and effective local and systemic treatment is available, should it occur [364,372,373].

Maintenance Therapy

The contribution made by the maintenance therapy in curing patients with ALL has only been debated in the past 20 years. Until higher remission rates were achieved, the overall survival of children at 1 year was of the order of 1 percent [376].

As the number of patients surviving for 5 years increases and the risk factors are identified more clearly, the question arises "How much is enough treatment". The increasing recognition of the long-term effects of chemoradiotherapy (vide infra) have led to a continual reappraisal of the treatment of the disease at all stages [362,377,378].

The Children's Cancer Study Group (CCSG) has recently reported the results of a randomised trial comparing 3 with 5 years' maintenance [369]. This study (CCG 141) compared 3 policies in a group of patients who had been in continuous complete remission for 3 years: (a) stop treatment (b) finish with a 4-week reinduction course consisting of prednisolone, vincristine and asparaginase (c) continue maintenance therapy with daily 6MP and weekly methotrexate for 2 years. The randomisation included over 100 patients in each arm but at 6 years following randomisation the percentage of patients in continuous complete remission was almost exactly the same in each arm (93%, 89% and 89%, respectively).

These results supported the findings of an earlier study (CCG - 101/143) which had also shown a poorer outcome for boys [379]. This may be explained by the fact that in the subsequent trial, wedge testicular biopsies were required at the final randomisation point (i.e., after 3 years in CCR). Boys who had positive biopsies were removed from the randomisation but for those who were biopsy negative there was no benefit from additional treatment.

The girls who continued to a total of 5 years did rather worse, suggesting that, at least in girls, treatment might actually be harmful.

Analysis of the MRC UKALL trials I-III showed that periods of 18 months or 2 years were as effective as 3 years for girls [377]. For boys the 18-month treatment was inferior but there was no difference between 2 and 3 years. Another report from St Jude's Hospital who treated their patients for 2.5 years showed no relapses beyond 4 years from stopping treatment [378]. The effect of the bioavailability of drugs on the duration of remission has again been raised by Koren et al. at the Hospital for Sick Children, Toronto, with respect to 6-mercaptopurine [380].

Treatment Following Relapse

The generally held view is that patients with HLA-compatible siblings should receive an allogeneic bone marrow transplant following intensive reinduction therapy (see A.M. Marmont's chapter in this volume). The arguments for and against transplantation have been reviewed [381-385].

The BFM German group [386] use very intensive reinduction and consolidation treatment. A recent report on 221 children and adolescents treated with 2 BFM protocols (studies 83 and 85) showed that 58% of the patients in each trial had relapsed within 6 months of stopping treatment and were designated "early relapses". This group received very intensive treatment; 64% achieved a second remission in the first study and 88% (52/59) in the ALL-REZ 85 study. Ninety-eight percent of the patients who relapsed late (>6 months C/R) achieved a second remission of which 50% (33/68) subsequently relapsed, a high proportion in the central nervous system.

The current MRC protocol for children with relapsed ALL is not as intensive as some recently described [386,387] because the evidence for an improved survival compared with more orthodox intensive reinduction and consolidation is not yet sufficiently convincing and the longer-term side effects may be unacceptable.

Patients with Ph-positive acute lymphoblastic leukaemia have a much poorer outlook but an encouraging report on the role of alpha interferon from Vienna and Ulm claims a good response in 2 children who had been heavily pretreated for ALL and had relapsed with CML. One obtained a stable remission with 2-4 x 10^6 units of interferon daily which was maintained for more than 2 years. A second achieved good control but subsequently relapsed [388].

Definition of Complete Remission

The criteria of a complete remission have been adopted uniformly for all forms of acute leukaemia (viz. a cellular bone marrow with <5% blast cells and peripheral blood counts showing Hb >12.5 G/dl, neutrophil count >1.0 x 10^9/l and platelet count >100 x 10^9/l). Haematologists have lived uneasily with this definition for some years as there is a wide range in the tumour load even when these guidelines are met.

Methods of demonstrating very small numbers of malignant cells have made it possible with some leukaemias to plan treatment strategies for the eradication of minimal residual disease [389-391].

The techniques for identifying residual leukaemia include immunophenotyping, DNA flow cytometry [392], cytogenetics [392], leukaemic colony assays [393] and analysis of gene rearrangements [394-397].

Fluorescent double staining with markers such as TdT and CALLA (CD10) for B-lineage cells and CD7 for T-lineage cells has made it possible to identify 1 in 10,000 leukaemia cells. Culture methods are also sensitive but relatively time consuming. Nevertheless, Estrov [393] was able to detect early relapse in 6 out of 13 patients with acute lymphoblastic leukaemia.

Immunoglobulin and T-cell receptor gene rearrangements have been used as markers for lineage and clonality and as markers of minimal residual disease. The sensitivity of the system is at the 0.1 level and, for the majority of patients, cannot be improved by means of the polymerase chain reaction because no consistent chromosomal translocation has occurred, as in low-grade lymphoma or CML [392,394]. In CML, the technique has been particularly valuable following bone marrow transplantation. In one series [396], 14 patients were investigated 3-63 months following allogeneic bone marrow transplantation. Five patients demonstrated rearranged *bcr/abl* mRNA, although all were in haematological remission and 13/14 were in cytogenetic remission. Two of the 5 positive cases became negative after 3 months.

A 2-step system employing "immune selection" with a panel of 5 monoclonal antibodies with predominantly myeloid specificity allows separation from the cells of interest on a fluorescence-activated cell sorter following labelling with fluorescin-conjugated goat-anti-mouse $(Fab)_2$ antiserum. Probes directed against the T-beta constant region and the joining region of the immunoglobulin heavy chain locus were used to identify rearrangements. The method made it possible to detect a very small percentage of abnormal cells in 4 out of 5 patients who relapsed out of a group of 11 in haematological remission at the time of the study [397]. There were no false positive results, i.e., gene arrangements found in a patient who did not relapse.

Adoption of this and similar techniques will enormously enhance our capacity to detect minimal residual disease and predict relapse before the burden of tumour is too great. We will have to wait to see what impact this has on the treatment policy and whether this can be translated into a higher percentage of patients cured of their disease.

Long-Term Effects of Treatment

When remission rates were low and survival beyond 5 years an exception, the issue of the delayed side effects of treatment was irrelevant.

The comparative success of the last 10-15 years in achieving durable remission has brought sequelae which could not have been imagined or taken into account earlier.

The incidence of clinically important endocrine morbidity has been estimated to be approximately 20%, with lack of growth being the most common [398]. This has been brought into sharp focus recently because of the availability of growth hormone.

Kirk et al. [399] measured growth patterns in 77 patients 3-9.5 years after intensive treatment for ALL in New South Wales. At 4 years after diagnosis, one-third of the survivors had fallen more than 1 standard below the normal and three-quarters were affected to the same degree after 6 years. Younger children and those tall for age at diagnosis were most affected: 30-46 patients tested had partial or complete growth hormone deficiency. "Prophylactic" cranial irradiation was proposed as the most important causative factor.

A later report on the same group of patients [400,401] confirmed the initial findings and demonstrated clear evidence of germ-cell damage, with marked increase in plasma levels of follicle-stimulating hormone and in the boys the absence of germ cells in the testicular biopsies combined with the small size of the testes for pubic hair stage.

Less than half the girls reaching puberty had measurable plasma inhibin levels indicating severe damage to the follicles, but plasma sex steroids were normal and girls reached the menarche at a mean of 1 year earlier than normal. Gonadal damage was independent of age at the time of treatment and may have resulted from the incorporation of cytosine arabinoside into the protocol.

The main consequences of gonadal damage may only appear in adulthood with sexual dysfunction, infertility, diminished bone mass and an increased risk of ischaemic heart disease being the major worries.

Early puberty also produces a more immediate problem because of the early closure of the epiphyses and restriction of growth.

Clayton [402] found a high proportion of patients with growth retardation in a group of 82 children in Manchester. The greatest reduction in yearly decrements was found in the first year following diagnosis, but growth increased significantly when treatment stopped, making the role of cranial irradiation less emphatic. In most of the children, the mean loss in height was not sufficiently great to justify long-term growth hormone therapy. This view was confirmed by the group at the Hospital for Sick Children, London [403]. They proposed that a trial of growth hormone should be reserved for the children below the tenth centile where growth is persistently poor, particularly when growth hormone deficiency has been demonstrated. They also included in this recommendation patients who had relapsed and had received further radiation treatment.

The incidence of clinically important endocrine morbidity has been estimated by Wheeler to be approximately 20% [404]. This was usually expressed by altered puberty or menarche, for although the onset of puberty in all patients in this review was within the normal range, there was again a greater proportion of children with early puberty. A similar detailed study by the CCSG group measured serum levels of follicle-stimulating hormone and luteinising hormone in 97 long-term survivors 7-10 years following intensive chemoradiotherapy which included, in some

patients, 12 Gy to the abdomen and gonads [405].
One-third of all the patients had elevated FSH and/or LH, but this included nearly all the patients receiving cranio-spinal plus abdominal irradiation, half of those who received cranio-spinal alone and only 1% of those receiving cranial irradiation.
Testicular hormonal function has not been severely affected by chemotherapy but impaired spermatogenesis is evident in some testicular biopsies [406].
The most worrying long-term neurological deficits are the learning difficulties which have become apparent. These cannot be identified by IQ tests alone, although the collective IQ values of 2 groups of children with and without learning difficulties reported by Wheeler were significantly different [404]. Early recognition is thought to be important, but the spoken word and numeracy seem to be more severely affected than pattern recognition and visual methods of perception and learning. Children under the age of 3 at the time of irradiation appear most vulnerable [407].
The educational standards in one group were at a level at which 20% were mentally retarded and required special educational assistance. The best clinical predictions of the IQ were the number of courses of irradiation, age, and the presence or absence of cerebral pathology, demonstrated on computerised axial tomography [408].
A contributory factor, however, is the high level of psychological and social problems within the families, in addition to a disturbed and possibly poor attendance record at school [409]. The incidence of learning problems in children with leukaemia has been estimated to be twice as high as in the school population as a whole [404].
No evidence has been found to suggest that cranial irradiation, intrathecal chemotherapy or systemic chemotherapy increases the risk of demyelination according to measurement of visual evoked potentials or EEG in patients with ALL compared with a normal group [410].
Another major worry for the long survivors is the susceptibility to second neoplasms. The largest review has been by Zarrabi [411], who documented 61 cases including 17 patients who developed another acute leukaemia - mainly M1 and M2 AML; 12 returned to a CML; 19 developed lymphomas of which nearly half were Hodgkin's disease and the majority of the remainder were apparently examples of histiocytic medullary reticulosis (HMR), which is an interesting finding in view of the proposed association of T-ALL and HMR through the production of lymphokines by neoplastic T lymphocytes [412]. Solid tumours developed in a further 13 patients 13 to 96 months after the diagnosis of ALL. The histological types described included hepatomas, thyroid malignancies, astrocytomas, glioblastoma, pancreatic adenocarcinoma, Ewing's sarcoma, Kaposi's sarcoma, rhabdomyosarcoma and liomyosarcoma. Secondary acute myeloid leukaemia developed in almost 0.2% of patients treated with intensive chemotherapy at St Judes Hospital [413] after a median follow-up of 3 years following diagnosis. At 3 years, the accumulative risk was 1.6%, at 6 years it was 4.7%. The incidence of secondary AML was much higher among patients with T-cell ALL. Cytogenetic studies identified entirely different karyotypes from the original pattern in the majority, with abnormalities in the 11q23 region in almost all the cases. There were no abnormalities of chromosome 5 or 7, which have been particularly common in AML associated with previous exposure to alkylating agents.
Nine brain tumours have also been described by Albo [414] as late effects in children treated with a single protocol. The subject has recently been reviewed extensively in a monograph [415].
Although the majority of children will not develop serious long-term effects as a result of their treatment, it is essential that patients, and children in particular, should continue to be followed up carefully.
The Late Effects Study Group of the Children's Cancer Research Group effectively coordinate the collection of this essential information in the U.S. and similar committees have been set up by other collaborative organisations in Europe.

Chronic Myeloid (Myelogenous) Leukaemia

Chronic Myeloid Leukaemia (CML) was the first of the leukaemias to be reported; the careful descriptions of the cases by Craigie and Bennett are models of case reports [1,2]. The condition has variously been called "stem cell leukaemia" and chronic granulocytic leukaemia (CGL). Although still used in some centres, the latter term is misleading while attempting to be more informative than the traditional "myeloid" nomenclature (i.e., blood resembling bone marrow).

Approximately 25% of patients are diagnosed before symptoms develop, but the classic features are splenomegaly, mild anaemia, thrombocytopenia or thrombocytosis and elevated white counts (sometimes very high) with a predominance of mature, later forms in the granulocytic series; basophilia is often a striking component of the circulating population.

The appearances of the bone marrow are characteristic but not specific. The features include hypercellularity, increased granulopoiesis with normal maturation but a left shift associated with increased megakaryocytes and some reduction in erythropoiesis: the value of examining the bone marrow in CML is to identify early transformation to a blastic stage which may not be apparent from the peripheral blood; it allows a greater chance of obtaining a successful cytogenetic preparation and a trephine biopsy gives a more accurate guide to the marrow cellularity. The PB and bone marrow characteristically show low leucocyte alkaline phosphatase (LAP) scores. The median age for diagnosis is 40-50 years.

Cytogenetic and enzyme studies have shown that the population of cells represent a monoclonal cell proliferation originating in the pluripotential stem cell so that the megakaryocytic and erythropoietic cell series are also involved in the neoplastic process [416].

The nature of the specific cytogenetic and molecular biological features which are so much part of the CML syndrome, are reviewed elsewhere in this monograph.

Suffice to recall here that the Philadelphia chromosome [417] is found in 85-90% of cases of CML [418] and the formation of the *bcr/abl* chimaeric gene expressed as a 8.5 Kd mRNA and a larger (210 Kd) protein with increased tyrosine kinase activity [419]. The normal functions of the c-abl and bcr genes are unknown but it has become clear that in Ph-negative CML there is often a transfer of varying amounts of the c-abl gene to the long arm of chromosome 22 without a reciprocal transfer of the bcr gene to chromosome 9 [420-427]. In Ph-positive ALL - more commonly found in adults - there may be a transfer of c-abl either to the bcr region or to an area outside the main bcr region with the formation of a smaller bcr/abl gene and a smaller (190 Kd) protein, but rearrangements outside the M-bcr occur in only about 5% of the cases [426]. Van Etten et al. [428] and Jackson et al. [429] have recently shown that the expression of the activating product of the mouse type IV c-abl gene is associated with movement to an intracytoplasmic site from its normal intranuclear position; CML can also be induced in irradiated mice following the transplantation of bone marrow from a syngeneic donor after the marrow had been infected with a retro-virus encoding $P210^{bcr/abl}$ [430]. These elegant studies present the most convincing evidence so far of the role of the $P210^{bcr/abl}$ gene in the pathogenesis of CML. The reliability of the application of the polymerase chain reaction (PCR) in the detection of leukaemia-specific transcripts following bone marrow transplantation has, however, thrown some doubt on the interpretation of some earlier reports. The group coordinating this important collaborative study warn of the hazards of the PCR method when used with a small number of target sequences [431].

Prognostic Factors and Staging in CML

There are few diseases in which the prognosis varies as much as it does in CML. In the chronic phase, treatment can be relatively straightforward if conducted by an experienced clinician and the patients quality of life is generally excellent.

In the transition to the accelerated and blastic phase, the disease takes an altogether differ-

Table 16. Univariate and multivariate analysis of the prognostic factors in CML in 678 patients (from Sokal et al. 1984) [435]

Feature (direction of worse prognosis)	**Prognostic significance** p value Univariate analysis	Multivariate regression
Sex (male)	0.5	0.06
Age (higher)	0.02	0.0009
Spleen size (larger)	0.000001	0.00003
Liver size (larger)	0.00001	0.09
Haematocrit (lower)	0.0004	0.7
WBC (higher)	0.001	0.6
Platelet count (higher)	0.001	0.001
Percentage blasts in blood (higher)	0.000001	0.00003

ent aspect and the outlook is very poor [418,432-434].

There have been several attempts to establish some guidelines which would be valuable in deciding on which therapeutic option to adopt and what may be expected of it.

Sokal has moved the emphasis in the prognostic methods to the early chronic stage and to the point before treatment begins. His analysis is based on more than 1600 patients with CML registered in the International CGL Prognosis Study [432].

At around the third year following diagnosis, the slope of the survival curve is linear with a 25% mortality rate per year. The median survival for all patients is approximately 3.5 years. A review of the prognostic features present at the time of diagnosis is shown in Table 16.

Four variables were important in the multivariate analysis. These were: age, spleen size, platelet count and percentage of circulating blasts. A Cox model was generated using the four variables and a hazard ratio function was calculated from the formula:

$$\lambda i(t)/\lambda o(t) =$$

$$\exp\left\{ 0.0116\,(\text{Age } 43.4) + 0.0345\,(\text{spleen} - 7.51) + 0.188\left[\left(\frac{\text{Plat.}}{700}\right)^2 - 0.563\right] + 0.0887\,(\text{blasts} - 2.1) \right.$$

Where $\lambda i(t)$ is the relative failure rate for the ith individual

and $\lambda o(t)$ is the relative failure rate for the overall group.

The model was tested on a further group of 361 patients [435] and produced similar subgroups using hazard ratios of 0.8 and 1.2 as boundaries. The median survival of 114 patients in the low-risk group (<0.8) was 60 months; that for the 102 patients in the high-risk group (>1.2) was 32 months, while the intermediate group of 145 patients had a median survival of 44 months.

The study was extended further to examine patients aged 5 to 45 who might be considered eligible for bone marrow transplantation [436,437]. Taking into account the risks of allogeneic transplantation, the model may help to select patients for whom this procedure would be the treatment of choice, i.e., a poor prognostic group with more than 30% chance of death from leukaemia within 2 years. Hazard ratios are not normally calculated, however, in discussing the role of allogeneic bone marrow transplantation in CML. The role for this treatment - the only one which can offer a relatively high chance of cure in CML - is discussed in another section by A.M. Marmont. The optimal time for a bone marrow transplant is not too well defined, but if an HLA-compatible donor is available, it should probably be carried out as soon as maximal cytoreduction has been achieved. A mathematical model has attempted to set upper and lower limits on the time; the factors involved in the calculations are complex but the conclusion of Simon et al. [438] is that the decision to transplant can be postponed in some patients longer than may generally be recommended.

Other valuable contributions to the interpretation of prognostic parameters in CML have been made by the Italian Cooperative Study Group on Chronic Myeloid Leukaemia. They addressed the question whether differences in the prognostic group as calculated by Sokal and others, represented intrinsic differences in the behaviour of the disease or merely earlier rather than later diagnosis. They calculated the range of intervals between the earliest possible diagnosis and the actual time of diagnosis [439,440]. The intervals ranged from 3-24 months and were the same for the different risk groups calculated using the 4-variable hazard ratio.

Treatment

Following the prolonged use of arsenic in chemotherapy of CML (vide supra), other forms of treatments were introduced in the early part of the century.

Splenic irradiation was first used in 1902 [441] and for over 50 years it remained the main form of treatment, notwithstanding Forkner and Scott's continued enthusiasm for arsenic, which they used in combination with radiotherapy [442].

The first effective drug in controlling the symptoms of CML was busulphan. The initial report by Galton et al. [443] in 1953 was accompanied by a paper by Haddow and Timmis [444] setting out the background to the development of 1.4-dimethanesulphonyloxybutane, which was known by the codename "GT41".

It has remained, for many, the treatment of choice for the treatment of CML ever since, either alone or in combination with other drugs such as 6-thioguanine.

An MRC study in which busulphan was compared with radiotherapy showed, busulphan to be superior in quality and duration of control.

Busulphan therapy carries certain risks. Unless the dosage is carefully monitored, severe myelosuppression can occur, making it unsafe to prescribe a supply of more than 4-6 weeks before rechecking the blood counts. Its main additional toxicity is a severe idiosynchratic pulmonary interstitial fibrosis known as "busulphan lung" [445].

Busulphan alone has been compared with busulphan plus 6-thioguanine in a recent MRC study to investigate the relative effectiveness of the 2 regimens in attaining smooth and extended control of the disease in the chronic phase.

This study follows an earlier report of smooth control after a rapid fall in white count [446].

There has been no improvement in survival with the combination and the long-term use of thioguanine has been hepatotoxic in some patients who have developed portal hypertension [447].

Hydroxyurea has recently gained increasing support as first-line treatment of CML. It is a cycle-specific inhibitor of DNA which was first manufactured in Germany 120 years ago [448], but its value in CML was not reported until nearly 100 years later [449].

Its advantages include rapid control of the leucocyte count and a relatively rapid reversal of the drug's effects, which decreases the risk of overdosage. The disadvantages of hydroxyurea include greater cost, the need for continuous therapy with relatively frequent blood counts and occasional difficulty in finding the dose that will maintain the white count in the range of 5-10 x 10^9/l. This may, in part, be due to unnecessary readjustments to the dose in response to slight fluctuations in the white count. Some patients develop nausea and rashes and stomatitis and almost all patients show quite florid macrocytosis of the red cells secondary to megaloblastic changes in erythropoiesis. Initial doses nec-

essary for control lie in the range 0.5-2 G daily, with maintenance doses between 0.5-1.5 G daily. A report by Bolin et al. [45] suggests that it may prolong the duration of the chronic phase.
Other drugs which have been used in the treatment of CML include dibromannitol (DBM), cyclophosphamide, 6-mercaptopurine and melphalan, but no treatment, however successful it may have been in controlling the symptoms of the disease and in reestablishing normal blood counts, has made any significant impact on the percentage of Philadelphia-positive cells in the bone marrow or on the rate of transition to an accelerated phase or to blast crisis.
This rather bleak prospect appears to have been improved by the remarkable reports of the action of alpha interferon in the chronic phase of CML. The initial report from Talpaz [451] used human leucocyte interferon from the Finnish Red Cross [452] and haematological remission was obtained in 5 patients. The rationale for using alpha interferon was based on earlier findings of the effect of interferon on cancer patients and *in vitro* work on normal and chronic myeloid leukaemia granulocytic progenitor cells [453,454].
In later reports in which recombinant alpha IFN2a was used to treat patients during the early phase of CML at a dose of 5×10^6 units/m^2 daily, a little over 40% of patients had significant suppression of the Ph chromosome (4/26 had suppression to 0% for more than 12 months) [455].
When combined with intensive chemotherapy with DOAP (daunorubicin; oncovin; Ara-C and prednisone) for 3 cycles followed by maintenance with alpha IFN at a dose of $3\text{-}9 \times 10^6$ units daily, the results were even more encouraging: 89% (25/28 patients) had Ph-suppression, 19 of them to less than 35% during induction therapy [456].
A curious phenomenon which has not yet been explained has been the unusually high percentage of lymphoblastic leukaemias when blast transformation has occurred. The projected 3-year survival for the group of patients receiving DOAP plus interferons is 82% at 3 years.
An Italian study of 65 patients with CML in chronic phase received 2 or 5×10^6 U/m^2 on 3 days/wk or daily, 68% of patients responded and 46% achieved complete haematological remission. Cytogenetic improvement was seen in 70% of the responders (median number of Ph-positive cells was 65%). The most impressive results in the study, in which interferon alpha 2B was used, were obtained in patients receiving daily doses of interferon.

Philadelphia-Negative CML

Approximatley 10-15% of patients with CML do not have the Philadelphia chromosome. Their survival is generally shorter but a closer study of this group shows it to be heterogeneous, consisting of patients who lack the Ph chromosome but are bcr positive [419-424] and a very small group who are negative for the Ph chromosome and the bcr rearrangement. A recent review by Kurzrock [425] at the MD Anderson Hospital found that patients who had classic features of chronic phase CML who were Ph negative and bcr negative represented only 3% of the patients referred to their institution. They all presented with fairly high white blood counts ($23 - 300 \times 10^9$/l) and other peripheral blood and clinical features which were indistinguishable from classic CML. The duration of survival was similar but the response to alpha interferon was relatively disappointing (33% remission rate compared with 75% for patients with classic CML treated with alpha interferon at their hospital). The patients with Ph-negative, bcr-negative CML were older (median age 60 years compared with a median of 46 for the Ph-positive cases).
The clinical course also was different in that none of the cases showed progression to the blast transformation phase but there was a gradual increase in the tumour load with progressive organomegaly and bone marrow failure. This course of events may, in part, explain the role of the *bcr/abl* gene in an intermediate stage towards clonal evolution with the appearance of other chromosome abnormalities such as trisomy of chromosome 8 as the disease enters the blastic phase. If the *bcr/abl* sequence is absent, the subsequent stages may not be possible. A further anomaly, however, is the so-called juvenile CML which has been found to be Ph-negative, bcr negative in the few cases so far studied.

This is an extremely rare form of CML first described by Hardisty in 1964 and reviewed later by others [457-460]. It is clearly distinguishable from true CML arising in childhood and the majority of patients are below the age of 5 years.
A regular finding has been the presence of persistently high levels of foetal haemoglobin [461], high serum immunoglobulin values, antinuclear antibodies and antibodies to human IgG.
Lymphadenopathy, splenomegaly, rashes and infected lesions dominate the clinical picture and survival is usually less than 1 year with respone to busulphan and splenic irradiation usually poor. The treatment which has been most successful has been of the type designed for the management of AML.

Complications of CML

The principal complications of the disease *per se* include splenic infarctions, which are often distressingly painful and require analgesia, rest and possibly splenic irradiation or splenectomy; thrombocytosis may be a dominant feature of the peripheral blood picture leading to the risks of arterial or venous thrombosis - 4mg busulphan daily appears to be more successful than lower doses in combination with 6-thioguanine in achieving a satisfactory response in the platelet count. Serious complications from a high platelet count are, however, rare, making it unnecessary to embark on heroic measures to reduce the platelet count.
Hyperviscosity is uncommon, in spite of the levels to which white counts may rise, although the two are correlated [462,463].
Priapism occurs in 1-2% of men with CML and was mentioned in one of the earliest descriptions of the disease [15]. If treated sufficiently, early direct aspiration may relieve the situation but surgical management is often necessary and this leads to loss of sexual function.
Hyperuricaemia is a potential problem, particularly after treatment has begun if the xanthine oxidase inhibitor allopurinol is not prescribed and hypercalcaemia, changes in the serum potassium level and the tumour lysis syndrome are less common than in acute lymphoblastic leukaemia.

Treatment of Blast Transformation

This is uniformly difficult, although transformations to ALL respond well to aggressive chemotherapy, sometimes with a return to the chronic phase of CML. The response rate is higher in the cases in which the blasts are both TdTand CD10 positive [464,465].
Muehleck [466] has shown that the response is better when the Ph chromosome is the only chromosomal abnormality in the lymphoblasts.

Chronic Lymphatic Leukaemia

Chronic lymphatic leukaemia (CLL) is the name given to a group of conditions associated with the accumulation of small, morphologically mature lymphocytes in the blood, bone marrow, lymph nodes and spleen. The term CLL is generally restricted to include only those cases derived from a B-cell lineage and T-CLL is used for tumours of the T lymphocyte. However, there are some similarities to other lymphoid neoplasms, the features of which are shown in Table 17.
The annual incidence of CLL is variously reported as being between 0.6 and 3.7 per 100,000 [467,468], but figures as high as 10/100,000 have been found in certain areas where the population consists of a large number of retired people [469,470].
There is no significant difference between white and black population, and males and females are also equally affected if allowance is made for the increased longevity of women; however, the male/female ratio for the mid sixties is approximately 2:1. CLL is unusual under the age of 40 and rare below the age of 20, but it has been reported in childhood [471]. It is far less common in the Orient, representing only 2.5% of all leukaemias, compared with about 30% of leukaemias in the Western world [472]. In Japan, B-CLL is rare but a T-cell form has been described in the southern part of the country near Kyushu [473,474].
There is some evidence, principally provided by Blattner et al. [475], of genetic susceptibility, although it has been pointed out by others that a relationship to alterations in immune

Table 17. Comparative features of chronic lymphatic leukaemia and variants of CLL

Clinical features	B-cell CLL "Common" type	B-cell CLL "Lymphosarcoma" type	B-cell type prolymphocytic	T-cell CLL Western type	T-cell CLL Japanese type (II-TLV)
Incidence	3/100,000	Less frequent leukaemic phase malignant lymphoma	Unusual	2-3% of all CLL	II-TLV related clusters, South Japan, Caribbean
Age range (yr)	Rare <30-40+	Rare < 20-30+	Not defined	Rare <30-40+	35-70
Alive peak (yr)	50-60	55-65	55-65	50-60	45-55
Sex ratio (m:f)	2:1	1:1	Almost always male	1:1	1:1
Symptoms	Often asymptomatic (many incidental)	Usual	Usual	Variable	Usual
Peripheral lymphadenopathy	None - too obvious and generalised	Usual	Usual but not prominent	Not prominent	Usual
Splenomegaly	Not prominent	Variable	Prominent to massive	Prominent to massive	Prominent
Skin infiltrate	Uncommon, may be seen in longstanding disease	Uncommon	Rare	Frequent	Frequent hyper-calcaemia, lytic bone lesions
Survival (yr)	2-40 (depends on clinical stage)	2 - 5	0.5 - 4	2.5	1
Laboratory findings					
Blood					
Lymphocytosis	$>5x10^9/l$	$>3x10^9/l$	$>100x10^9/l$	$>5x10^9/l$	$>5x10^9/l$
Common range	10-150	10-100	80-500	5-300	50-700
Lymphocyte morphology	Small, mature cell, condensed chromatin	Variable size and shape, folded nucleus, prominent nucleolus	Large cell, less chromatin condensation, prominent nucleolus	Mature lymphocyte, folded nucleus, azurophilic granules in ample cytoplasm	
Cell surface markers	B cell	B cell	Usually B cell, rarely T cell	T cell	T cell
Bone marrow infiltration	>30% nucleated cells	Variable	Almost complete replacement by prolymphocytes	Moderate lymphocyte	Moderate lymphocyte

Adapted from: Sawitsky A and Rai KR: The chronic lymphoid leukaemias. In: Whittaker JA and Delamone IW (eds) Leukaemia. Blackwell Science Publ, Oxford 1987

function in families may be at least as important [470].
The advent of immunological techniques in the 1970s opened up new insights into the nature of the B-cell lymphoproliferative disorders. The sensitivity of the methods used has been enhanced further by the use of monoclonal antibodies against cell surface proteins. These techniques have been applied by the FAB (French, American, British) Group to set out a classification of the B- and T-cell leukaemias [478], based on the examination of specimens from 110 patients with various forms of chronic lymphoid leukaemias. The marker characteristics of the chronic B and T cell forms are shown in Tables 18A, 18B and 18C.

Table 18A. Monoclonal antibodies for the study of B-cell disorders

CD No.	Reactivity	Commonly used monoclonal antibodies
CD 5	Mature T cells, (strong) B CLL cells and some NHL cells (weak expression)	Leu 1, T101, T1, OKCLL, UCHT2
CD10	Common ALL antigen, early B cells and some NHL (follicular lymphoma)	J5, OKB-CALLA, VIL-A1, NU-N1, anti-CALLA
CD19	All B lymphocytes from early to late maturation stages	B4, Leu 12
CD20	Most B lymphocytes	B1, Leu 16, RFB7, NU-B2
CD21	Restricted to intermediate	B2, RFB6, BA-5
CD22	Late B cells, hairy cells	B3, Leu 14, TO15, RFB4, CLB/BLy 1
FMC7*	Late B cells, hairy cells, B prolymphocytes	FMC7
CD24	Most B lymphocytes	BA1
CD25	Activated B and T cells; hairy cells	Anti-Tac, Tac 1, IL-2 R1
CD 38	Activated B and T cells; plasma cells	OKT10
Anti-class II MHC antigens*	All B lymphocytes up to plasma cells; activated T cells and haemopoietic precursors maturation stages	HLA-Dr, OK1a, GRB1, FMC4

* Not allocated to a particular cluster of differentiation; FMC7 is probably distinct from CD22, although findings in some of the B-cell leukaemias suggest that both appear on the cell membrane at a relatively late stage of B-cell maturation

Table 18B. Markers in chronic B-cell leukaemias

Marker	CLL	PLL	HCL
SmIg	weak	<----------strong----------	>
CyIg	-	-/+	-/+
M-rosettes	++	-	-/+
CD5	++	-/+	-
CD19/20/24	++	++	++
Anti-class II	++	++	++
FMC7/CD22	-/+	++	++
CD10	-	-/+	-
CD25	-	-	++
CD38	-	-	-/+

\+ indicates incidence at which a marker is positive in >30% of cells in a particular B-cell tumour (++ 80-100%; + 40-80%; -/+ 10-40%; - 0-9% of cases)

Table 18C. Markers in chronic (mature) T-cell leukaemia

Marker	T-CLL	T-PLL	ATLL	Sezary's syndrome
TdT	-	-	-	-
CD1a	-	-	-	-
E-rosettes	++	++	++	++
CD2	++	++	++	++
CD3	++	+	++	++
CD4	-	+	++	++
CD5	-	++	++	++
CD7	-	++	-	-
CD8	++	-/+	-	-
CD25	-	-	++	-
CD38	-	-	-	-

\+ indicates rate at which a marker is positive in >30% of cells in particular T-cell leukaemias (++ 80-100%; -/+ 10-40%; - 0-9% of cases)

Clinical Features

The clinical features of CLL vary considerably. At least 20% of patients are asymptomatic and have early disease with no physical signs. Symptoms of anaemia are present in a minority, but the cardinal features of B-CLL are lymphadenopathy, splenomegaly, hepatomegaly, anaemia and thrombocytopenia. The clinical signs and haematological parameters have formed the basis for the Rai staging system on which many therapeutic decisions are based [479]. An alternative staging system has been proposed by Binet and has been adopted, with slight modifications, by the Leukaemia workshop on CLL [480] on the grounds that (i) there are fewer groups (3 vs 5) and therefore greater statistical power; (ii) better discrimination of the intermediate groups, e.g., Rai I and II; (iii) the lack of difference in prognosis between Rai stages III (anaemia) and IV (thrombocytopenia) (Table 19).

Apart from the classic manifestations of CLL, there are less common features which may present difficult therapeutic problems.

Altered immunity is common with hypogammaglobulinaemia as the most frequent feature. However, other immune disorders may dominate the clinical picture in a significant proportion of patients. Autoimmune haemolytic anaemia occurs in about 10%-20% [481] and is usually due to a warm anti-IgD antibody; immune thrombocytopenia (ITP) also occurs in 1%-2% [482].

Table 19. Definitions of staging and progressive disease

Stage	Organ enlargement*	Hb** (g/dl)	Platelets ** (x 10^9/l)
A	0, 1 or 2 areas	≥10	≥100
B	3, 4 or 5 areas	≥10	≥100
C	not considered	< 10 and/or	< 100

* Each of the following counts as one area: lymph nodes >1 cm in the neck, axillae, groins, spleen liver

** Secondary causes of anaemia (iron deficiency, folate or B12 deficiency) must be identified and treated before staging. Patients with autoimmune cytopenias will be randomised after treatment for this complication

The combination of autoimmune haemolytic anaemia and thrombocytopenia (Evans-Duane syndrome) [485] was first described in 1951 and may occur, according to some estimates, in half the patients with B-CLL [484]. ITP is associated with the production of a platelet-associated IgG [485] and may, in common with the haemolytic process, be triggered by radiotherapy or treatment with alkylating agents [486,487]. Treatment with steroids is usually effective, but high-dose intravenous immunoglobin can be a valuable alternative [488].

Autoimmune neutropenia is rare [489] and pure red-cell aplasia is more commonly associated with T-CLL than B-CLL phenotypes; when it occurs in B-CLL, it may be possible to demonstrate antibodies to developing erythroblasts [490].

Rare associations of CLL with systemic lupus erythematosis, rheumatoid arthritis, Sjogren's syndrome, allergic vasculitis, nephrotic syndrome and pernicious anaemia have been reported, but the aetiological links between these conditions and CLL are uncertain [491,492].

Although most antibodies are of the IgG class and polyclonal, monoclonal immunoglobulins are detected on serum electrophoresis in 5-10% of patients with CLL. In the majority of cases, the monoclonal antibody is of the IgM class and has been associated with mu-heavy chain disease [493].

The most common immunological complication of B-CLL, however, is hypogammaglobulinaemia, which occurs in 50-75% of patients with the disease. The severity is closely correlated with the Rai staging and affects most patients in clinical stage III or stage II [494] (Table 20).

The consequence of prolonged hypogammaglobulinanaemia is a marked increase in the susceptibility to infections which accounts for the fact that overwhelming sepsis is the principal cause of death in approximately half the patients with B-CLL [495-498]; immune deficiency can also impair the patient's quality of life substantially when recurrent debilitating infections follow one upon another [499].

Table 20. Serum Immunoglobulin levels according to CLL

Clinical Stage	Immunoglobulin levels (median) G/L		
Stage	IgG	IgA	IgM
0	9.2	1.0	0.6
1	9.0	0.98	0.46
2	7.2	1.05	0.38
3	5.7	0.5	0.33
4	6.0	0.7	0.6
Normal range	8-18	0.9-4.5	0.6-2.8

Bacterial infections, including bronchopneumonia, urinary tract infections, sinusitis, staphylococcal diseases and skin infection form the majority [491], while the most commonly documented viral infection is herpes zoster which occasionally can result in a disseminated varicella zoster infection.

Exposure to DNA viruses (herpes simplex, herpes zoster, cytomegalovirus etc.) may lead to a histiocytic medullary reticulosis-like syndrome. Patients deteriorate rapidly with the development of fever and jaundice in the presence of large numbers of marrow macrophages exhibiting active haemophagocytosis [500].

The availability of high-quality immunoglobulin preparations has lead to clinical trials of the value of regular intravenous immunoglobulin in the prevention of recurrent infections in B-CLL. Patients are randomised in a double-blind study to receive either intravenous immunoglobulin or a 0.1% albumin preparation at intervals of 3-4 weeks. Two such studies are currently being conducted in Britain and similar trials have been set up in Europe and the United States.

Treatment

There have been many different opinions on the indications for treating CLL and the choice of drugs has until fairly recently remained relatively narrow.

The guidelines established by staging the disease and the assignment to prognostic groups has produced a more structured approach to the care of patients with this condition and a greater awareness of the potential problems [501].

Patients in the low-risk group (Stage 0 in the Rai staging) generally have a disease which takes an indolent course. Early treatment with an alkylating agent has not conferred any advantage in survival compared with a group of patients who have merely been observed carefully. At least half of these patients will die from causes unrelated to the disease. Furthermore, the clinical stage at the time the patient is first seen does not take into account the rate of change in an individual case. Rai and his colleagues have therefore recommended a period of observation for all patients with CLL [501] and have incorporated this philosophy into their protocol.

The principal drug used in the treatment of CLL for the last 30 years has been chlorambucil administered traditionally at a dose of 0.05-0.15 mg/kg daily until maximal clinical and haematological response has been maintained [502]. It has gained popularity because it is a relatively easy drug to use and in Britain at least it has in the past often been prescribed by general physicians rather than haematologists. Recently, there has been a vogue for intermittent short courses of treatment at doses in the range of 1.0-2.5 mg/kg for 1-4 days each month. High-dose intermittent therapy is thought to be less myelosuppressive and less immunosupressive than the low-dose continuous regimen and may prove more effective.

Although it is effective in controlling the disease, it is unlikely that it has ever resulted in a complete cure. Furthermore, in common with other alkylating agents, it is leukaemogenic; Galton found a 10% incidence of AML among patients who have received chlorambucil for more than 3 years [502].

Patients with Stage I or Stage II disease fall into a group for which there are no defined guidelines [503,504]. However, it is generally accepted that patients with symptoms from the disease should be treated. In a British MRC trial which entered 660 patients with-CLL up to 1984 [504], those with Rai Stage I and II were observed for a period of up to a year after diagnosis and then classified as static or progressive. The latter was defined by a persistent downward trend in either haemoglobin or platelets, with either a significant increase in physical signs or a consistent upward trend in the lymphocyte counts (doubling time 12 months or less) or constitutional symptoms. Apart from the stage at the time of diagnosis, age, sex (females fared better than males) and response to treatment were significant prognostic features. However, one third of the deaths during this study were ascribed to factors other than activity of the CLL and included disseminated carcinomas and cardiovascular accidents.

A recent report from the French Cooperative Group on chronic lymphocytic leukaemia [505] has also investigated the policy of managing patients with Stage A disease either with observation alone or with immediate chemotherapy. The overall survival was slightly better for the untreated group at 5 years (82% for the untreated group and 75% in the chlorambucil group). Chlorambucil was able to slow down progression to Stage B and response to chlorambucil was correlated with a prolonged survival; however, patients whose disease progressed while receiving chlorambucil therapy had a very short survival. There was also a significant increase in epithelial cancers in the chlorambucil-treated group (33/303) compared with the no-treatment group (19/309), causing deaths in 13 and 3 patients, respectively.

They concluded that patients with haemoglobin values >12 G/L and lymphocyte count <30×10^9/l had a survival which was not significantly different from a sex- and age-matched French population. These patients, accounting for approximately 50% of all cases of chronic lymphatic leukaemia, should not be treated unless the disease progresses.

Prednisolone has been added to chlorambucil as an additional lympholytic agent. It is particularly useful when bone marrow failure is advanced and was recommended as initial therapy alone for the first 4 weeks for patients with Stage III or IV disease in the MRC first CLL trial [504]. While steroids alone may produce dramatic shrinkage in the size of the spleen and lymph nodes, the lympocyte count may rise very substantially [506-508]. However, the long-term use of steroids in CLL is not recommended because of its well-known side effects, not least immunosuppression leading to severe infections. There is no evidence that more intensive therapy is beneficial in patients in earlier forms of the disease. Even those patients with stage B disease gain no advantage compared with patients treated with chlorambucil [509].

A Danish study comparing CHOP with chlorambucil plus prednisolone in patients with stage B and C diseases showed more complete remissions with the CHOP regimen (63% vs 29%), but no overall difference in survival after a relatively short follow-up period [510].

In more advanced disease, combinations of drugs generally include cyclophosphamide, hydroxydaunorubicin, vincristine, prednisone and cytosine arabinoside. One of the most recent reports has come from the French Cooperative Group [511,512]. Patients with stage C disease were randomised to COP (cyclophosphamide, oncovin and prednisolone) vs CHOP (addition of adriamycin). The 3-year survival rates were 71% in the CHOP group and 28% in the COP group (median survivals 62 months and 22 months, respectively). Their subsequent trial (CLL 85) has extended the use of CHOP in comparison with chlorambucil plus prednisolone for patients with stage B disease.

A combination of 5 drugs, including cyclophosphamide, adriamycin, cytosine arabinoside, vincristine and prednisolone (POACH), was used to treat a group of untreated and previously treated patients at the MD Anderson Hospital [513]. The majority (71%) of patients fell into stage B or C. Forty-seven percent of untreated patients compared with 29% of previously treated patients had clearance of their disease. The response/lack of response to therapy provided the strongest indication for survival [513].

The toxicity of combination therapy, particularly in the older populations of patients, continues to present major problems which need to be justified by the therapeutic response and quality of life.

Low-dose splenic irradiation has been used for many years [514] and was included as a potentially valuable form of treatment in the MRC CLL 1 trial; it has recently been retried, with success, in a group of patients in London [515].

A flow diagram of the third MRC CLL trial is shown in Figure 3.

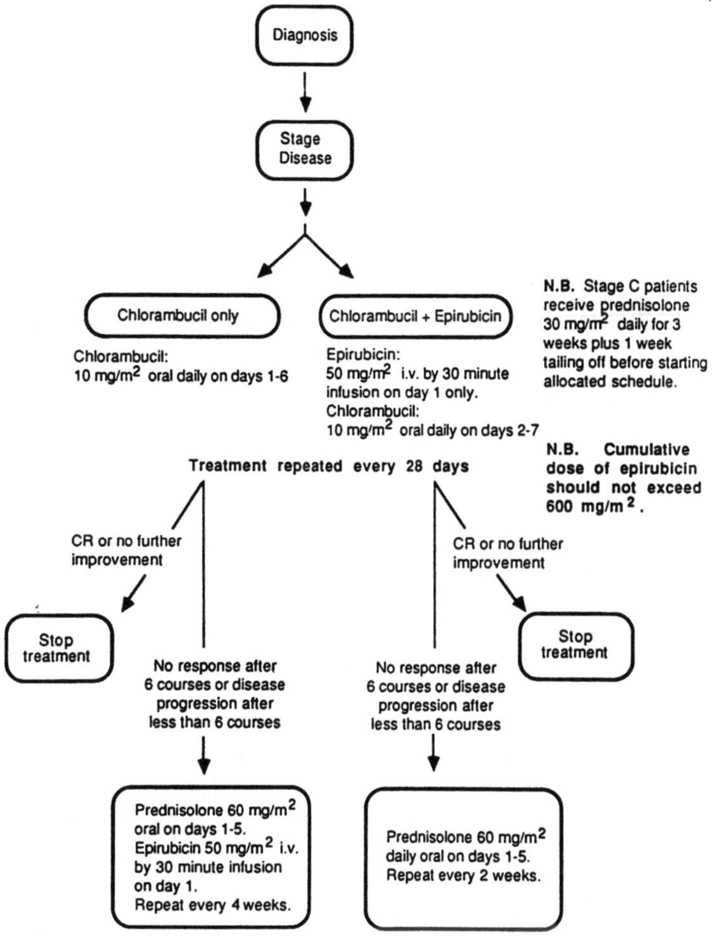

Fig. 3. Third MCR CLL trial

Other Forms of Treatment

Fludarabine

The clinical use of the purine analogue arabinosyladenine (Ara A) in cancer treatment is limited, because it is rapidly metabolised by adenosine deaminase (ADA). An ADA-resistant analogue was developed, 2-fluoro-Ara A (2F-Ara A), but it was poorly soluble in water and therefore of little value for clinical use; the monophosphate (2F-ara AMP, fludarabine) is, however, soluble [516,517]. The structural relationships of this group of drugs is shown in Figure 4.

The mode of action of fludarabine is probably similar to Ara-A [517], it is phosphorylated and subsequently converted into its triphosphate, which is a potent inhibitor of ribonuleotide reductase and the DNA polymerases. Fludarabine is purely an inhibitor of DNA synthesis and has no effect on RNA or protein synthesis [516,517].

Earlier work with adenine arabinoside had provided evidence that it could be an effective anti-leukaemic agent and subsequent studies with fludarabine on patients with lymphoma had confirmed its possible value [518]. The halogenated derivative of Ara-A is not a substrate for human adenosine deaminase [519]. It therefore obviates the need for combining Ara-A with an adenosine deaminase inhibitor such as deoxycoformycin, which is also active in CLL although currently principally used in HCL. Fludarabine had produced lymphopenia in patients being treated for solid tumours [520] before Keating et al. [521] reported on 68 patients with previously treated CLL who received 25 mg/m^2 or 30 mg/m^2 daily for 5 days. Forty-three percent of patients in Rai stage 1-3 and 19% of patients in Rai stage 4 returned to Rai stage 0. The response was rapid, with 92% of the

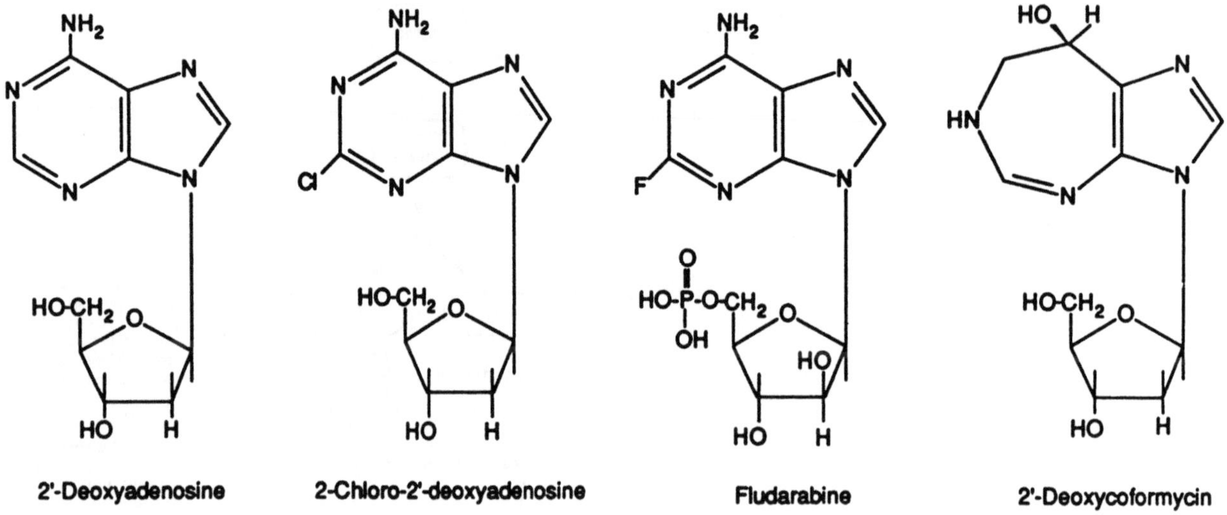

Fig. 4. Structural relationship of purine inhibitors

responders achieving at least a partial response following the first 3 courses. The tolerance was excellent, with little toxicity, apart from that associated with infection. The overall response was superior to the multidrug combination (POACH) used in the same centre (see ref. 513).

At the higher doses used in a group of patients with acute leukaemia (up to 150mg/m^2/day for 7 days) [522], severe central nervous toxicity developed; this included optic neuritis, blindness, seizures, paralysis and coma. The experiences of this phase II study were not unique [523-525], but the future development of the drug for CLL is very exciting and could represent the first important therapeutic advance for many years.

Monoclonal Antibodies

The treatment of CLL with monoclonal antibodies directed against surface immunoglobulin idiotypes has produced only short-term responses because of the development of various escape mechanisms of which immune modulation is the most important [526,527].

The majority of the early trials of the use of unconjugated monoclonal antibodies were interesting rather than impressive in their responses [528-531].

It was soon recognised that the therapeutic effect can be limited by the antiglobulin response which appears in about 10 days in most patients, apart from those severely immunosupressed by terminal disease or previous therapy. The initial effectiveness of the antibody is probably determined by the ability to activate human effector mechanisms such as complement binding, antibody-dependent cell-mediated cytotoxicity and opsonisation. These, in turn, are affected by the distribution and density of the target antigen, its tendency to modulate, the species and isotype of the antibody and the extent to which natural effector mechanisms are compromised by disease or other therapeutic agents. Dyer et al. have treated patients with a series of monoclonal antibodies in the CAMPATH series [532].

The IgM (CAMPATH-IM) produced transient depletion of blood lymphocytes with consumption of complement; transfusions of fresh frozen plasma were required to replete the complement stores.

A further development of the antibody structure resulted in a variant designated IgG2b. Unlike the earlier forms of the antibody, the IgG2b molecule was able to achieve prolonged clearance of lymphocytes from the peripheral blood of 2 patients whose B-CLL had advanced to a prolymphocytic stage. There was, however, no substantial effect on the lymph nodes (Fig. 5).

The structure of the CAMPATH antibody has been humanised, using the hypervariable

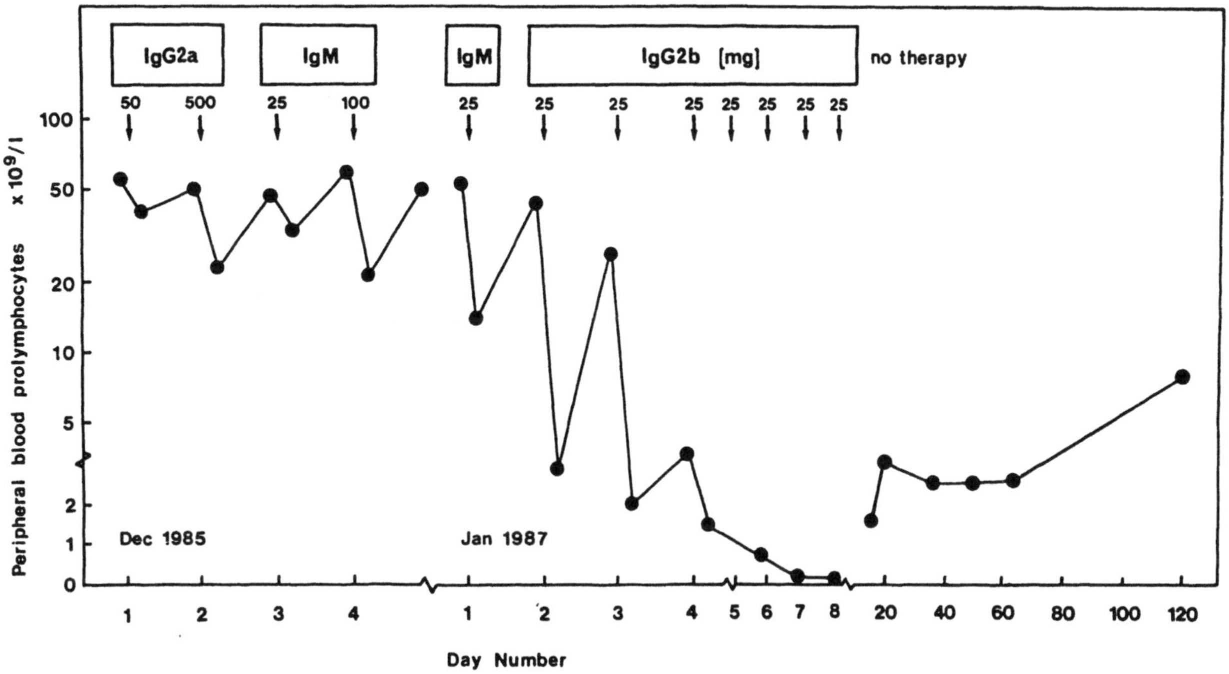

Fig. 5. Response to monoclonal antibodies in CLL

region of CAMPATH-IG [533], and has entered clinical trials in B-cell lymphoid malignancies [534].

Another possible future application of such antibodies may be in the treatment of minimal residual disease in patients receiving bone marrow transplantation for lymphoid malignancies.

Prolymphocytic Leukaemia

Prolymphocytic leukaemia (PLL) was first described as a distinct variant of CLL by Galton [535]. The relationship between these 2 conditions has been comprehensively reviewed in a series of papers by Melo et al. [536-539]. It is important to recognise the condition because of the very different prognosis for patients presenting with or progressing to PLL. Melo defined 3 groups, separated by the percentage of PLL cells in the circulation. "Typical" CLL has less than 10% prolymphocytes (PROL) in the circulation. An intermediate group CLL/PL has 11-55% PROL and PLL has >55% PROL.

There was no significant difference in survival between the first 2 groups (CLL and CLL/PL), but the PLL group had a much shorter survival (median 3 years) compared to the patients with the other 2 groups continued (median 8 years).

Richter's Syndrome

In 1928, Richter [540] described the development of a large cell lymphoma in a patient who had previously had CLL; it arises in 3-5% of patients with CLL. The clinical features include unexplained fever, night sweats, weight loss, increased lymphadenopathy, particularly in the retroperitoneal group, and lymphocytopenia [541]. The histological findings are characterised by the presence of multinucleate giant cells and a pleomorphic infiltrate, alongside areas with classical features of CLL. The lymphoma cells are positive for SmIg and some of the other markers for CLL. The progressive changes are not related to previous chemotherapy as the clinical picture may develop soon after the diagnosis is made in some patients.

Evidence from the analysis of immunoglobulin gene rearrangements suggests that, in some cases, there are distinct genetic events associated with the development of the lymphoma, which are not a development of an earlier gene rearrangement in the preceding CLL [542,543], whereas other studies have shown modification of the CLL pattern [544,545]. The syndrome is often associated with a monoclonal paraprotein in the serum and free light chain in the urine.
The response to treatment is very poor and the majority of patients die within 6 months of the transformation [546,547].

Hairy Cell Leukaemia (Leukaemic Reticuloendotheliosis)

The first description of leukaemic reticuloendotheliosis has been ascribed by Bouroncle [548] to Ewald [549] in 1923, though subsequently a variety of terms were used to describe what appears to have been the same condition [550-552]. Bouroncle's detailed review in 1958 set out the essential clinical features of hairy cell leukaemia and earns the title of a "classic report" - the terms in which she referred to it in a later review [553]. Her description of a "lace-like" outline to the cell membrane on electron microscopy sadly was not taken up by later authors to introduce the name "lace-like leukaemia" and the all-Greek designation of "tricholeukocyte leukaemia" [554] did not achieve any popular appeal outside France.
The term "hairy cells" was first used by Schrek and Donnelly in 1966 [555] in their description of 2 patients with features similar to those described by Bouroncle in a review of 26 cases of leukaemic reticuloendotheliosis. The description of the cells avoided "any commitment in regard to classification". Their reluctance to enter the debate was a remarkably adroit decision in view of the subsequent debate on the nature of the normal counterpart of the hairy cell.
Before the condition was more widely accepted as a distinct haematological malignancy, many had been misdiagnosed as cases of chronic lymphatic leukaemia.

Incidence

Hairy cell leukaemia (HCL) is a disease of middle age; the male/female ratio is approximately 4:1 [553,556,557]. It is, however, not rare in patients under 40 or over 70 years of age and represents about 2% of all leukaemias.

Clinical Features

Anaemia is one of the presenting symptoms and splenomegaly is found in 80% of cases. Hepatomegaly is present in half of the patients, but lymphadenopathy is very rare.
Infections occur in about 30% of patients and represent the major cause of morbidity; those patients who do not develop infections have a significantly longer survival [557,558]. The incidence of infections does not appear to correlate closely with the degree of neutropenia or monocytopenia present at diagnosis, but, in addition to the more common infections with gram-v_e micro-organisms such as E.Coli and Pseudomonas Aeruginosa, mycobacterial infections such as M. Kansasii present a particular problem in HCL.
The explanation for the high incidence of mycobacterial infections [559,560] may lie in the degree of monocytopenia which leads to impaired granuloma formation. Pyrexial episodes which occur in a patient with HCL must be investigated very fully and a trial of antituberculosis drugs has been advocated as empirical antibiotic treatment when no organism has been isolated [561].
Although the classic combination of splenomegaly and pancytopenia is the most common finding, other features which have been described include vasculitis, presenting as a polyarteritis nodosa and associated with joint pains and fever [562,563].
This complication is more frequently seen in patients who have undergone splenectomy, suggesting a decreased ability to clear immune complexes [564,565].
Osteolytic lesions have been described by several authors [566-568]. These are usually found at the upper end of the femur but are not associated with hypercalcaemia. Paraproteinaemia is rare but is of the IgG type when present, and an intriguing association with myelomatosis or amyloidosis may illus-

trate the similarity in the ontogeny of the B-cell lineage [569].
Some of the more unusual presentating features of hairy cell leukaemia have been reviewed by Bouroncle [570].
Bone marrow aspirates are notoriously difficult to obtain and trephine biopsies are required in the majority of patients. The diagnosis is normally confirmed by the finding of hairy cells in the circulation, which demonstrate tartrate-resistant acid phosphatase (TRAP) staining [571], but a variety of monoclonal antibodies have been produced which allow more accurate diagnosis and monitoring of the response to chemotherapy [572-575].
The recognition of the presence in very high concentrations in the serum of the IL-2 receptor p55 chain (the Tac antigen) in a soluble form (sIL-2R) in HCL (concentrations up to 50,000 U/ml) has made it possible to distinguish it from other forms of B-cell proliferative disorders, although high levels are also found in adult T-cell leukaemia [576-579]. The correlation with tumour burden gives a very valuable, non-invasive method of monitoring HCL during treatment [577-580].
Monoclonal antibodies which are diagnostically useful in frozen sections include the B-Ly7. CD22 and CD11c, particularly when they are used in combination. An extension of the application of these techniques in paraffin sections uses fixation-resistant B-cell related epitopes; cells which have a combination of L26+, LN1+ MT2+ are not normally seen in the bone marrow and can confidently be identified as hairy cells. The introduction of more specific antibodies has been of great value because inaccurate assessment of the degree of infiltration of the bone marrow and other organs with hairy cells may account for the varying responses to treatment which have been reported.
A staging system has been proposed by Jansen et al. [582], based on haemoglobin levels and spleen size at the time of diagnosis in 291 patients from a European international collaborative group. The system has not been widely used, however, partly because of the introduction of new therapy since the method was devised.
The median survival has been 5-6 years [581], but more recent treatment methods bring hope of a very substantial improvement in the prognosis.

Treatment

The traditional method of treating patients with HCL has been with supportive care, chlorambucil and splenectomy [583,584].
The timing of splenectomy in HCL has not easily been resolved and the benefits have been restricted to a group of patients with large spleens (>4 cm below costal margin) and pancytopenia. Jansen's retrospective analysis of patients from 22 European centres could show no benefit for patients aged >60, symptoms >12 months, haemoglobin values >12 g/dl, neutrophils >0.5 x 10^9/l or platelets >100 x 10^9/l, but overall there was a highly significant difference in survival between the non-splenectomised patients, who had a median survival of 21 months, compared with 89 months for the splenectomised patients [582]. Complete responders to splenectomy were defined as the group in which all 3 haematological parameters improved (haemoglobin, white count and platelets).
In another collaborative study, 75% of the patients were alive at 5 years; one useful prognostic assessment of the possible value of splenectomy in this group of patients was the reticulocyte count - a value of less than 2% predicting a poor response to splenectomy [584].
In the light of subsequent developments in the therapy of HCL, it is not worthwhile dwelling too long on earlier efforts at achieving remissions. Chlorambucil at relatively low dose produced satisfactory responses, particularly in the platelet count, in some patients [581,583].

Interferon

The management of HCL was revolutionised by the advent of interferon and has made splenectomy a relatively uncommon choice of treatment.
Quesada was the first to report the effect of interferon in the treatment of HCL, using a partially purified leucocyte preparation [585,586]. Until that time, the drug had enjoyed a period of popularity for the treatment of lymphomas and acute lymphoblastic leukaemia, but in the

late 1970s and early 1980s there was a general feeling among physicians that interferon - which by this time had become much more widely available - was a drug looking for a disease to treat. Hairy cell leukaemia was a remarkable and at the time unexpected model on which a drug would earn its reputation.

Quesada reported a 100% response in 7 patients, and a subsequent report on 22 patients confirmed the encouraging results [587].

The early studies in England [588] were conducted with a purified human lymphoblastoid interferon produced by challenging cells in tissue culture with Sendai virus. It contains at least 8 naturally occurring alpha interferons and is more similar to the purified leucocyte interferon than to the recombinant preparations which contain a single form. This may be important in the incidence of antibodies to various interferons discussed later.

Quesada subsequently published his results on the treatment of 93 patients with either the partially purified alpha interferon or a recombinant IFN [587].

There was a higher incidence of complete remissions in untreated patients (i.e., non-splenectomised) and the remission rate increased with time (62% after 2 years' treatment compared with 22% at 1 year). The median time to complete remission was 16 months, using 3 mega-units of interferon daily.

None of the 23 patients treated with the purified IFN-alpha had relapsed while receiving treatment, whereas a small number had relapsed while receiving the recombinant preparation because they developed antibodies.

Following the initial encouraging reports, a large number of studies were set up using various forms of interferon. Both interferon alpha-2a and interferon alpha-2b have received product licences in the United States for the treatment of hairy cell leukaemia.

Many of the larger trials were reported in 1987 [589-591] and reviewed by Cheson in that year [592]; more recently, the role of biotherapy in HCL and other conditions has been reviewed by Figlin [593].

The apparent variations in response were in part due to differences in the criteria for complete remission. Golomb [594,595], in reporting one of the larger series, laid down strict criteria for a complete response: <5% hairy cells in the bone marrow biopsy; improvement in the peripheral blood counts to a haemoglobin >12G/dl, platelets $>100\times10^9$/l and neutrophils $>1.5\times10^9$/l. Only 4% of 128 patients achieved this, but over 80% of patients had substantial improvements in their blood counts (complete and partial remissions).

Following the discontinuation of therapy, there was often a further rise in the haemoglobin and platelet counts, but these were usually reversed after 3-4 months [596]. There was no significant fall in the counts in the next year and only 1 of 24 patients required further therapy during this period.

The optimal duration of treatment has not been established. A recent randomised study comparing 12 months treatment with 19 months of interferon alpha-2b given 3 times weekly subcutaneously at a dose of 2×10^6U/m^2 showed no significant difference in the clinical course of the disease in the 2 groups, but responses were maintained while patients received therapy [594]. There was also a high incidence of fatigue among the patients continuing treatment for an additional 6 months. The conclusion was that therapy could be discontinued after 12 months in asymptomatic patients.

Magnetic resonance images have been found useful in assessing response and predicting relapse. This could be helpful in some centres in planning the duration of treatment [597].

The main side effects of alpha-interferon are now well recognised [590,598]. Constitutional symptoms such as flu-like symptoms, fatigue and anorexia are the most troublesome and can be sufficiently distressing for a patient to refuse further treatment. The symptoms are minimised by administering IFN in the late evening with paracetamol [599,600].

Gastrointestinal symptoms include nausea, vomiting and diarrhoea in 30% and neurological toxicity may take the form of peripheral neuropathies, memory loss and depression.

Raynaud's phenomenon associated with reversible cryoglobulinaemia has been described in a patient with myeloma and in another with chronic myeloid leukaemia. The symptoms disappeared when the interferon was stopped [601].

Local inflammation at injection sites, dry skin, seborrhaic dermatitis, vasculitis, alopecia and liver dysfunction have also been reported, but Schilsky found no adverse effects on gonadal and sexual dysfunction in male patients receiving recombinant interferon [602].

The effect on bone marrow fibrosis has been variable. Coci et al. [603] found it was not influenced by human lymphoblastoid interferon but Dupuy reported an improvement following the correction of a defect in platelet-derived growth factor and thromboglobulin [604].

The mechanism of action of interferon has remained unclear but recent evidence has gone some way to clarifying the situation [605].

Investigations on one case of HCL and 8 cases of B-cell chronic lymphatic leukaemia (B-CLL) provide evidence that interferon alpha can interrupt the production of tumour necrosis factor (TNF). Earlier work from the same group had shown that tumour necrosis factor can also act as a tumour growth factor, maintaining HCL and B-CLL cell survival *in vitro* and inducing proliferation without terminal differentiation [606,607].

The production of growth factors is achieved by reducing the accumulation of mRNA for IL-1a and b, TNF alpha and IL-6. Interferon alpha also increases the expression of mRNA for the enzyme 2-5A synthetase, a ribonuclease activator.

It is suggested that interferon alpha works by reducing endogenous growth factor production rather than by enhancing antileukaemic host cytotoxic mechanisms. However, a direct enhancing role for interferon alpha on host cytotoxic effector mechanisms has been proposed by Roth [600], while other studies have found a reduction in plasma levels of soluble CD8 antigen and IL-2 receptor antigen, suggesting an effect on the suppressor/cytotoxic cells.

Clinical resistance to the interferons has recently been described in several series [608-611].The incidence of antibody production varies with the clinical setting, being higher in patients receiving IFN for renal cell carcinoma and AIDS-associated Kaposi's sarcoma. Early reports suggested that in HCL this was more likely to occur with the recombinant interferon alpha-2a preparation and a lower incidence was found among patients receiving the interferon alpha-2b [612].

Steis et al. found antibodies to interferon in 31 out of 51 patients with HCL who had been treated for a median of 7 months with interferon alpha-2a. In 15 of the 31 cases, the antibody was non-neutralising but in the remaining 16 the antiviral effect of the antibody was active *in vitro*. It was not active against purified natural alpha interferon. Clinical resistance of varying degrees was seen in 6 out of 16 patients having neutralising antibodies.

Antibodies to recombinant interferon alpha-2b in HCL have not been reported until a single case was described recently at the Michael Reese Medical Centre in Chicago [613].

In a series of 75 patients with HCL treated with lymphoblastoid interferon in a multi-centre study in England, no neutralising activity was detected in any of the cases, in spite of the high accumulated doses the patients had received - median 780 x 10^6 units (range 24-2688).

An interesting combination of interferon with recombinant G-CSF has apparently increased the rate of recovery in the neutrophil and platelet counts in one study, and G-CSF has been used alone in gradually increasing doses in a small phase I/II study to determine its value in raising the neutrophil counts in patients with HCL and neutropenia. A brisk response in absolute neutrophil counts was seen within 2 weeks with values ranging from <0.9 x 10^9/l to >4.0 x 10^9/l. The authors concluded that GM-CSF may be a useful adjunct to definitive treatment of hairy cell leukaemia with interferon or pentostatin [614].

2-Deoxycoformycin

An alternative form of treatment for HCL was proposed by Spiers et al. [615], who reported the results of a study with 2-deoxycoformycin (pentostatin). He obtained a 59% complete remission rate and a 37% partial remission rate in 27 patients - only 1 patient showed no response. A dose of 5 mg/m^2/day for 2 consecutive days every 2 weeks was as effective as higher doses.

None of the patients with a complete response relapsed during a median follow-up period of 9 months. Some myelosuppression occurred but renal and hepatic toxicity was rare and the drug was well tolerated [616].

A later report on the use of low-dose pentostatin [617] - 4 mg/m^2 every other week - resulted in complete remission in 9 out of 10 patients. A further update on the study has confirmed the earlier results on 23 patients [618]. Treatment was not continued once complete remission had been achieved by 20 patients, but 15 of these remained in remission for an average of 12.6 months. A study carried out by the National Cancer Institute of Canada on 31 patients showed a high complete remission rate with 4 mg/m^2 weekly for 3 weeks every 8 weeks. The toxicity has generally been mild and reversible but includes nausea and vomiting, conjunctivitis and rash. Renal failure, a severe problem at higher doses [610,619,620] was not seen at the lower dose used by Kraut.

Pentostatin has also been shown to be very effective in patients who have HCL which is refractory to interferon. A collaborative EORTC (European Organisation for Research and Treatment of Cancer) group have reported the response of 33 patients with IFN-resistant disease who subsequently received 4 mg/m^2 weekly for 3 weeks followed by 4 mg/m^2 alternate weeks for 3 cycles. Eleven of the 33 patients achieved complete remission and 15 partial remission, giving an overall response rate of 88%. The median duration of response was 11.5 months [621].

The studies on HCL followed earlier work on other leukaemias and lymphomas by Smyth and his co-workers in Edinburgh [622,623].

The rationale for investigating the activity of adenosine deaminase (ADA) inhibitors followed the acknowledged importance of ADA for normal lymphocyte function and the demonstration of greatly elevated ADA activity in human malignant lymphocytes [623]. They hypothesised at that time that the pharmacological inhibition of ADA might be of value in the treatment of lymphoid neoplasia and have reviewed their results recently [624].

The mechanism of action is not entirely clear although the accumulation of intracellular deoxyadenosine triphosphate (dATP) is thought to have a central role [625-627], with DNA-ligase the probable target for the inhibition of DNA synthesis [628]. Side effects include nausea and vomiting, conjunctivitis, lethargy, rash and renal and central nervous system toxicity. It may also produce prolonged reduction of CD4 T lymphocytes [629].

2-Chlorodeoxadenosine

Exceptional results have also been described recently in 12 patients treated at the Scripps Clinic, La Jolla, using the deoxyadenosine analogue 2-chloro-deoxyadenosine [630]. At a dose of 0.1 mg per kilogram daily by continuous infusion for 7 days, complete remissions were obtained in 11 of the 12 patients. No relapses have occurred and the median duration of remission is 15 1/2 months.Unlike deoxycoformycin, it is not an adenosine deaminase inhibitor, although both drugs increase the intranuclear levels of deoxy-nucleotides, and it is independent of cell division. It has no direct effect on S-adenosyl-L-homocysteine metabolism [631] or adenosine receptors, which may account for its remarkable lack of toxicity. The drug is not yet commercially available as the supply used in this study was synthesised at the Scripps Clinic and Research Foundation. When larger quantities are available, controlled trials in comparison with deoxycoformycin should prove very interesting.

A recent editorial entitled "What is the choice of treatment for hairy cell leukaemia?" reviews the situation very succinctly. It emphasises that there is no single "first choice" treatment for HCL and that perhaps 10% of newly diagnosed patients may never require any treatment [632].

Splenectomy still has a role if the spleen is large and the patient has severe cytopenia, although this procedure carries the highest risk in the very situation in which it may be most valuable.

It is premature to abandon the alpha interferons in favour of pentostatin, in spite of the great promise shown by this drug and randomised trials comparing alpha-IFN and pentostatin have begun. Meanwhile, pentostatin is not widely available and interferon will remain the treatment of choice - or because of a lack of choice - for many patients in the next few years.

REFERENCES

1 Bennett JH: Case of hypertrophy of the spleen and liver in which death took place from suppuration of the blood. Edin Med Surg J 1845 (64):413-415
2 Craigie D: Case of disease of the spleen in which death took place in consequence of the presence of purulent matter in the blood. Edin Med Surg J 1945 (64):400-401
3 Virchow R: Weisses Blut. N Notiz Geb Nat Heilk 1845 (36):151-153
4 Barth J: Alteration du sang remarquable par la predominance des globules blancs ou muquex; hypertrophie considerable de la rate. Bull et Mem Soc Méd Hôp Paris 1856 (3):55-56
5 Donné A: Cours de Microscopie Complémentaire des Etudes Médicales, Anatomie Microscopique et Physiologique des Fluides de l'Economie. JB Baillière, Paris 1844 pp 132
6 Fuller HW: Particulars of a case in which enormous enlargement of the spleen and liver, together with dilataion of the blood vessels of the body were found coincident with a peculiarly altered condition of the blood. Lancet 1846 (ii):43-44
7 Bennett JH: Leucocythaemia, or White Cell Blood, in relation to the physiology and pathology of the lymphocytic glandular system. Sutherland & Cox, Edinburgh 1852
8 Virchow R: Die Leukaemie. In: Gesammelte Abhandlungen zur wissenschäftlichen Medizin. Meidinger Sohn & Comp, Frankfurt 1856 pp 190
9 Barthez F: Procès verbal de la séance du 9 janvier 1856 (Discussion on leukocythemia). Bull et Mem Soc Méd Hôp Paris 1856 (3):59-61
10 Neumann E: Ueber die bedeutung des Knochenmarkes für die Blutbildung. Centrabl Med Wiss 1868 (6):689-691
11 Neumann E: Ueber myelogene Leukaemie. Berliner Klin Wochenschr 1878 (15):69-71
12 Bizzozero G: Sulla funzione ematopoietica del midollo delle ossa R.C.R. 1st Lomb Sci Lett 1868 (2 ser 1):815-818
13 Bizzozero G: Su di un nuovo elemento morfologico del sangue dei mammiferi e della sua importanza nella trombosi e nella coagulazione. Osservatore 1882 (17):785-787 (transl into German in Virchows Arch Path Anat 1882 (90):261-332
14 Tavassoli M, Yoffey JM: Bone Marrow Structure and Function. Alan R Liss Inc, New York 1983
15 Lissauer H: Zwei fälle von Leukämie. Berliner Klin Wochenschr 1865 (2):403-404
16 Forkner CE and Scott TFM: Arsenic as therapeutic agent in chronic myelogenous leukaemia: preliminary report. JAMA 1931 (97):3-5
17 Gunz FW: Leukaemia in the past. In: Henderson E and Lister TA (eds) Leukaemia. WB Saunders & Co, Philadelphia 1990
18 Muratet L: Faure-Fremiet. Confidential report of the French Gas Service, 1918
19 Zunz G: Report to the Interallied Gas Conference, Paris 1918
20 Stewart MJ: Report on cases of poisoning by "mustard gas" (dichlorethyl sulphide) with special reference to the histological changes and to the alterations on the leucocyte count. Report of the Chemical Warfare Committee, Great Britain, Med Res Com Rep No 17, 1918
21 Krumbhaar EB: Role of the blood and the bone marrow in certain forms of gas poisoning. I. Peripheral blood changes and their significance. JAMA 1919 (72):39-41
22 Pappenheimer AM and Vance M: The effects of intravenous injections of dichloroethyl sulphide in rabbits, with special reference to its leucotoxic action. J Exp Med 1920 (31):71-94
23 Gilman A and Phillips FS: Biological actions and therapeutic applications of B-chloroethylamines and sulfides. Science 1946 (103):409-415
24 Gilman A: Symposium on advances in pharmacology resulting from war research: therapeutic applications of chemical warfare. Fed Proc 1946 (5):285-292
25 Goodman LS, Wintrobe MM, Damashek W et al: Nitrogen mustard therapy: use of methyl-bis-(B-chloroethyl) amine hydrochloride and tris-(B-chloroethyl) amine hydrochloride for Hodgkin's disease, lymphosarcoma, leukaemia and certain allied and miscellaneous disorders. JAMA 1946 (132):126-132
26 Freireich EJ: Nitrogen mustard therapy (landmark perspective). JAMA 1984 (251):2262-2269
27 Heilman FR and Kendall EC: The influence of 11 dehydro-17-hydroxycorticosterone (Compound E) on the growth of a malignant tumor in the mouse. Endocrinology 1944 (34):416-420
28 Rhoads CP, Barker WH: Refractory Anaemia: analysis of 100 cases. JAMA 1938 (110):794-796
29 Hamilton-Paterson JL: Preleukaemic anaemia. Act Haematol 1949 (2):309-316
30 Rheingold JJ, Kaufman R, Adelson E, Lear A: Smouldering acute leukaemia. N Engl J Med 1963 (268):812-815
31 Dameshek W, Gunz FW: Classification of leukemia. In: Leukemia. Grune & Stratton, New York 1958 p16
32 Linman JW, Sarni MI: The preleukemic syndrome. Semin Haematol 1974 (11):93-100
33 Greenberg PL, Mana B: The preleukemic syndrome. Am J Med 1979 (66):951-958
34 Cohen JR, Gregen WP, Greenberg PL, Schrier SL: Subacute myeloid leukemia. Am J Med 1979 (66):959-966
35 Bjorkman SD: Chronic refractory anaemia with sideroblastic bone marrow. A study of four cases. Blood 1956 (ii):250-259
36 Gruneberg H: The anaemia of flexed-tail mice (Mus musculus L) II siderocytes: J Genetics 1942 (44):246-272
37 Dreyfus B, Rochant H, Sultan C et al: Les anemies refractaires avec exces de myeloblastes dans la moelle: Etude de onze observations. Nouv Presse Medecin 1970 (78):359-364

38 Linman JW: Myelomonocytic leukaemia and its preleukaemic phase. J Chronic Disease 1970 (22):49-60

39 Bennett JM, Catovksy D, Daniel M-T et al: Proposals for the classification of the acute leukaemias. Br J Haematol 1976 (33):451-458

40 Bennett JM, Catovsky D, Daniel M-T et al. Proposals for the classification of the myelodysplastic syndromes. Br J Haematol 1982 (51):189-199

41 Groupe Français de Morphologie Hématologique, French Registry of Acute Leukemia and Myelodysplastic Syndromes: Age distribution and hemograin analysis of the 4,496 cases recorded during 1982-1983 and classified according to FAB criteria. Cancer 1987 (60):1385-1394

42 Todd WM, Pierre RV: Preleukaemia: a long term prospective study of 326 patients. Scand J Haematol 1986 (36):114-120

43 Coiffier B, Adeleine P and Viala JJ: Dysmyelopoietic syndromes: a search for prognostic factors in 193 patients. Cancer 1983 (52):83-90

44 Foucar K, Langdon II RM and Armitage JO et al: Myelodysplastic syndromes: a clinical and pathological analysis of 109 cases. Cancer 1985 (56):553-561

45 Vallespi T, Torrabadella M, Julia A et al: Myelodysplastic syndromes: a study of 101 cases according to the FAB classification. Br J Haematol 1985 (61):83-92

46 Oscier DG: Myelodysplastic Syndromes. Bailliere's Clin Haematol 1987 (1):389-425

47 Cartwright RA, Alexander FE, McKinney PA et al: Leukaemia and lymphoma: an atlas of distribution within areas of England and Wales. Leukaemia Research Fund, London 1990 pp 32-40

48 Stott H, Fox W, Girling DJ et al: Acute leukaemia after busulphan. Br Med J 1977 (ii):1513-1517

49 Buckman R, Cuzick J, Galton DAG: Long term survival in myelomatosis: a report to the MRC Working Party on Leukaemia in Adults. Br J Haemat 1982 (52):589-599

50 Cuzick J, Erskine S, Edelman D, Galton DAG: A comparison of the incidence of the myelodysplastic syndrome and acute myeloid Leukaemia following melphalan and cyclophosphamide treatment. Br J Cancer 1987 (55):523-529

51 Bloomfield CD: Chromosome abnormalities in secondary myelodysplastic syndromes. Scand J Haematol 1986 (36 Suppl 45):82-90

52 Prchal JT, Trockmorton DW, Carroll AJ et al: A common progenitor for myeloid and lymphoid cells. Nature 1978 (274):590-591

53 Raskind WH, Tirumali N, Tacobson R, et al: Evidence for a multistep pathogenesis of a myclodysplastic syndrome. Blood 1984 (63):1318-1323

54 Abkowitz JL, Ott RM, Holly RD and Adamson JW: Clonal evolution following chemotherapy induced stem cell depletion in cats heterozous for glucose-6-phosphate dehydrogenase. Blood 1988 (71):1687-1692

55 Hirai H, Kobayashi Y, Mano H et al: A point mutation at codon 13 of the N-ras oncogene in myelodysplastic syndrome. Nature 1987 (327):430-432

56 Bos JL, Toksoz D, Marshall CJ et al: Amino acid substitutions at codon 13 of the N-ras oncogene in human acute myeloid leukaemia. Nature 1985 (315):726

57 Needlemann SW, Kraus MH, Scrivastava SK et al: High frequency of N-ras activation in acute myelogenous leukaemia. Blood 1986 (67):753-757

58 Bos JL, Verlan-de Vries M, Vander Eb AJ et al: Mutations in N-ras predominate in acute myeloid leukemia. Blood 1987 (69):1237-1241

59 Lyons J, Janssen JWG, Bartram C et al: Mutations of Ki-ras and N-ras oncogenes in myelodysplastic syndromes. Blood 1988 (71):1707-1712

60 Forrester K, Almoguera C, Han K et al: Detection of high incidence of K-ras oncogene during human colon tumourigenesis. Nature 1987 (327):298-303

61 Robenhuis S, van de Wetering ML, Mooi WJ et al: Mutational activation of the K-ras oncogene: A possible pathogenetic factor in adenocarcinoma of the lung. N Engl J Med 1987 (317):929-935

62 Albino AP, Le Strange R and Oliff AT: Transforming ras genes from human melanoma: A manifestation of tumour heterogeneity? Nature 1984 (308):69-72

63 Barbacid M: Mutagens, oncogenes and cancer. Trends Genet 1986 (2):188

64 Padua RA, Carter G, Hughes D et al: RAS mutations in myelodysplasia detected by amplification, oligonucleotide hybridization and transformation. Leukemia 1988 (2):503-510

65 Shen WP, Aldrich TH, Venta-Perez G: Expression of normal and mutant ras proteins in human acute leukemia. Oncogene 1987 (1):157-165

66 Klein G, Klein E: Evolution of tumours and the impact of molecular oncology. Nature 1985 (315):190-195

67 Ridge SA, Worwood M, Oscier D et al: FMS mutations in myelodysplastic, leukemic and normal

subjects. Proc Natl Acad Sci 1990 (87):1377-1380
68 Russell NH and Reilly IAG: Role of autocrine growth factors in the leukemic transformation of the myelo-dysplastic syndromes. Leukemia 1989 (3):83-84
69 Pierre RV, Catovsky D, Mufti GJ et al: Clinical-cytogenetic correlations in myelodysplasia (preleukemia). In: Report of the 6th International Workshop on Chromosomes in Leukemia. London 1987. Cancer Genet Cytogenet 1989 (40):149-161
70 Second International Workshop on Chromosomes in Leukaemia 1979: Chromosomes in preleukemia. Cancer Genet Cytogenet 1980 (2):108-113
71 Third MIC Cooperative Study Group: Recommendations for a morphologic, immunologic and cytogenetic (MIC) working classification of the primary and therapy-related myelodysplastic syndromes. Cancer Genet Cytogenet 1988 (32):1
72 Knapp RH, Dewald GW, Pierre RV: Cytogenetic studies in 174 consecutive patients with preleukemic or myelodysplastic syndromes. Mayo Clin Proc 1985 (60):507-516
73 Van den Berghe H: The 5q- syndrome. Scand J Haematol 1986 (36):78-81
74 Pedersen-Bjergaard J, Vindelov V, Phillip P et al: Varying involvement of peripheral granulocytes in the clonal abnormality 7 in bone marrow cells in preleukemia secondary to treatment of other malignant tumours: cytogenetic results compared with results of flow cytometric DNA analysis and neutrophil chemotaxis. Blood 1982 (60) 172-179
75 Scheres JMJC, Hustinx TWJ, Geraedts JPM et al: Translocation 1;7 in hematologic disorders: a brief review of 22 cases. Cancer Genet Cytogenet 1985 (18):207-213
76 Nowell PC: Cytogenetics of preleukemia. Cancer Cytogenet 1982 (5):265-278
77 Yunis JJ, Rydell RE, Oken MM et al: Refined chromosome analysis as an independent prognostic indicator in de novo myelodysplastic syndromes. Blood 1986 (67):1721-1727
78 Bloomfield CD, Garson OM, Volin L et al: t(1;3)(p36;q21) in acute non lymphocytic leukaemia: a new clinicopathological association. Blood 1986 (68):320-322 (letter)
79 de la Chapelle A, Knuutila W and Elonen E: Translocation (2;11)(p21;q23) in acute non lymphocytic leukaemia: a non-random assocation. Scand J Haematol 1986 (36 Suppl 45):91-97
80 Le Beau MM, Westbrook CA, Diaz Mo et al: Evidence for the involvement of GM-CSF and FMS in the deletion (5q) in myeloid disorders. Science 1986 (231) 984-987
81 Nienhuis AW, Bunn HF, Turner PH et al: Expression of the human cfms proto oncogene in hemopoietic cells and its deletion in the 5q-syndrome. Cell 1985 (42):421-428
82 Tricot G, De Wolf -Peeters C, Vlietinck R, Verwilghen RL: Bone marrow histology in myelodysplastic syndromes II. Prognostic value of abnormal localisation of immature precursors in MDS. Br J Haematol 1984 (58):217-225
83 Frisch B, Bartl R: Bone marrow histology in myelodysplastic syndromes. Scand J Haematol 1986 (36 Suppl 45):21-37
84 Mufti GJ, Steven JR, Oscier DG et al: Myelodysplastic syndromes: a scoring system with prognostic significance. Br J Haematol 1985 (590):425-433
85 Tricot G, Vlietinck R, Verwilghen RL: Prognostic factors in the myelodysplastic syndromes: A Review. Scand J Haematol 1986 (36 Suppl 45):107-113
86 Koeffler HP: Myelodysplastic syndromes (Preleukemia). Sem Haematol 1986 (23):284-299
87 Weisdorf DJ, Oken MM, Johnson GJ, Rydell RE: Chronic myelodysplastic syndrome: short survival with or without evolution to acute leukemia. Br J Haematol 1983 (55):691-700
88 Worsley A, Oscier DG, Stevens J et al: Prognostic features of chronic myelomonocytic leukaemia: a modified Bournemouth score gives the best prediction of survival. Br J Haematol 1988 (68):17-21
89 Solal-Celigny P, Desaint B, Herrera A et al: Chronic myelomonocytic leukaemia according to FAB classification :analysis of 35 cases. Blood 1984 (63):634-638
90 Allessandrino EP, Orlandi E, Brusamolino E et al: Chronic myelomonocytic leukaemia:clinical features, cytogenetics and prognosis in 30 consecutive cases. Haematol Oncol 1985 (3):147-155
91 Fenaux P, Jouet JP, Zandecki M et al: Chronic and subacute myelomonocytic leukaemia in the adult: a report of 60 cases with special reference to prognostic factors. Br J Haematol 1987 (65):101-106
92 Ruutu T, Partenen S, Lintula R et al: Erythroid and granulocyte - macrophage colony function in myelodysplastic syndromes. Scand J Haematol 1984 (32):395-402
93 Zittoun R: Subacute and chronic myelomonocytic leukaemia: a distinct haematological entity. Br J Haematol 1976 (32):1-7
94 Varela BL, Chuang C, Woll JE: Modifications in the classification of primary myelodysplastic

syndromes. The addition of a scoring system. Haematol Oncol 1985 (3):55-63
95 Kerhofs H, Hermans J, Haak HL and Leeksma CHW: Utility of the FAB classification for myelodysplastic syndromes, investigation of prognostic features in 256 cases. Br J Haematol 1987 (65):73-81
96 Major P, Egan EM, Beardsley G et al: Lethality of human myeloblasts correlates with the incorporation of Ara-C into DNA. Proc Nat Acad Sci 1981 (78):3235-3238
97 Griffin JD, Munroe D, Major P, Kufe D: Induction of differentiation of human myeloid leukemic cells by inhibitors of DNA synthesis. Exper Haematol 1982 (10):744-781
98 Weinstein HJ, Griffin JW, Feeney J et al: Pharmacokinetics of continuous intravenous and subcutaneous infusions of cytosine arabinoside. Blood 1982 (59):1351-1353
99 Spriggs D, Sokal J, Griffin J, Kufe D: Low dose Ara-C administration by continuous subcutaneous infusion: a pharmacologic evaluation. Cancer Drug Delivery 1986 (3):211-216
100 Griffin JD, Spriggs D, Wisch JS et al: Treatment of preleukemic syndromes with continuous intravenous infusion of low dose cytosine arabinoside. J Clin Oncol 1985 (3):982-991
101 Castaigne S, Daniel MT, Tilly H et al: Does treatment with Ara-C in low dosage cause differentiation of leukemic cells? Blood 1983 (62):85-86
102 Ishikuna H, Sawada H, Okazaki T et al: The effect of low dose ara-c in acute nonlymphoblastic leukemias and atypical leukemia. Br J Haematol 1984 (58):9-18
103 Tricot G, De Bock R, Dekker AW et al: Low dose cytosine arabinoside (ara-C) in myelodysplastic syndromes. Br J Haematol 1984 (58):231-240
104 Winter JN, Variakojis D, Gaynor ER et al: Low dose cytosine arabinoside (ara-C) therapy in the myelodysplastic syndromes and acute leukemia. Cancer 1985 (56):443-449
105 Roberts JD, Ershler WB, Tindle BH, Stewart JA: Low dose cytosine arabinoside in the myelodysplastic syndromes and acute myelogenous leukemia. Cancer 1985 (56):1001-1005
106 Degos L, Castaigne S, Tilly H et al: Treatment of leukemia with low dose ara-C: a study of 160 cases. Semin Oncol 1985 (12 Suppl 3):196-199
107 Bolwell BJ, Cassileth PA, Gale RP: Low dose cytosine arabinoside in myelodysplasia and acute myelogenous leukemia: A review. Leukemia 1987 (1):575-579
108 Lishner M, Curbis JE, Minkin S, McCulloch EA: Interaction between retinoic acid and cytosine arabinoside affecting the blast cells of acute myeloblastic leukaemia. Leukemia 1989 (3):784-788.
109 Castaigne S, Chomienne C, Ballerine P et al: All-trans retinoic acid: A novel differentiation therapy for acute promyelo-cytic leukaemia. Blood 1989 (74 Suppl 1):434 (abstract)
110 Gallagher RE, Said F, Pua I et al: Expression of retinoic acid receptor . mRNA in human leukaemia cells with variable responsiveness to retinoic acid. Leukemia 1989 (3):789-795
111 Elias L, Hoffman R, Boswell S and Bonnem E: A trial of recombinant alpha-2 interferon in the myelodysplastic syndrome. Blood 1985 (66 Suppl):675 (abstract)
112 Herberman RB, Holden HT: Natural killer cells as antitumour effector cells. JNCI 1979 (62):441-445
113 Djeu JY, Heinbaugh JA, Holden HT, Herberman RB: Augmentation of mouse natural killer cell activity by interferon and interferon inducers. J Immunol 1979 (122):175-181
114 Haliotis T, Roder J, Klein M et al: Chediak-Higashi gene in humans. J Exper Med 1980 (151):1039-1048
115 Tayaki S, Kitagawa S, Takeda A et al: Natural killer-interferon system in patients with preleukemic states. Br J Haematol 1984 (58):71-81
116 Sorskaar D, Forre O, Albrechtsen D et al: Decreased natural killer cell activity versus normal killer cell markers in mononuclear cells from patients with smouldering leukaemia. Scand J Haematol 1986 (37):154-161
117 Kerndup G, Mayer K, Ellegard J et al: Natural killer (NK) activity and antibody dependent cellular cytotoxicity (ADCC) in primary preleukaemic syndrome. Leuk Res 1984 (8):239-247
118 Pedersen-Bjengaard J, Haahr S, Philip P et al: Abolished production of interferon by leucocytes of patients with the aquired cytogenetic abnormalities 5q-or -5 in seconday and de novo acute non-lymphocytic leukaemia. Br J Haematol 1980 (46):211-223
119 Goldstein D, Laszlo J: Interferon therapy in Cancer from imaginon to interferon. Cancer Res 1986 (46):4315-4329
120 Taylor-Papadimitriou J, Rozengurt E: Interferons as regulators of cell growth and differentiation. In: Taylor-Papadimitriou J (ed) Interferons: Their Impact in Biology and Medicine. Oxford University Press, Oxford 1985 pp 81-98
121 Elias L, Van Epps DE, Smith KJ et al: A trial of recombinant alpha2 interferon in the

myelodysplastic syndrome:2 characterisation and response of granulocyte and platelet dysfunction. Leukemia 1987 (1):111-115
122 Galvani DW, Cawley JC, Nethersall A, Bottomley JM: Alpha interferon in myelodysplasia. Br J Haematol 1987 (66):145-146
123 Elias L, Hoffman R, Boswell S et al: A trial of recombinant alpha interferon in the myelodysplastic syndromes. 1:Clinical results. Leukemia 1987 (1):105-110
124 Gisslinger H, Chott A, Linkesch W: Long-term interferon therapy in myelodysplastic syndromes. Leukemia 1990 (4):91-94
125 Vadhan-Raj S, Keating M, Le Maistre A et al: Effects of recombinant human granulocyte-macrophage colony stimulating factor in patients with myelodysplastic syndromes. N Engl J Med 1987 (317):1545-1552
126 Ganser A, Volkers B, Greher J et al: Recombinant human granulocyte macrophage colony-stimulating factor in patients with myelodysplastic syndromes - A phase I/II trial. Blood 1989 (73):31-37
128 Groopman JE, Mitsuyasu RT, De Leo MJ et al: Effect of recombinant human granulocyte-macrophage stimulating factor on myelopoiesis in the acquired immune deficiency syndrome. N Engl J Med 1987 (317):593-598
129 Antin JH, Smith BR, Holmes W and Rosenthal DS: Phase I/II study of recombinant human granulocyte-macrophage colony stimulating factor in aplastic anaemia and myelodysplastic syndrome. Blood 1988 (72):705-713
130 Negrin RS, Haenber DH, Nagler A et al: Treatment of myelodysplastic syndromes with recombinant human granulocytic colony-stimulating factor: a phase I/II trial. Ann Intern Med 1989 (110):976-984
131 Groopman JE, Molina JM and Scadden DT: Hemopoietic growth factors: Biology and clinical applications. N Engl J Med 1989 (321):1449-1459
132 Koeffler HP, Hirji K, Itra L et al: 1,25 Dihyroxyvitamin D3; in vivo and vitro effects on human preleukaemic cells. Cancer Treat Rep 1985 (69):1399-1407
133 Oscier DG, Worsley A, Hamblin TJ, Mufti GJ: Treatment of chronic myelomonocytic leukaemia with low dose etoposide. Br J Haematol 1989 (72):468-471
134 Johnson E, Parapia LA: Successful oral chemotherapy with Idarubicin in Refractory Anaemia. Eur J Haematol 1987 (39): 278-281
135 De Witte T, Zwaan F, Gratwohl A et al: Allogeneic bone marrow transplantation in secondary leukaemias and myelodysplastic syndromes. Bone Marrow Transpl 1988 (3 Suppl 1):142-143
136 Appelbaum FR, Storb R, Rainberg RE: Treatment of preleukemic syndromes with marrow transplantation. Blood 1987 (69):92-96
137 Bessis M: Blood Smears Reinterpreted. Springer Verlag, Berlin/Heidelberg 1977
138 Bennett JM, Catovsky D, Daniel M-T et al: Prepared revised criteria for the classification of acute myeloid leukaemia: a report of the French-American-British Cooperative GroupAm J Med 1985 (103): 620-629
139 Hayhoe FGJ: A modern classification of the acute non-lymphoblastic leukaemias. Bone Marrow Transplant 1989 (4 Suppl 1):70-72
140 Hayhoe FGJ: Classification of the acute leukaemias. Blood Reviews 1988 (2):186-193
141 Report of the MIC Cooperative Study Group: Morphologic, immunologic and cytogenetic (MIC) working classification of the acute myeloid leukaemias. Br J Haematol 1988 (68):487-494
142 Selvin S, Levin LI, Merrill DW, Winkelstein W Jr: Selected epidemiologic observations of cell-specific leukaemia mortality in the United States 1969-1977. Am J Epidemiol 1983 (117):140-152
143 Gilliam AG: Age, sex and race selection at death from leukaemia and the lymphomas. Blood 1953 (8):693-702
144 Freireich EJ: Methods for evaluating response to treatment on adult acute leukaemia. Blood Cells 1983 (9):5-20
145 Amaki I, Hattoni K, Bennett JM et al: FAB classification of acute leukaemias correlates with response to chemotherapy. Acta Haematol Jpn 1984 (47):206-238
146 Preisler HD: Prediction of response to chemotherapy in acute myelocytic leukaemia. Blood 1980 (56): 361-367
147 Curtis JE, Messner HA, Hasselback R et al: Contributions of host and disease-related attributes to the outcome of patients with acute myelogenous leukaemia. J Clin Oncol 1984 (2):253-259
148 Yunis JJ and Brunning RD: Prognostic significance of chromosomal abnormalities in acute leukaemia and myelodysplastic syndromes. Clin Haematol 1986 [15]:597-620
149 Grier HE, Gelber RO, Camilta BM et al: Prognostic factors in childhood acute myelogenous leukaemia. J Clin Oncol 1987 (5):1026-1030
150 Ritter J, Crentzig V, Schellong G: Improved treatment results in the myelocytic subtypes FAB M1-M4 but not in FAB M5 after intensification of induction therapy: results of the German childhood

AML studies BFM-78 and BFM-83. Haematol Blood Transf 1990 (33):185-192
151 Amadori S, Mandelli A, Ceci A et al: Results of the Italian AIEOP/LAM 8204 study for the treatment of childhood AML: an update. Bone Marrow Transpl 1989 (4):114-115
152 Chessels JM, O'Callaghan U and Hardisty RM: Acute myeloid leukaemia in childhood: clinical factors and prognosis. Br J Haematol 1986 (63):555-564
153 Stuber CP, Cuthbert SJ, Ravindranath Y et al: Therapy of childhood acute non lymphocytic leukaemia: the Pediatric Oncology Group Experience (1977-1988). Haematol Blood Transf 1990 (33):188-209
154 Kalwinski D, Mirro J Jr, Schell M et al: Early intensification of chemotherapy for childhood acute nonlymphoblastic leukaemia: improved remission induction with a fine drug regimen including etoposide. J Clin Oncol 1988 (6):1134-1143
155 Yates J, Glidewell O and Wiernik P: Cytosine arabinoside with Daunorubicin or Adriamycin for therapy of Acute Myelocytic Leukaemia: A CALGB Study. Blood 1982 (60): 454-462
156 Vogler WR, Winton EF, Gordon DS et al: A randomised comparison of post remission therapy in acute myelogenous leukaemia: a Southeastern Cancer Study Group Trial. Blood 1984 (63):1039-1045
157 Rees JKH and Gray R: Remission induction and post remission therapy in acute myelogenous leukaemia: British MRC Study. Haematol Blood Transf 1990 (33):243-248
158 Petti MC, Broccia G, Carona F et al: Therapy of acute myelogenous leukaemia in adults. Haematol Blood Transf 1990 (33):240-253
159 Kurrle E, Ehninger E, Fackler-Schwalbe E et al: Consolidation therapy with high dose cytosine arabinoside: Experience of a prospective study in Acute Myeloid Leukaemia. Haematol Blood Transf 1990 (33):254-260
160 Buchner T, Hiddemann W and Blasuis S: Adult AML: The role of chemotherapy intensity and duration. Two studies of the AML Cooperative Group. Haematol Blood Transf 1990 (33):261-266
161 Cassileth PA, Harrington DP and Hines JD: Comparison of post remission therapies in adult acute myeloid leukaemia: preliminary analysis of an ECOG study. Haematol Blood Transf 1990 (33):267-270
162 Hayat M, Zittoun R and Strychmans P: EORTC Leukaemia Group Trials in Acute Myeloid Leukaemia. Haematol Blood Transf 1990 (33):271-276
163 Labar B, Nemet D, Minigo H et al: Aclarubicin in the treatment of de-novo acute myelocytic leukaemia. New Trends in the Treatment of Acute Leukaemia, Dubrovnik 1989
164 Jehn U, Zittoun R, Suciu S et al: Randomised comparison of intensive maintenance treatment for adult acute myelogenous leukaemia using either cyclic alternating drugs or repeated courses of the induction-type chemotherapy: AML6 Trial of the EORTC Cooperative Group. Haematol Blood Transf 1990 (33):277-289
165 Amadori S, Ceci A and Connelli A: Therapy of childhood acute myelogenous leukaemia. An update of the AIEOP/LAM 8204 study. Blood Transf 1990 (33):222-225
166 Grier HE, Gelber RE and Claver LA: Intensive sequential chemotherapy for children with acute myelogenous leukaemia. Haematol Blood Transf 1990 (33):193-197
167 Steuber CP, Culbert SJ, Ravindranath Y et al: Therapy of childhood acute nonlymphocytic leukaemia. The Pediatric Oncology Group Experience (1977-1988). Haematol Blood Transf 1990 (33):198-209
168 Lampkin BC, Woods WG, Buckley JD et al: Preliminary results of intensive therapy of children and adults with acute non lymphocytic leukaemia. A Childrens' Cancer Study Group report. Haematol Blood Transf 1990 (33):210-214
169 Ritter J, Creutzig U and Schellong G: Improved treatment results in the myelocytic subtypes FAB M1-4 but not in FAB M5 after intensification of induction therapy: Results of the German Childhood AML Studies BFM-78 and BFM-83. Haematol Blood Transf 1990 (33):185-192
170 The Toronto Leukaemia Study Group: Results of chemotherapy for unselected patients with acute myeloblastic leukaemia: effect of exclusion or interpretation of results. Lancet 1986 (i):786-788
171 Copplestone JA, Smith AG, Oscier DG and Hamblin T: True outlook in acute myeloblastic leukaemia. Lancet 1986 (i): 1104 (letter)
172 Preisler HD: Failure of remission induction in acute myelogenous leukaemia. Med Pediatr Oncol 1978 (4):275-276
173 Estey EH, Keating MJ, McCredie KB et al: Causes of initial remission induction failure in acute myelogenous leukaemia. Blood 1982 (60): 309
174 Rees JKH, Gray R, Hayhoe FGJ: The Ninth British Medical Research Council Trial for the Treatment of Acute Myeloid Leukaemia. Haematol Blood Trans 1987 (30):35-37
175 Bodey GP, Buckley M, Sathe YS et al: Quantitative relationships between circulating leukocytes and

infection in patients with acute leukaemia. Ann Int Med 1986 (64):328-240
176 Gaya H: Antimicrobial therapy in neutropenic patients with malignant disease. In: Klastersky J (ed) Clinical Use of Combinations of Antibiotics. Hodden & Staughton, London 1975 pp 117-125
177 Rubin M, Hathorn JW and Pizzo PA: Controversies in the management of febrile neutropenic cancer patients. Cancer Invest 1986 (6): 167-184
178 Rubin M, Walsh T, Butler K et al: The febrile neutropenic patient: newer options for emperical therapy. Haematol Blood Transf 1990 (33):531-538
179 Walsh TJ and Pizzo PA: Noxcomial fungal infections. Ann Rev Microbiol 1988 (42):517-545
180 Gold JW: Opportunistic fungal infections in patients with neoplastic disease. Am J Med 1984 (76):458-463
181 Meunier F and Klastersky J: Recent development in prophylaxis and therapy of invasive fungal infections in granulocytopenic cancer patients. Eur J Cancer and Clin Oncol 1988 (24):539-544
182 Crumbacker II CS: Molecular targets of antiviral therapy. N Engl J Med 1989 (321):163-172
183 Hughes WT, Rivena GK, Sohell MJ et al: Successful intermittent chemoprophylaxis for pneumocystis carinii pneumonitis. N Engl J Med 1987 (316):1627-1632
184 Schimpff SC, Young VM, Green WH et al: Origin of infection in acute non-lymphocytic leukaemia: significance of hospital acquisition of potential pathogens. Ann Intern Med 1972 (77):707-714
185 Young LS: Double a-lactam therapy in the immunocomprised host. J Automicrob Chemo 1985 (16):4-6
186 Infections in haematology. In: Prentice HG (ed) Clinics in Haematology. WB Saunders & Co, London, Philadelphia, Toronto 1984
187 Brandt SJ, Peters WP, Atwater SK et al: Effect of recombinant human granulocyte-macrophage colony stimulating factor or haemopoietic reconstitution after high dose chemotherapy and autologous bone marrow transplantation. N Engl J Med 1988 (318):869-876
188 Gabrilone JL, Jakubowski A, Scher H et al: Effect of granulocyte stimulating factor on neutropenia and associated morbidity due to chemotherapy for transitional-cell carcinoma of the urathelium. N Engl J Med 1988 (318):1414-1422
189 Antman KS, Griffin JD and Elias A: Effect of recombinant human granulocyte-macrophage colony stimulating factor or chemotherapy induced myelosuppression. N Engl J Med 1988 (319):594-598
190 Buchner T, Hiddemann W, Koenigsman M et al: Recombinant human granulocyte colony-stimulating factor after therapy for acute leukaemias at higher age or after relapse. Haematol Blood Transf 1990 (33):724-731
191 Hermann F, Schulz G, Wieser M et al: Effect of granulocyte-macrophage stimulating factor on neutropenia and related morbidity induced by myelotoxic chemotherapy. Haematol Blood Transf 1990 (33):717-723
192 Andreef M, Tafuni A, Hegewisch-Becker S: Colony-Stimulating factors (rhG-CSF, rhGM-CSF, rh1L-3 and BCFG) recruit myeloblastic and lymphblastic leukemic cells and enhance the cytotoxic effects of cytosine arabinoside. Haematol Blood Transf 1990 (33):747-762
193 Vellenga E, Young DC, Wagner K et al: The effects of GM-CSF and G-CSF in promoting growth of clonagenic cells in acute myeloblastic leukemia. Blood 1987 (69):1771-1776
194 Schipperus MR, Vink N, Lindemans J et al: In vitro growth kinetics of myeloid progenitor cells of myelodysplastic patients in response to granulocyte macrophage colony stimulating factor and Interleukin 3. Haematol Blood Transf 1990 (33):98-102
195 Schrader C, Reuter M, Mempel K et al: In vitro effects of G-CSF, GM-CSF and 1L-3an Leukemic cells of children with acute non lymphoblastic leukemia. Haematol Blood Transf 1990 (33):95-97
196 Estey EH, Kantaryian HM, Beran M et al: Treatment of poor prognosis newly diagnosed acute myelagenous leukemia with high dose Cytosine Arabinoside (Ara-C) and rHUGM-CSF. Haematol Blood Transf 1990 (33):732
197 Brittingham TE, Chaplin H: Febrile transfusion reactions caused by sensitivity to donor leukocytes and platelets. JAMA 1975 (165):819-825
198 Brubaker DB: Immunologically mediated immediate adverse effects of blood transfusions. Plasma Ther Transf Technol 1985 (6):19-30
199 Class FHJ, Smeenk RJT, Schmidt R et al: Alloimmunisation against the MLC antigens after platelet transfusion is due to contaminating leukocytes in the platelet suspension. Exp Haematol 1981 (90):84-89
200 Lang DJ, Ebent PA: Reduction of post perfusion cytomegalovirus infections following the use of leukocyte depleted blood: a comparison of filtration techniques. Transfusion 1977 (17):391-395
201 Mijovic V, Brozovic B, Hughes ASB, Davies TD: Leukocyte depleted blood: a comparison of filtration techniques. Transfusion 1983 (23):30-32

202 Cassileth PA, Begg CB, Silber R: Prolonged unmaintained remission after intensive consolidation therapy in adult acute nonlymphocytic leukemia. Cancer Treat Rep 1987 (71):137-140
203 Preisler HD, Raza A, Early A: Intensive remission consolidation therapy in the treatment of acute nonlymphocytic leukemia. J Clin Oncol 1987 (5):722-730
204 Tricot G, Boogaents MA, Vlietinck R: The role of intensive remission induction and consolidation therapy in patients with acute myeloid leukaemia. Bri J Haematol 1987 (66):37-44
205 Champlin R, How Winston D et al: Treatment of adults with acute myelogenous leukemia: Prospective evaluation of high dose cytarabine in consolidation chemotherapy and with bone marrow transplantation. Semin Oncol 1987 (14 Suppl1):1-6
206 Wal SN, Herzig RH, Phillips GL: High dose cytosine arabinoside and daunorubicin as consolidation therapy for acute nonlymphocytic leukemia in first remission: An update. Semin Oncol 1987 (14 Suppl):12-17
207 Eastey E, Keating MJ, Plunkett W: Continuous infusion high-dose cytosine arabinoside without antraycyclines as induction andintensification therapy in adults under age 50 with newly diagnosed acute myclogenous leukemia. Semin Oncol 1987 (14 Suppl):58-63
208 Capizzi RL, Pole M, Cooper MR et al: Treatment of poor risk acute leukemia with sequential high dose Ara-C and asparaginase. Blood 1984 (63): 694-700
209 Kurrle E, Ehninge G, Fackler-Schwalbe E et al: Consolidation therapy with high-dose cytosine Arabinoside: Experiences of a prospective study in acute myeloid leukemia. Haematol Blood Transf 1990 (33):254-260
210 Zittoun R, Marie JP, Zittoun J et al: Modulation of Cytosine Arabinoside (Ara-C) and high dose Ara-C in acute leukemia. Semin Oncol 1985 (12):139-143
211 Plunkett W, Heinemann V, Estey E, Keating MJ: Pharmacologically directed design of Leukemia Therapy. Haematol Blood Transf 1990 (33):610-613
212 Plunkett W, Liliemark JO, Estey E, Keating MJ: Saturation of Ara-CTP accumulation during high dose Ara-C therapy: Pharmacologic rationale for intermediate dose Ara-C. Semin Oncol 1987 (14):159-166
213 Karp JE, Donehower RC, Dole GB and Burke PJ: Correlation of drug-perturbed marrow cell growth kinetics and intracellular 1-B-D-arabinofuranosylcytosine metabolism with clinical response in adult acute myelogenous leukaemia. Blood 1987 (69): 4, 1134-1140
214 Bernard J, Lasnanet J, Chome J et al: A cytological and histological study of acute promyelocytic leukaemia. J Clin Path 1963 (16):319-325
215 Bennett, J., Catovsky D., Daniel, M-T et al: A variant form of hypergranular promyelocytic leukaemia (M3). Ann Int Med 1980 (92):261 (letter)
216 Rosenthal RL: Acute promyelocytic leukaemia associated with hypofibrinogenemia. Blood 1963 (21):495-500
217 Didsheim P, Thrombold JS, Vandervoot RLE et al: Acute promyelocytic leukaemia with fibrinogen and factor V deficiencies. Blood 1964 (23):717-728
218 Gralnick HR and Sultan C: Acute promyelocytic leukaemia, haemorrhagic manifestations and morphologic criteria. Br J Haematol 1975 (29): 373-376 (Annotation)
219 Gonault-Heilmann M, Chardon E, Sultan C et al: The procoagulant factor of leukaemic promyelocytes: Demonstration of immunologic cross reactivity with human brain tissue factor. Br J Haematol 1975 (30):151-158
220 Sultan C, Gonault-Heilmann M and Tulliez M: Relationship between blast cell morphology and occurrence of a syndrome of disseminated intravascular coagulation. Br J Haematol 1973 (24):255-259
221 Bernard J, Weil-Boiron M et al: Acute promyelocytic leukaemia: results of treatment by daunorubicin. Blood 1973 (41):489-496
222 Marty M, Ganem G, Fischer J et al: Leucémie aigue promyelocytaire: étude rétrospective de 119 malades traités par Daunorubicine. Nouv Rev Fr Hematol 1984 (26):371-378
223 Cordonnier C, Vernaut JP, Brun B et al: Acute promyelocytic leukaemia in 57 primarily untreated patients. Cancer 1985 (55):18-25
224 Collins AJ, Bloomfield CD, Peterson BA et al: Acute promyelocytic leukaemia: management of the coagulopathy during Daunorubicin-prednisone remission induction. Arch Int Med 1978 (138):1677-1680
225 Goldberg MA, Ginsberg D, Mayer RJ et al: Is heparin administration necessary during induction chemotherapy for patients with acute promyelocytic leukemia? Blood 1987 (69):187-191
226 Venook AP, Shuman MA and Corash L: Prophylactic heparin in APL. Blood 1987 (70):886-887
227 Hoyle CF, Swirsky DM, Freedman L and Hayhoe FGJ: Beneficial effects of heparin in the management of patients with APL. Br J Haematol 1988 (68):283-298
228 Avvisati G, Buller HR, Wouter ten Cate J and Mandelli F.: Transexamic acid for control of

haemorrhage in promyelocytic leukaemia. Lancet 1989 (ii):122-124
229 Ogston D (ed) Antifibrinolytic Drugs. Chemistry, Pharmacology and Clinical Usage. John Wiley, Chicester 1984 pp 81-83
230 Sandler RM, Liebman HA, Patch MJ et al: Antithrombin III and anti activated factor X activity in patients with acute promyelocytic leukaemia and intravascular coagulation treatment with heparin. Cancer 1983 (51):681-685
231 Chabner BA: The oncologic end game: Karnofsky memorial lecture. J Clin Oncol 1986 (4):625-638
232 Kartner N and Ling V: Multidrug resistance in cancer. Sci Am 1989 (iii):26-33
233 Piller GJ: Leukaemia Research Fund International Research Symposium on cytotoxic drug resistance in leukaemia and other malignancies. Leukaemia 1989 (3):461-467
234 Pastan I and Gottesman M: Multidrug resistance in human cancer. N Engl J Med 1987 (316):1388-1393
235 Juranka PF, Zastawny RI and Ling V: P-glycoprotein: multidrug resistance and a superfamily of membrane-associated transport proteins. FASEB 1989 (3):2583-2592
236 Ma DDF, Schurr RD, Davey RA et al: Detection of a multidrug resistant phenotype in acute non lymphoblastic leukaemia. Lancet 1987 (i):135-137
237 Kartner N, Evernden-Porelle D, Bradley G and Ling V: Detection of P-glycoprotein in multidrug resistant cell lines by monoclonal antibodies. Nature 1985 (316):820-823
238 Bell DR, Trent JM, Willard HF et al: Chromosomal location of human P-glycoprotein gene sequences. Cancer Genet Cytogenet 1987 (25):141-148
239 Wilson CM, Serrano AE and Wasley A: Amplification of a gene related to mammalian MDR genes in drug-resistant plasmodium falciparum. Science 1989 (244):1184-1186
240 McGrath JP and Varshavsky A: The yeast STE 6 gene encodes a homologue of the mammalian multidrug resistance P-glycoprotein. Nature 1989 (340):400-404
241 Tsuruo T, Lida H, Tsukagoshi S, Sakurai Y et al: Overcoming of vincristine resistance in P388 leukaemia in vivo and in vitro enhanced cytotoxicity of vincristine and vinblastine by verapamil. Cancer Res 1981 (41):1967-1972
242 Maruyama Y, Murohashi I and Nava N: Effects of verapamil on the cellular accumulation of daunorubicin in blast cells and on the chemosensitivity of leukaemic blast progenitors in acute myelogenous leukaemia. Br J Haematol 1989 (72):357-362
243 Twentyman PR, Fox NE and White DJG: Cyclosporin A and its analogues as modifiers of adriamycin and vincristine resistance in multidrug resistant human lung cancer cell line. Br J Cancer 1987 (56):55-57
244 Twentyman PR: Resistance modification by non-immunosuppressive cyclosporins. Br J Cancer 1988 (57):254-258
245 Twentyman PR, Fox NE and Rees JKH: Chemosensitivity testing of fresh leukaemic cells using the MTT colorimetric assay. Br J Haematol 1989 (71):19-24
246 Arrick BA and Nathan CF: Glutathione metabolism as a detriment of therapeutic efficacy: a review. Cancer Res 1984 (44):4224-4232
247 Russo A, Carmichael J, Friedman N et al: The roles of intracellular glutathione in antineoplastic chemotherapy. Int J Radiat Oncol Biol Phys 1986 (12):1347-1354
248 Tew KD, Schisselbauer JC, Clapper ML and Kuzmich S: Glutathione S-transferases and resistance to alkylating agents. Hayes JD, Pickett CB, Mantle TJ (eds) Proc 3rd Int GST Conf, Edinburgh 1989 pp 309-318
249 Tew KD, Bomber AM and Hoffman SF: Ethacrynic acid and Piriton as enhancers of cytotoxicity in drug-resistant and sensitive cell lines. Cancer Res 1988 (48):3617-3625
250 Clapper ML, Dwyer PJ and Tew KD: Sensitisation of tumours to alkylating agents using inhibitors of glutathione S-transferases. Hayes JD, Pickett CB, Mantle TJ (eds) Proc 3rd Int GST Conf, Edinburgh 1989 pp 451-459
251 McVie JG: DNA topoisomerases in cancer treatment. Br Med J 1988 (296):1145-1146
252 Potsmeil M, Hsiang YH and Liu LF: DNA topoisomerase 11 as a potential factor in drug resistance of human malignancies. NCI Monographs 1987 (4):105-109
253 Ogawa M, Ikebuchi K, Leary AG: Humoral regulation of stem cell proliferation. Ann NY Acad Sci 1989 (554):185-191
254 Tavassoli M, Yoffey JM: Bone marrow structure and function. Alan Liss Inc, New York 1983
255 Francis GE, Pinsky CP: Growth and differentiation control. In: Pinedo HM, Chabner BA and Longo DL (eds) Cancer Chemotherapy and Biological Response Modifiers. Elsevier, Amsterdam 1988 pp 507-544
256 Bagby GC Jr: Interleukin-1 and haematopoiesis. Blood Rev 1989 (3):152-161
257 Broxmeyer HE, Moore HAS: Communication between white cells and the abnormalities of this in

Leukaemia. Biochem. Biophys Acta. 1978 (516) 129-166
258 Fliender TM, Steinbach KH: Repopulating potential of haemopoietic precursor cells. Blood Cells 1988 (14):393-410
259 Pantel K, Nakeff A: Lymphoid cell regulation of haematopoiesis. Int J Cell Cloning 1989 (7):2-12
260 McCulloch EA: Stem cells in normal and leukaemic haemopoiesis. Blood 1983 (62):1-13
261 McCulloch EA, Minden MD, Miyanchi J et al: Stem cell renewal and differentiation in acute myeloblastic leukaemia. J Cell Sci 1988 (10):267-281
262 Sieff CA: Haematopoietic growth factors. JNCI 1987 (79):1549-1557
263 Bagby GC Jr: Production of multilineage growth factors by haemopoitic stromal cells: an intercellular regulatory network involving mononuclear phagocytes and interleukin-1. Blood Cells 1987 (13):147-159
264 Wright EG, Lord BI: Production of stem cell proliferation regulators by fractionated haemopoietic stem cell suspensions. Leuk Res 1979 (3):15-22
265 Lord BI, Lu LF, Pojda Z, Spooncer E: Inhibitor of haemotapoietic CFU-S proliferation: assay production, sources and regulatory mechanisms. In: A Najman A, Guigon M, Gorin NC, Mary JY (eds) The Inhibitors of Haematopoiesis. John Libbey Eurotext 1987 (162):227-240
266 Sainteny F, Fache MP, Dumenil D, et al: Further studies of the biological activity of the CFU-S inhibitor peptide ACSDKP. Leukemia Res 1989 (13 Suppl 1):15-19
267 Gordon MY, Dowding CR, Riley GP, Greaves MF: Characterisation of stroma-dependent blast colony-forming cells in human marrow. J Cell Physiol 1987 (130):150-156
268 Roberts R, Gallagher J, Spooner E: Heparan sulphate-bound growth factors: a mechanism for stromal cell mediated haemopoiesis. Nature 1988 (332):376-378
269 Gordon MY, Riley GP, Clarke D: Heparan sulphate is necessary for adhesive interactions between human early haemopoietic progenitor cells and the extracellular matrix of the marrow microenvironment. Leukaemia 1988 (2):804-809
270 Guigon M, Najman A: The inhibitors of haematopoiesis. Int J Cell Cloning 1988 (6):69-75
271 Broxmeyer HE, Bagnacki J, Ralph P et al: Monocyte-macrophage-derived acidic isoferritins: normal feedback regulators of granulocyte-monophage progenitor cells in vitro. Blood 1982 (60):595-607
272 Broxmeyer HE, Williams DE, Lu L et al: Biomolecules associated with suppression of myelopoiesis in normal conditions and during myeloid leukaemia and other related disorders In: Najman A, Guigon M, Gorin NC, Mary JY (eds) The Inhibitors of Haematopoiesis. John Libbey Eurotext 1987 (162):139-148
273 Gentile PS, Pelus LM: In vivo modulation of myelopoiesis by prostaglandin E2. II. Inhibition of CFU-GM cycle rate. Exper Haematol 1987 (15):119-123
274 Murphy M, Louden R, Kobayashi M, Trinchieri G: Gamma - interferon and lymphotoxin, released by activated T cells, synergise to inhibit granulocyte/macrophage colony formation T Exp Med 1986 (164):263-268
275 Delwel R, Salem M, Pellens C, Dorssers L et al: Growth regulation of human acute myeloid leukaemia: effect of five recombinant haemopoietic factors in a serum-free culture system. Blood 1988 (72):1944-1949
276 Wu MC, Zaun MR, Wu FM: Inhibition of myeloid differentiation by inhibitors of ADP-ribosylation. FEBS Letters 1989 (244):338-342
277 Broxmeyer HE, Williams DE: The production of myeloid blood cells and their regulation during health and disease. CRC Critical Reviews in Oncol/Haematol 1988 (4):173-226
278 Metcalf D: The Haemopoietic Colony Stimulating Factors. Elsevier, Amsterdam 1984
279 Steinberg HN: Suppression of normal haemopoiesis in Leukaemia: in vivo and in vitro studies. In: Najman A, Guigon M, Gorin NC, Mary JY (eds) The Inhibitors of Haematopoiesis. John Libbey Eurotext 1987 (162):163-175
280 Steinberg HN, Tsiftsoglou AS, Robinson SH: Loss of suppression of normal bone marrow colony formation by leukaemia cell lines after differentiation is induced by chemical agents. Blood 1985 (65):100-106
281 Dorner MH, Broxmeyer HE, Silverstone A, Andreeff M: Biosynthesis of ferritin subunits from different cell lines of HL-60 human promyelocytic leukaemia cells and the release of acidic isoferritin: inhibitory activity against normal granulocytic-macrophage progenitor cells. Br J Haematol 1983 (55):47-52
282 Petrides PE, Dittman K: Leukaemic cells HL-60 release a polypeptide which disturbs the interaction of various target cells with their extracellular matrix. Exper Haematol 1989 (17):534
283 Michaelewicz R, Taheri MR, Katz F, Hoffbrand AV: The effect of the leukaemic cell line HL-60 and acute myeloblastic leukaemic cells before and after induction of differentiation on normal pluripotent

haemotopoietic progenitors (CFU-GEMM). Leukaemia Res 1985 (9):441-448
284 Stevens VL, Owens NE, Winter EF et al: Modulation of retinoic acid-induced differentiation of human leukemia (HL- 60) cells by serum factors and sphinganine. Cancer Res 1990 (50):222-226
285 Sartorelli AC: Malignant cell differentiation as a potential therapeutic approach. Br J Cancer 1985 (52):293-302
286 Hassan HT and Rees JKH: Triple combination of retinoic acid + low concentration of cytosine arabinoside + hexamethylene bisacetamide induces differentiation of human AML blasts in primary culture. Haematol Oncol 1989 (7):429-440
287 Goodman D: Vitamin A and retinoid in health and disease. N Engl J Med 1984 (310):1023-1031
288 Sporn M, Roberts A: The role of retinoids in differentiation and carcinogenesis. Cancer Res 1983 (43):3034-3040
289 Hoffman SJ, Robinson WA: Use of differentiation-inducing agents in myelodysplastic syndromes and acute lymphocytic leukaemia. Am J Haematol 1988 (28):124-127
290 Mufti GJ, Oscier DG, Hamblin TJ, Bell AJ: Low dose cytarabine in the treatment of myelodysplastic syndromes and acute myeloid leukaemia. N Engl J Med 1983 (309):1653-1654
291 Flynn PJ, Miller WJ, Weisdorf DJ et al: Retinoic acid treatment of acute promyelocytic leukaemia: in vitro and in vivo observations. Blood 1983 (62):1211-1217
292 Nilsson B: Probable in vivo induction of differentiation by retinoic acid of promylocytes in acute promylocytic leukaemia. Br J Haematol 1984 (57):365-371
293 Degos L, Shroot B, deThé H et al: Retinoic acid in hematopoietic differentiation. Nouv Rev Fr Hématol 1990 (32):25-38
294 Chomienne C, Ballerini P, Huang M et al: In vitro effects of retinoic acid. Nouv Rev Fr Hématol 1990 (32):32-34
295 Giguere V, Ong ES, Segui P, Evans RM: Indentification of a receptor for the morphogen retinoic acid. Nature 1987 (330):624-629
296 Brand N, Petkovich M, Krust A et al: Identification of a second human retinoic acid receptor. Nature 1988 (332):850-853
297 Zelent A, Krust A, Petkovich M et al: Cloning of alpha and beta retinoic acid receptors and a novel receptor predominantly expressed in the skin. Nature 1989 (339):714-717
298 Ragsdale CW Jr, Petkovich M, Gates PB: Identification of a novel retinoic acid receptor in regenerative tissues of the newt. Nature 1989 (341):654-657
299 Meng-er H, Yu-Chen Y, Shu-song C et al: Use of All-Trans retinoic acid in the treatment of acute promyelocytic leukaemia. Blood 1988 (72):567-572
300 Castaigne S, Chomienne C, Ballerini P et al: All-trans retinoic acid: a novel differentiation therapy for acute promyelocytic leukaemia. Blood 1989 (74 Suppl 1) abstr 434
301 Chomienne C, Ballerini P, Balitrand N et al: Retinoic acid therapy for promyelocytic leukaemia. Lancet 1989 (ii):746-747
302 Castaigne S, Chomienne C, Daniel M-T et al: Retinoic acids in the treatment of acute promyelocytic leukaemia. Nouv Rev Fr Hématol 1990 (32):36-38
303 Hassan HT, Rees J: Triple combination of retinoic acid + 6 Thioguanine + hexamethylene bisacetamide induces differentiation of human AML blasts in primary culture. Leuk Res 1990 (14):109-117
304 Ishikura H, Okazaki T, Mochizuki T: Effects of antimetabolites and thymidine blockage on the induction of differentiation of HL-60 cells by retinoic acid or 1,25 - dihydroxy-vitamin D3. Exper Haematol 1985 (13):981-988
305 Matzner Y, Gavison R, Rachmilewitz EA, Fibach E: Expression of granulocytic functions by leukaemic promyelocytic HL-60 cells: differential induction by dimethyl sulphaxide and retinoic acid. Cell Differentiation 1987 (21):261-269
306 Hemmi H, Breitman TR: Combinations of recombinant human interferons and retinoic acid synergistically induce differentiation of the human promyelocytic leukaemia cell line HL-60. Blood 1987 (69):501-507
307 Francis GE, Mufti GJ, Knowles SM et al: Differentiation induction in myelodysplasia and acute myeloid leukaemia: use of synergistic drug combinations. Leuk Res 1987 (11):971-977
308 Lie SO and Slordahl SH: High-dose cytosine arabinoside and retinol in the treatment of acute myelogenous leukemia in childhood. Haematol and Blood Transf 1987 (30):399-402
309 Zuckerman SH, Surprenant YM, Tang J: Synergistic effect of GM-CSF and Vitamin D-3 on the differentiation of the human monocytic cell line U937. Blood 1988 (71):619-624
310 Kelsey SM, Newland AC, Makin HLJ: Vitamin D and Human Leukaemia. Br J Haematol 1989 (71):173-176
311 Dawson DM, Rosenthal DS, Moloney WC: Neurological complications of acute leukemia in

adults: Changing rate. Ann Int Med 1979 (79):541-544
312 Law IP, Blom J: Adult acute leukaemia: Frequency of central nervous system acute leukemia in adults. Cancer 1981 (47):184-196
313 Steward DJ, Keating MJ, McCredie KB et al: Natural history of central nervous system acute leukemia in adults. Cancer 1981 (47):184-196
314 Bennett JM, Cassileth P, Begg C: Central nervous system involvement in the acute myeloid leukemias (AML): the Eastern Cooperative Oncology Group (ECOG) experience. Blood 1984 (64):144a
315 Rees JKH, Gray R, Swirsky D, Hayhoe FGJ: Principal results of the Medical Research Council's 8th acute myeloid leukaemia trial. Lancet 1986 (ii):1236-1241
316 Weinstein HJ, Mayer RJ, Rosenthal DS et al: Treatment of acute myelogenous leukemia in children and adults. N Engl J Med 1980 (303):473-478
317 Holmes R, Keating MJ, Cork A et al: A unique pattern of central nervous system leukemia in acute myelomonocytic leukemia associated with INV(16)(P13q22). Blood 1985 (65):1071-1078
318 Sakurai M, Kaneko Y, Abe R: Further characterisation of acute myelogenous leukaemia with t(8;21) chromosome translocation. Cancer Genet Cytogenet 1982 (6):143-152
319 Andrew W: The Anatomy of Aging in Man and Animals. Grune & Stratton, New York 1971
320 Goldstein S, Harley CB, Moerman EJ: Some aspects of cellular aging. J Chron Dis 1983 (36):103-116
321 Richey DP, Bender AD: Pharmacokinetic consequences of aging. Ann Rev Pharmacol Toxicol 1977 (17):49-65
322 Editorial: Pharmacokinetics in the elderly Lancet 1983 (i) 568-569
323 Moutamat SC, Cusack BJ, Vestal RE: Management of drug therapy in the elderly. N Engl J Med 1989 (321):303-309
324 Bricker H: Estimate of overall treatment results in acute nonlymphocytic leukaemia based on age-specific rates of incidence and of complete remission. Cancer Treat Rep 1985 (69):5-11
325 Cheson BD, Jasperse DM, Simon R, Friedman MA: A critical appraisal of low-dose cytosmi arabinoside in patients with acute non-lymphocytic leukaemia and myelodysplastic syndromes. J Clin Oncol 1986 (4):1857-1864
326 Powell BL, Capizzi RL, Muss HB: Low dose Ara-C therapy for acute myelogenous leukaemia in elderly patients. Leukemia 1989 (3):23-28
327 Sebban C, Archimband Coiffier B et al: Treatment of acute myeloid leukemia in elderly patients. Cancer 1988 (61):227-231
328 Walters RS, Kantavjian HM, Keating MJ et al: Intensive treatment of acute leukemia in adults 70 years of age and older. Cancer 1987 (60):149-155
329 Berman E, Witties RE, Leyland-Jones B et al: Phase I and clinical pharmacology studies of intravenous and oral administration of 4-demethoxydaunorubicin in patients with advanced cancer. Cancer Res 1983 (43):6096-6101
330 Resegotti L, Mandelli F, Amadori S et al: An Italian multicentre phase III trial of Idarubicin plus Ara-C vs daunorubicin plus Ara-C in elderly patients with acute non-lymphoid leukaemia. Proc 4th Int Symp Ther Acute Leuk, Rome 1987 pp 42-49
331 Waterhouse J, Muir C, Shanmugaratnum K et al: Cancer incidence in five continents. WHO 1982 (IV), IARC Lyon
332 Young YH, Miller RW: Incidence of malignant tumors in US children. J Pediatr 1975 (86):254
333 Bennett JM, Catovsky D, Daniel MT et al: The morphological classification of acute lymphoblastic leukemia: concordance among observers and clinical correlations. Br J Haematol 1981 (47):553-561
334 Mauer AM and Simone JV: The current status of the treatment of childhood acute lymphoblastic leukaemia. Cancer Treat Rev 1976 (3):17-41
335 Report to the Council by the Working Party on Leukaemia in Childhood: Improvement in treatment for children with acute lymphoblastic leukaemia. The Medical Research Council UKALL Trials 1972-84, Lancet 1986 (i):408-411
336 Bloomfield CD: Classification and prognosis of acute lymphoblastic leukaemia. Prognostic Clinical and Biological Research 1981 (58):167-183
337 Lilleyman JS, Hann IM, Stevens RF, Eden OB and Richards SM: French American British (FAB) morphological classification of childhood leukaemia and its clinical importance. J Clin Path 1986 (39):998-1002
338 Bloomfield CD, Goldman AI, Alimena G et al: Chromosomal abnormalities identify high risk and low risk patients with acute lymphoblastic leukaemia. Blood 1986 (67):415-420
339 Robinson LL, Nesbit ME, Sather HN and Hammond GD: Assessment of the interrelationship of prognostic factors in childhood acute lymphoblastic leukaemia. A report from Children's Cancer Study Group. Am J Pediat Haemat Oncol 1986 (2):5-3
340 Baccarani M, Corbelli G, Amadori S et al: Adolescent and adult acute lymphoblastic

leukaemia: prognostic features and outcome of therapy. A study of 293 patients. Blood 1982 (60): 677-684

341 Bloomfield CD: The clinical relevance of lymphocytic surface markers in adult acute lymphoblastic leukaemia. In: CD Bloomfield (ed) Adult Leukaemias. Martinus Nijhoff Publ, The Hague 1982 pp 265-308

342 Garay G, Pavlovsky S, Eppinger-Helft M, Cavagnaro F et al: Long term survival in acute lymphoblastic leukaemia: evaluation of prognostic factors. Proc Am Soc Clin Oncol 1982 (1):137 (abstr)

343 Mertelsmann R, Moore MAS and Claubron B: Leukaemia cell phenotype and prognosis: an analysis of 519 adults with acute leukaemia/ Blood Cells 1982 (8):561-583

344 Hoelzer D, Thiel E, Loffler H, Buchner T et al: Prognostic factors in multicentre study for treatment of acute lymphoblastic leukaemia in adults. Blood 1988 (71):123-131

345 Shuster JJ, Falletta JM, Pullen DJ: Prognostic factors in childhood T-cell acute lymphoblastic leukemia: A pediatric oncology group study. Blood 1990 (75):166-173

346 Clarkson B, Ellis S, Little C, Gee T et al: Acute lymphoblastic leukaemia in adults. Semin Oncol 1985 (12):160-179

347 Henze G, Langermann HJ, Ritter J, Schellong and Riehm H: Treatment strategy for different risk groups in childhood acute lymphoblastic leukaemia: a report from the BFM Study Group. Haematol Blood Transf 1981 (26):87-93

348 Gingrich RD, Burns CP, Armitage JO et al: Long term relapse-free survival in adult acute lymphoblastic leukaemia. Cancer Treat Rep 1985 (69):153-160

349 Sobol RE, Royston I, Le Bien TW, Minowada J et al: Adult acute lymphoblastic leukaemia phenotypes defined by monoclonal antibodies. Blood 1985 (65):730-735

350 Van den Berghe H: Cytogenetics in leukaemia. In: Whittaker J and Delamore IW (eds) Leukaemia. Blackwell Scient Publ, Oxford 1987 pp 137-151

351 Secker-Walker LM, Lawler SD and Hardisty RM: Prognostic implications of chromosomal findings in acute lymphoblastic leukaemia at diagnosis. Br Med J 1978 (2):1529-1530

352 Swansbury GJ, Secker-Walker LM, Lawler SD et al: Chromosomal findings in acute lymphoblastic leukaemia of childhood: an independent prognostic factor. Lancet 1981 (ii):249-250

353 Williams DL, Tsiatis A, Braden GM et al: Diagnostic importance of chromosome numbers in 136 untreated children with acute lymphoblastic leukaemia. Blood 1981 (60):864-871

354 Frei E III, Karan M, Levin R and Freireich EJ: The effectiveness of combinations of antileukaemic agents in inducing and maintaining remission in children with acute leukaemia. Blood 2965 (26):642-656

355 Freireich EJ, Gehan E, Frei E et al: The effect of 6-mercaptopurine on the duration of steriod-induced remissions in acute leukaemia: a model for evaluation of other potentially useful therapy/ Blood 1963 (21):699-716

356 Selawry OS and Frei E III: Prolongation of remission in acute lymphocytic leukaemia by alteration in dose schedule and route of administration of methotrexate/ Clin Res 1964 (2):230-235

357 Pinkel D: Curing children with leukaemia. Charles F Kettering Prize Oration 1986. Cancer 1987 (59):1683-1691

358 Lennard L and Lilleyman JS: Are children with lympoblastic leukaemia given enough 6-mercaptopurine? Lancet 1987 (ii):785-787

359 Lennard L and Lilleyman JS: Variable mercaptopurine metabolism and treatment outcome in childhood lymphoblastic leukaemia. J Clin Oncol 1989 (7):1816-1823

360 DeVita VT: Dose response is alive and well. J Clin Oncol 1986 (4):1157-1159

361 Riehm H, Gadner H and Henze G: Results and significance of six randomised trials in four consecutive ALL-BFM studies. Haematol Blood Transf 1990 (33):439-450

362 Buchner T, Henze G, Hoffmann J, Reiter A et al: Central nervous system relapse prevention in 1165 standard risk children with acute lymphoblastic leukaemia in five BFM finals. Haematol Blood Transf 1990 (33):500-503

363 Nesbit ME, Sather HN, Robison LL et al: Presymptomatic central nervous system therapy in previously untreated childhood lymphoblastic leukaemia: Comparison of 1800 Rads and 2400 Rads. Lancet 1981 (i):461-465

364 Gimema Cooperative Group: Gimema ALL0183: a multicentre study on adult acute lymphoblastic leukaemia in Italy. Br J Haematol 1989 (71):377-386

365 Byrd RL, Chatten J, Raney RB, Littman P et al: Testicular leukaemia incidence and management results. Med Pediat Oncol 1981 (9):493-500

366 Land VJ, Berry DH, Henson J et al: Long term survival in childhood acute leukaemia: "late" relapses. Med Pediat Oncol 1979 (7):19-24

367 Baum E, Sather H, Nachman J et al: Relapse rates following cessation of chemotherapy during complete remission of acute lymphoblastic leukaemia. Med Pediat Oncol 1979 (7):25-34
368 Medical Research Council: Testicular disease in acute lymphoblastic leukaemia in childhood. Br Med J 1978: (1):334-338
369 Miller DR, Leikin SL, Albo VC et al: Three versus five years of maintenance therapy are equivalent in childhood acute lymphoblastic leukemia: A report from the childrens Cancer Study Group. J Clin Oncol 1989 (7):316-325
370 Nesbit ME, Robison LL, Ortega JA et al: Testicular relapse in childhood acute lymphoblastic leukaemia: association with pretreatment patient characteristics and treatment. Cancer 1980 (45):2009-2016
371 Sullivan MP, Perez CA, Herson J et al: Radiotherapy (2500) Rads) for testicular leukaemia, local control and subsequent clinical events: A South Western Oncology Group Study. Cancer 1980 (46):508-515
372 Oakhill A, Mainwaring D, Hill FG et al: Management of leukaemic infiltration of the testis. Arch Dis Child 1980 (55):564-566
373 Tiedemann K, Chessells JM and Sandland RM: Isolated testicular relapse in boys with acute lymphoblastic leukaemia: treatment and outcome. Br Med J 1982 (285):1614-1616
374 Pui C-H, Dahl GV, Bowman WP et al: Elective testicular biopsy during chemotherapy for childhood leukaemia is of no clinical value. Lancet 1985 (ii):410-412
375 Eden DB: Extramedullary leukaemia. In: Willoughby M and Siegel B (eds) Paediatric Haematology and Oncology. Butterworth Med Rev 1982 pp 47-79
376 Burchenal JH: Long term survivors in acute leukaemia and Burkitt's tumour. Cancer 1968 (21):595-599
377 Medical Research Council: Duration of therapy in childhood ALL. Med Pediat Oncol 1982 (10):511-520
378 George SL, Aur RJA, Mauer AM and Simone JV: A reappraisal of the results of stopping therapy in childhood leukaemia. N Engl J Med 1979 (300):269-273
379 Nesbit ME, Sather HN, Robinson LL et al: Randomised study of 3 years versus 5 years chemotherapy in childhood acute lymphoblastic leukaemia. J Clin Oncol 1983 (1):308-316
380 Koren G, Ferranzani G, Hassan S et al: Systemic exposure to mercaptopurine as a prognostic factor in acute lymphocytic leukemia in children. N Engl J Med 1990 (323):17-21
381 Woods WG, Nesbit ME, Ramsay NKC et al: Intensive therapy followed by bone marrow transplantation for patients with acute lymphoblastic leukaemia in second or subsequent remission: determination of prognostic factors (A report from the University of Minnesota Bone Marrow Transplantation Team). Blood 1983 (61):1182-1189
382 Rivera GK, Buchanan G, Boyett JM et al: Intensive retreatment of childhood acute lympoblastic leukaemia in first bone marrow relapse: a paediatric oncology group study N Engl J Med 1986 (315):273-278
383 Chessells JM, Leiper AD, Plowman PN et al: Bone marrow transplantation has a limited role in prolonging second marrow remission in childhood lymphoblastic leukaemia. Lancet 1986 (i):1239-1241
384 Butturini A, Bortin MM Rivera G et al: Which treatment for childhood acute lymphoblastic leukaemia in second remission? Lancet 1987 (i):429-432
385 Saunders JE, Thomas ED, Buckner CD et al: Marrow transplantation for children with acute lymphoblastic leukaemia in second remission Blood 1987 (70):324-326
386 Henze G, Fengler R, Hartmann R et al: BFM Group treatment results in relapsed childhood acute lymphoblastic leukemia. Haematol Blood Transf 1990 (33):619-626
387 Steinberz PG, Gaynon P, Miller DR et al: Improved disease free survival of children with acute lymphoblastic leukaemia at high risk of early relapse with the New York Regime - a new intensive therapy protocol: a report from the Children's Cancer Study Group. J Clin Oncol 1986 (4):744-752
388 Haas OA, Mor W, Gadner H and Bartram CR: Treatment of Ph-positive acute lymphoblastic leukaemia with alpha- Interferon. Leukaemia 1987 (i):555 (letter)
389 Swanson G, Hu E, Sklar J et al: A prospective assessment of residual clonal disease in adult ALL utilising immunoglobulin gene rearrangement (IgR). Blood 1985 (66):246a (abstract)
390 Wright JJ, Poplack DG, Dakhshi A: Gene rearrangements as markers for clonal variation and minimal residual disease in acute lymphoblastic leukaemia. J Clin Oncol 1987 (5):735-741
391 Korsmeyer SJ: Antigen receptor genes as molecular markers for lymphoid neoplasms. J Clin Invest 1987 (79):1291-1295
392 Lee MS Chang KS Caanillas et al: Detection of minimal residual cells carrying the t(14:18) by DNA

sequence amplification/ Science 1987 (23):175-178
393 Estrov Z, Grunberger T, Dube ID et al: Detection of residual acute lymphoblastic leukaemia cells in cultures of bone marrow obtained during remission. N Engl J Med 1986 (315):538-542
394 Lee MS, Chang KS, Freireich EJ et al Detection of immunal residual bcr/abl transcripts by a modified polymerase chain reaction. Blood 1988 (72):893-897
395 Zehnbauer BA, Pardoll DM, Burke PJ et al: Immunoglobulin gene rearrangements in remission bone marrow specimens from patients with acute lymphoblastic leukaemia. Blood 1986 (67):835-838
396 Delfau M-H, Kerckaert J-P, d'Hooghe MC et al: Detection of minimal residual disease in chronic myeloid leukaemia patients after bone marrow transplantation by polymerase chain reaction. Leukemia 1990 (4): 1-5
397 Bregni M, Siena S, Neri A et al: Minimal residual disease in acute lymphoblastic leukemia detected by immune selection and gene rearrangement analysis. J Clin Oncol 1989 (7):338-343
398 Robison LL, Nesbit ME, Sather HN et al: Height of children successfully treated for acute lymphoblastic leukaemia. A report from the Late Effects Study Group of the Childrens Cancer Study Group. Med Pediatr Oncol 1985 (13):14-21
399 Kirk JA, Raghupathy P, Stevens MM et al: Growth failure and growth hormone deficiency after treatment for acute lymphoblastic leukaemia. Lancet 1987 (i): 190-193
400 Quigley C, Cowell C, Jimenez M et al: Normal or early development of puberty despite gonadal damage in children treated for acute lymphoblastic leukaemia. N Engl J Med 1989 (321):143-151
401 Civin CI: Reducing the cost of the cure in childhood leukaemia. N Engl J Med 1989 (321):185-187 (editorial)
402 Clayton PE, Shalet SM, Morris-Jones PH and Price DA: Growth in children treated for acute lymphoblastic leukaemia. Lancet 1988 (i):460-462
403 Leiper AD, Wheeler K and Chessells JM: Growth in children treated for acute lymphoblastic leukaemia. Lancet 1988 (i):943 (letter)
404 Wheeler K, Leiper AD, Jannoun L and Chessells JM: Medical cost of curing childhood acute lymphoblastic leukaemia. Br Med J 1988 (296):162-166
405 Hamre MR, Robinson LL, Nesbit ME et al: Effects of radiation on ovarian function in long term survivors of childhood acute lymphoblastic leukemia: A report from the Children's Cancer Study Group. J Clin Oncol 1987 (5) 1759-1765
406 Ise T, Kishi K, Imashuku S et al: Testicular histology and function following long-term chemotherapy of acute leukemia in children and outcome of the patients who received testicular biopsy. Am J Pediat Haematol Oncol 1986 (8):288-293
407 Jannoun L: Are cognitive and educational development affected by the age at which prophylactic therapy is given in acute lymphoblastic leukaemia? Arch Dis Childh 1983 (58):953-958
408 Mulhern RK, Ochs J and Fairclough D: Intellectual and academic achievement status after CNS relapse: a retrospective analysis of 40 children treated for acute lymphoblastic leukaemia. J Clin Oncol 1987 (5):933-940
409 Maguire P, Comaroff J, Ramsell PJ and Morris-Jones PH: Psychological and social problems in families of children with leukaemia. In: Morris Jones PH (ed) Topics in Paediatrics. I. Haematology and Oncology. Pitman Medical, Tunbridge Wells 1979 pp 141-149
410 O'Hare AE, McInnes A, Clarke M and Eden OB: The latency of visual evoked potential as an index of myelin disturbance in children treated for acute lymphoblastic leukaemia. Clin Electroencephalography 1987 (18):68-71
411 Zarrabi MH, Rosner F, Grunwald HW: Second neoplasms in acute lymphoblastic leukaemia. Cancer 1983 (52):1712-1719
412 Rosner K and Grunwald HW: Association of T-cell acute lymphoblastic leukaemia and histiocytic medullary reticulosis. Am J Med 1984 (77):910-914
413 Pui CH, Behm FG and Raimondi SC: Secondary acute myeloid leukaemia in children treated for acute lymphoid leukaemia. N Engl J Med 1989 (321):136-142
414 Albo V, Miller D, Leiken S et al: Nine brain tumours as a late effect in children 'cured' of acute lymphoblastic leukaemia (ALL) from a single protocol/ Proc Am Soc Clin Oncol 1985 (4):172 (abstr)
415 Green DM (ed) Long Term Complications of Therapy for Cancer in Childhood and Adolescence. The Johns Hopkins University Press, Baltimore 1989 pp 171
416 Fialkow PJ: Clonal development and stem cell origin of leukaemias and related disorders. Gunz FW and Henderson ES (eds) Leukaemia 4th Ed. Grune & Stratton, New York 1983 pp 63-76
417 Nowell PC and Hungerford DA: A minute chromosome in human chronic granulocytic leukaemia. Science 1960 (132):1497 (abstract from Nat Acad Sci, autumn meeting)

418 Canellos GP: Chronic granulocytic leukaemia. Med Clin North Am 1976 (60):1001-1018
419 Kurzrock R, Shtalrid M, Gutterman JU, Talpaz M: The molecular diagnostics of chronic myelogenous leukemia and philadelphia positive acute leukemia. Cancer Cells 1989 (7):9-13
420 Shtalrid M, Talpaz M, Blick M et al: Philadelphia-negative chronic myelogenous leukemia with breakpoint cluster rearrangement: Molecular analysis, clinical characteristics and response to therapy. J Clin Oncol 1988 (6):1569-1575
421 Bartram CR, Kleihauer E, de Klein A et al: C-abl and bcr are rearranged in a Ph-negative patient. EMBO J 1985 (4):683-686
422 Wiedemann LM, Karhi KK, Shivjim KK et al: The correlation of breakpoint cluster region rearrangement and P210 bcr/abl expression with morphological analysis of Ph-negative chronic myeloid leukemia and other myeloproliferative diseases. Blood 1988 (71):349-355
423 Bartram CR: Rearrangement of the C-abl and bcr genes in Ph-negative CML and Ph- CML and Ph-positive acute leukemia. Leukemia 1988 (2):63-64
424 Van der Plas DC, Hermans ABC, Soekarman D et al: Cytogenetic and molecular analysis in Philadelphia negative CML. Blood 1989 (73):1038-1044
425 Kurzrock R, Kantarjian M, Shtalrid M: Philadelphia chromosome negative chronic myelogenous leukemia without breakpoint cluster rearrangements: A chronic myeloid leukemia with a distinct clinical course. Blood 1990 (75):445-452
426 Goldman JM, Grooveld G, Baltimore D et al: Chronic myelogenous leukemia: the unfolding saga. Leukemia 1990 (4):163-167
427 Rassool F, Martiat P, Taj A et al: Interstitial insertion of varying amounts of abl-containing genetic material into chromosome 22 in Ph-negative CML. Leukemia 1990 (4):273-277
428 Van Etten R, Jackson P, Baltimore D: The mouse type IV c-abl gene product is a nuclear protein and activation of transforming ability is associated with cytoplasmic localisation. Cell 1989 (58):669-678
429 Jackson P, Baltimore D: N-terminal mutations activate the leukemogenic potential of the myristoylated form of c-abl. EMBO J 1989 (8):449-456
430 Daley GQ, Van Etten RA, Baltimore D: Induction of chronic myelogenous leukemia by the P210 bcr/abl gene of the Philadelphia chromosome. Science 1990 (247):824-830
431 Hughes T, Janssen JWG, Morgan G et al: False positive results with PCR to detect leukaemia-specific transcript. Lancet 1990 (i):1037-1038
432 Karanas A and Silver RT: Characteristics of the terminal phase of chronic granulocytic leukaemia. Blood 1968 (32):445-459
433 Theologides A: Unfavourable signs in patients with chronic myelocytic leukaemia. Ann Int Med 1972 (76):95-99
434 Shaw MT: Clinical and haematological manifestations of the terminal phase. In: Shaw MT (ed) Chronic Granulocytic Leukaemia. Praeger Publishers, Eastbourne 1982 pp 169-188
435 Sokal JE, Cox EB and Baccarani M et al: Prognostic discrimination in 'good risk' chronic granulocytic leukaemia. Blood 1984 (63):789-799
436 Sokal JE, Baccarani M, Tura S et al: Prognostic discrimination among younger patients with chronic granulocytic leukaemia: relevance to bone marrow transplantation. Blood 1985 (66):1352-1357
437 Sokal JE: Prognosis in chronic myeloid leukaemia: biology of the disease vs treatment. In: Goldman JM (ed) Bailliere's Clinical Haematology (Chronic Myeloid Leukaemia). Bailliere Tindall 1987 (1):907-929
438 Simon W, Segel GB, Lichtman A: Upper and lower time limits in the decision to recommend marrow transplantation for patients with chronic myelogenous leukaemia. Br J Haematol 1988 (70):31-36
439 Italian Cooperative Study Group on Chronic Myeloid Leukaemia. Timing of the haematological diagnosis of Ph positive chronic myeloid leukaemia. Eur J Haematol 1987 (38):75-79
440 Italian Cooperative Study Group on Chronic Myeloid Leukaemia. Prospective confirmation of a prognostic classification for Ph-positive chronic myeloid leukaemia. Br J Haematol 1988 (69):436-466
441 Pusey WA: Report of cases treated with roentgen rays. JAMA 1902 (38):911-919
442 Forkner CE and Scott TF: Arsenic as a therapeutic agent in chronic myelogenous leukaemia. JAMA 1931 (97):3-5
443 Galton DAG: Myleran in chronic myeloid leukaemia: results of treatment. Lancet 1953 (i):208-213
444 Haddow A and Timmis GM: Myleran in chronic myeloid leukaemia: chemical constitution and biological action. Lancet 1953 (i):207-208
445 Burns WA, McFarland W and Matthews MJ: Toxic manifestations of busulfan therapy. Med Ann DC 1971 (40):567-569
446 Allan NC, Duvall E, Stockdill G: Combination therapy for chronic granulocytic leukaemia. Lancet 1978 (ii):523 (letter)
447 Key NS, Emerson PM, Allan NC, Kelly PMA et al: Oesophageal varices associated with busulphan-

thioguanine combination therapy for chronic myeloid leukaemia. Lancet 1987 (ii):1050-1052
448 Dresler WF and Stein R: Veber den Hydroxylharnstoff. Justus Liebig's Ann Chem Pharm 1869 (150):242-245
449 Kennedy BJ and Yarboro JW: Metabolic and therapeutic effects of hydroxyurea in chronic myeloid leukaemia. JAMA 1966 (195):1038-1043
450 Bolin RW, Robinson WA, Sutherland J and Hamman RF: Busulfan versus hydroxyurea in long-term therapy of chronic myelogenous leukaemia. Cancer 1982 (50):1683-1686
451 Talpaz M, McCredie KB, Mavligit GM and Gutterman JV: Leukocytic interferon - induced myeloid cytoreduction in chronic myelogenous leukaemia. Blood 1983 (62):689-692
452 Cantell K and Hirvonnen S: Large scale production of human leucocyte interferon containing 10 units per ml. J Gen Virol 1978 (39):541-543
453 Neumann HA and Fauser AA: Effect of interferon on pluripotent haemopoietic progenitors (CFU-GEMM) derived from human bone marrow. Exp Haematol 1982 (10):587-590
454 Williams CK, Svet-Moldavskaya I and Vilcek J: Inhibitory effects of human leucocyte and fibroblast interferons on normal and chronic myelogenous leukaemia granulocytic progenitor cells. Oncology 1981 (38):356-360
455 Talpaz M, Kantarjian HM, McCredie K et al: Hematologic remission and cytogenetic improvement induced by recombinant human Interferon alpha in chronic myelogenous leukaemia. N Engl J Med 1986 (314):1065-1069
456 Kantarjian HM, Talpaz M, Kurzrock R and Keating MJ: Intensive combination chemotherapy and interferons in the management of chronic myelogenous leukaemia. Acta Haemat 1987 (78 Suppl 1):70-74
457 Hardisty RM, Speed DE, Till M: Granulocytic leukaemia in childhood. Br J Haematol 1964 (10):551-556
458 Weatherall DJ, Brown MJ: Juvenile chronic myeloid leukaemia. Lancet 1970 (i):526
459 Fox AM: Case of juvenile chronic myeloid leukaemia. Lancet 1970 (i):368-369
460 Shapira Y, Polliack A, Cividalli G, Rachmilewitz EA: Juvenile chronic myeloid leukemia with fetal erythropoiesis. Cancer 1972 (30):353-357
461 Maurer HS, Vida LN, Honig GR: Similarities of the erythrocytes in juvenile chronic myelogenous leukemia and fetal erythrocytis. Blood 1972 (39):778-784
462 Goldman JM and Baughan ASJ: Chronic granulocytic leukaemia. In: Goldman JM and Preisler HD (eds) Leukemias. Butterworth International Medical Reviews 1984 pp 239-265
463 Allan NC, Shepherd PCA: Treatment of chronic myeloid leukaemia. In: Goldman JM (ed) Bailliere's Clinical Haematology 1. Bailliere Tindall 1987 (1):1031-1054
464 Janossy G, Woodruff RK, Pippard MJ et al: Relation of 'Lymphoid' phenotype and response to chemotherapy incorporating vincristine-prednisolone in the acute phase of PL-positive leukaemia. Cancer 1979 (43):426-434
465 Griffin JD, Ttodd RF, Ritz J et al: Differentiation patterns in the blastic phase of chronic myeloid leukemia. Blood 1983 (61):85-91
466 Muehleck SD, McKenna RW and Arthur DC: Transformation of chronic myelogenous leukemia: clinical morphologic and cytogenetic features. Am J Clin Path 1984 (82):1-14
467 Office of Population Censuses and Surveys. Cancer Statistics. Registration series in B1 No 14 and mortality statistics DH2 No 9. HMSO, London 1982
468 Linet MS and Blattner WA: The epidemiology of chronic lymphatic leukaemia. In: Polliack A and Catovsky D (eds) Chronic Lymphatic Leukaemia. Harwood Academic Publishers, New York 1988 pp 11-32
469 Sawitsky A and Rai K: The chronic lymphoid leukaemias. In: Whittaker J and Delamore IW (eds) Leukaemia. Blackwell Science Publishers, Oxford 1983 pp 386-406
470 Hamblin TJ: Chronic lymphocytic leukaemia. Baillere's Clin Haematol 1987 (i):449-491
471 Casey TD: Chronic lymphatic leukaemia in a child presenting at the age of 2 years and 8 months. Austr Ann Med 1968 (17):70-74
472 Gunz FW: Epidemiology of leukaemia. In: Gunz FW and Henderson ES (eds) Leukaemia 4th Ed. Grune & Stratton, New York 1983 pp 27-28
473 Uchiyama T, Yodoi J et al: Adult T-cell leukaemia: clinical and haematological features of 16 cases. Blood 1977 (50):481-492
474 Hattori T, Uchiyama T, Toibana T, Takatsuki K and Uchino H: Surface phenotype of Japanese adult T-cell leukaemia cells characterised by monoclonal antibodies. Blood 1981 (58):645-647
475 Blattner WA, Strober W, Muchmore AV, Blaese RM et al: Familial chronic lymphocytic leukaemia. Immunologic and cellular characterisation. Annal Int Med 1976 (84):554-557
476 Williams RC, Erickson JL, Polesky HF, Swann WR: Studies of monoclonal immunoglobulins (M-components) in various kindreds. Ann Int Med 1967 (67):309-327

478 Bennett JM, Catovsky D, Daniel M-T, Flandrin G et al: Proposals for the classification of chronic (mature) B and T lymphoid leukaemias. J Clin Pathol 1989 (42):567-584
479 Rai KR, Sawitsky A, Cronkite KP, Chanana EP et al: Clinical staging of chronic lymphocytic leukaemia. Blood 1975 (46):219-234
480 Binet JL, Catovsky D, Chandra P et al: Report from the International Workshop on CLL Chronic Lymphatic Leukaemia: proposals for a revised prognostic staging system. Br J Haematol 1981 (48):365-367
481 Sweet DC Jr, Golomb HM and Ultmann JE: The clinical features of chronic lymphocytic leukaemia. Clinics in Haematology 1977 (6):185-202
482 Ebbe S, Wittels B and Damashek W: Autoimmune thrombocytopenic purpura (ITP type) with chronic lymphocytic leukaemia. Blood 1962 (19):23-27
483 Evans RS, Takahaski K, Duane RT et al: Primary thrombocytopenic purpura and acquired haemolytic anaemia. Arch Int Med 1951 (87):48-65
484 Kaden BR, Rosse WF and Hauch TW: Immunothrombocytopenia in lymphoproliferative diseases. Blood 1979 (53):545-551
485 Hegde UM, Williams K, Devereux S, Bowes A et al: Platelet associated IgG and immune thrombocytopenia in lymphoproliferative and autoimmune disorders. Clin and Lab Haematol 1983 (5):9-15
486 Rosse WF: The acquired haemolytic anaemias In: Hoffbrand AV and Lewis SM (eds) Postgraduate Haematology, 2nd Ed. W Heinemann Medical Books Ltd, Oxford 1981 pp 229-268
487 Lewis FB, Schwartz RS and Dameshek W: X-radiation and alkylating agents as possible "trigger" mechanisms in the autoimmune complications of malignant lymphoproliferative disease. Clin Exp Immunol 1966 (1):3-11
488 Ritch PS, Anderson T: Reversal of autoimmune hemolytic anemia associated with chronic lymphocytic leukemia following high-dose immunoglobulin. Cancer 1987 (60):2637-2740
489 Rustagi P, Han T, Ziolkowski L et al: Antigranulocyte antibodies in chronic lymphocytic leukemia and other chronic lymphoproliferative disorders. Blood 1983 (62 Suppl 1):106 (abstract)
490 Abelhoff MD and Waterbury MD: Pure red cell aplasia and chronic lymphocytic leukaemia. Arch Int Med 1974 (134):721-724
491 Miller DG: Patterns of immunological deficiency in leukaemias and lymphomas. Ann Int Med 1962 (57):703-715
492 Damashek W: Chronic lymphocytic leukaemia - an accumulative disease of immunologically incompetent lymphocytes. Blood 1967 (29): 566-584
493 Franklin EC: MU chain disease. Arch Int Med 1975 (135):71-72
494 Rai KR and Sawitsky A: Studies in clinical staging, lymphocyte function and markers as an approach to the treatment of chronic lymphocytic leukaemia. Silber R et al (eds) Contemporary Haematology/Oncology. Plenum, New York 1981 pp 227-262
495 Shaw RK, Szwed D, Boggs DR et al: Infection and immunity in chronic lymphocytic leukaemia. Arch Int Med 1960 (106):467-478
496 Miller DG and Karnofsky DA: Immunological factors and resistance to infection in chronic lymphatic leukaemia Am J Med 1961 (31):748-757
497 Cone L and Uhr JW: Immunological deficiency disorders associated with chronic lymphocytic leukaemia and multiple myeloma. J Clin Invest 1964 (43):2241-2248
498 Chapel H and Bunch C: Mechanisms of infection in chronic lymphocytic leukaemia. Semin Haematol 1987 (24):291-296
499 Boggs DR, Sofferman SA, Wintrobe MM and Cartwright GE: Factors influencing the duration of survival in chronic lymphocytic leukaemia. Am J Med 1966 (40):243-254
500 Manoharan A, Catovsky D, Lampert I A et al: Histiocytic medullary reticulosis complicating chronic lymphocytic leukaemia: malignant or reactive? Scand J Haematol 1981 (26):5-13
501 Rai KR and Sawitsky A: Diagnosis and treatment of chronic lymphocytic leukaemia. In: Wiernik PH, Canellos GP, Kyle RA and Schiffer CA (eds) Neoplastic Diseases of the Blood. Churchill Livingstone, New York 1985 pp 105-120
502 Galton DAG: Chronic lymphocytic leukaemia: treatment. In: Goldman JM and Preisler HD (eds) Haematology/Leukaemias. Butterworths, London 1984 pp 299-321
503 Hansen MM: Chronic lymphocytic leukaemia: clinical studies based on 189 cases followed for a long time. Scand J Haemat 1973 (18):3-28
504 Catovsky D, Fooks J and Richards S: Prognostic factors in chronic lymphocytic leukaemia: the importance of age, sex and response to treatment on survival. Br J Haematol 1989 (72):141-149
505 French Cooperative group on CLL: Two clinical trials in CLL and clinical staging. Bone Marrow Transpl 1989 (4):158
506 Sawitsky A, Rai KR, Glidewell O, Silver RT et al: Comparison of daily versus intermittent chlorambucil and prednisone therapy in the

treatment of patients with chronic lymphocytic leukaemia. Blood 1977 (50):1049-1059
507 Freymann JG, Vancer JB, Marler EA and Meyer DG: Prolonged corticosteroid therapy of chronic lymphocytic leukaemia and the closely allied malignant lymphomas. Br J Haematol 1960 (6):303-323
508 Galton DAG, Wiltshaw E, Szur L and Dacie JV: The use of chlorambucil and steroids in the treatment of chronic lymphocytic leukaemia. Br J Haematol 1961 (7):73-98
509 Chastang C, Travade P, Benichou J, Dighiero G and Binet J-L: Patients accrual and interim statistical analysis in long-term clinical trials: the French chronic lymphocytic leukaemia CLL 80 protocol as a case study. Statistics in Medicine 1986 (5):465-473
510 Hansen MM, Anderson E, Christensen BE, Christiansen I et al: CHOP versus prednisolone + chlorambucil in chronic lymphocytic leukaemia: preliminary results of a randomised multicentre study. Nouv Rev Fr Hématol 1988 (30):433-436
511 French Cooperative Group: Effectiveness of CHOP regimen in advanced untreated chronic lymphocytic leukaemia. Lancet 1986 (i):1346-1349
512 French Cooperative Group on Chronic Lymphocytic Leukaemia: Long-term results of the CHOP regimen in stage C chronic lympocytic leukaemia. Br J Haematol 1989 (73):334-340
513 Keating MJ, Scouros M, Murphy S and Kantarjian H et al: Multiple agent chemotherapy (POACH) in previously treated and untreated patients with chronic lymphocytic leukaemia. Leukaemia 1988(2):157-164
514 Rubin P, Bennett JM, Begg C, Bozdech MJ and Silber R: The comparison of total body irradiation vs chlorambucil and prednisone for remission induction of active chronic lymphocytic leukaemia: an ECOG study. Part I: Total body irradiation. Response and toxicity. Int J Rad Oncol Biol Physics 1981 (7):1623-1632
515 Singh AK, Bates T, Wetherley-Mein G: A preliminary study of low-dose irradiation for the treatment of chronic lymphocytic and prolymphocytic leukaemia. Scand J Haematol 1986 (37):50-58
516 Riscoe MK, Brouns MC, Fitchen JH Purine metabolism as a target for leukemia chemotherapy. Blood Rev 1989 (3):162-173
517 Tseng WC, Derse D, Cheng YC et al: In vitro biological activity of 9-B-D arabinofuranosyl-2-fluoroadenine and the biological actions of its triphosphate on DNA polymerase and ribonucleotide reductase from HeLa cells. Mol Pharmacol 1982 (21):474-477
518 Leiby JM, Snider KM, Kraut EH, Metz EN et al: Phase II trial of 9-a-d-arabinofuranosyl-2-fluoradenine 5'monophosphate in non-Hodgkin's lymphoma. Prospective comparison of responses with deoxycytidine kinase activity. Cancer Res 1987 (47):2719-2722
519 Lee WW, Benitz A, Goodman A and Baker BR: Potential anticancer agents XL: synthesis of the B-anomer of 9-(d-arabino- furanosyl) adenine. J Am Chem Soc 1960 (82):2648-2649
520 Boldt DH, von Hoff DD, Kuhn JG and Hersch M: Effects on human peripheral lymphocytes of in vivo administration of 9-a-d- arabinofuranosyl-2-fluoradenine-5'-monophosphate (NSC 312887), a new purine antimetabolite. Cancer Res 1984 (44):4661-4666
521 Keating MJ, Kantarjian H, Talpaz M and Redman J et al: Fludarabine: a new agent with major activity against chronic lymphocytic leukaemia Blood 1989 (74): 19-25
522 Warrell RP Jr, Berman E: Phase I and II study of fludarabine phosphate in Leukaemia: therapeutic efficacy with delayed central nervous system toxicity J Clin Oncol 1986 (4):74-79
523 Harvey WH, Fleming TR, Beltran G et al: Phase II study of fludarabine phosphate in previously untreated patients with hepatoma: a Southwest Oncology Group Study. Cancer Treat Rep 1987 (71):1111-1112
524 Spriggs DR, Stopa E, Mayer RJ et al: Fludarabine phosphate (NSC212878) infusions for the treatment of acute leukemia: phase I and neuropathological study. Cancer Res 1986 (46):5953-5958
525 Merkel DE, Griffin NL, Kagan-Hallet K, von Hoff DD: Central nervous system toxicity with fludarabine. Cancer Treat Rep 1986 (70):1449-1450
526 Hamblin TJ, Abdul-Ahad AK, Gordon J and Stevenson FK et al: Preliminary evidence in treating lymphocytic leukaemia with antibody to immunoglobulin idiotypes on the cell surface. Br J Cancer 1980 (42):495-502
527 Gordon J, Abdul-Ahad AK, Hamblin TJ and Stevenson FK: Barriers to successful immunotherapy with anti-idiotype antibody. Br J Cancer 1984 (49):547-557
528 Ritz J and Schlossman SF: Utilisation of monoclonal antibodies in the treatment of leukaemia and lymphoma. Blood 1982 (59):1-11
529 Levy R and Miller RA: Biological and clinical implications of lymphocytic hybridisations: Tumour

therapy with monoclonal antibodies. Ann Rev Med 1983 (34): 107-116
530 Bertram JH, Gill PS, Levine AM, Boquiren D et al: Monoclonal antibody T101 in T-cell malignancies: a clinical, pharmacokinetic and immunologic correlation. Blood 1986 (68):752-761
531 Press OW, Appelbaum F, Ledbetter J, Martin PJ et al: Monoclonal antibody IF5 (anti-CD20) serotherapy of human B cell lymphomas. Blood 1987 (69): 584-591
532 Dyer MJS, Hale G, Hayhoe FGJ and Waldman H: Effects of CAMPATH-1 antibodies in vivo in patients with lymphoid malignancies: Influence of antibody isotype. Blood 1989 (73):1431-1439
533 Riechmann L, Clark MR, Waldmann H and Winter G: Reshaping human antibodies for therapy. Nature 1988 (332):323-327
534 Hale G, Dyer MJS, Clark MR and Phillips JM et al: Remission induction in non-Hodgkin's lymphoma with the reshaped human monoclonal antibody CAMPATH-IH. Lancet 1988 (ii):1394-1399
535 Galton DAG, Goldman JM, Wiltshaw E et al: Prolymphocytic leukaemia. Br J Haematol 1974 (27):7-23
536 Melo J, Catovsky D and Galton DAG: The relationship between chronic lymphocytic leukaemia and prolymphocytic leukaemia. I. Clinical and laboratory features of 300 patients and characterisation of an intermediate group. Br J Haematol 1986 (63):377-387
537 Melo J, Catovsky D and Galton DAG: The relationship between chronic lymphocytic leukaemia and prolymphocytic leukaemia. II. Patterns of evolution of 'prolymphocytoid' transformation. Br J Haematol 1986 (64):77-86
538 Melo J, Wandle J, Chitty M and England J: The relationship between chronic lymphocytic leukaemia and prolymphocytic leukaemia. III. Evaluation of cell size by morphology and volume measurements. Br J Haematol 1986 (64):469-478
539 Melo J, Catovksy D, Gregory WM and Galton DAG: The relationship between chronic lymphocytic leukaemia and prolymphocytic leukaemia. IV. Analysis of survival and prognostic features. Br J Haematol 1987 (65):23-29
540 Richter MH: Generalised reticular sarcoma of lymph nodes associated with lymphatic leukemia. Am J Path 1928 (4):285-292
541 Lortholary P, Boiron M, Ripault P et al: Leucémie lymphoide chronique secondairment associée a une réticulopathie maligne; syndrome de Richter. Nouv Rev Fr Hematol 1964 (4):621-644
542 Van Dongen JJM, Hooijkaas H, Michels JJ et al: Richter's syndrome with different immunoglobulin light chains and different heavy chain gene rearrangements. Blood 1984 (64):571-575
543 McDonnel JM, Beschorner WE, Staal SP et al: Richter's syndrome with two different B-cell clones. Cancer 1986 (58):2031-2037
544 Delsol G, Laurent G, Kuhlein E et al: Richter's syndrome. Evidence for the clonal origin of the two proliferations. Am J Clin Path 1981 (76):308-315
545 Baumann MA, Libnoch JA, Patrick CW et al: Prolonged survival in Richter's syndrome with subsequent reemergence of CLL. Am J Hematol 1985 (20):67-72
546 Harousseau JL, Flandrin G: Malignant lymphoma supervening in chronic lymphocytic leukemia and related disorders. Richter's syndrome: a study of 25 cases. Cancer 1981 (48):1302-1308
547 Galton DAG: Terminal transformation in B-cell chronic lymphocytic leukaemia. Bone Marrow Transpl 1989 (4 Suppl 1):156-157
548 Bouroncle BA, Wiseman BK and Doan CA: Leukaemic reticuloendotheliosis. Blood 1958 (13):609-630
549 Ewald O: Die Leukamische reticuloendotheliose. Deutsches Arch Klin Med 1923 (142):222-229
550 Rosenthal N and Lee SL: Reticulum cell leukaemia: A clinical and morphological entity. Report of 16 cases. Proc of 13th Annual Meeting of Am Soc Clin Path 1951
551 Belding HW, Dalard GA, Parker F: Histiocytic and monocytic leukemia. A clinical, hematological and pathological differentiation. Cancer 1955 (8):237-252
552 Dameshek W: Proliferative disease of the reticulo-endothelial system. II. Aleukemic reticulosis. Folia Haematol 1933 (49):64-67
553 Bouroncle BA: Leukemic reticuloendotheliosis (Hairy Cell Leukaemia). Blood 1979 (53):412-436
554 Flandrin G, Daniel MT, Fourcade M and Chelloul N: Leucemie a "Tricholeucocyte" (Hairy cell leukaemia): etude clinique et cytologique de 55 observations. Nouv Rev Fr Hematol 1973 (13):609-640
555 Schrek R, Donnelly WJ: "Hairy" cells in blood in lymphoreticular neoplastic disease and "flagellated" cells of normal lymph nodes. Blood 1966 (27):199-211
556 Golomb HM, Catovsky D, Golde DW: Hairy cell leukaemia - A clinical review on 71 cases Ann Int Med 1978 (89):677-683
557 Cawley JC, Burns GF, Hayhoe FGJ: Hairy cell leukaemia. Recent Results in Cancer Research. Springer-Verlag, Berlin, Heidelberg 1980 (72)

558 Golomb HM and Hadad LJ: Infectious complications in 127 patients with hairy cell leukaemia. Am J Haematol 1984 (16):393-401

559 Marie JP, Degos L and Flandrin G: Hairy cell leukemia and tuberculosis. N Engl J Med 1977 (297):1354 (letter)

560 Weinstein RA, Golomb HM, Grumet G et al: Hairy cell leukemia: association with disseminated atypical mycobacterial infection. Cancer 1981 (48):380-383

561 Rice L, Shenkenberg T, Lynch EC et al: Granulomatous infections complicating hairy cell leukaemia. Cancer 1982 (49):1924-1928

562 Elkon KB, Hughes GRV, Catovsky D et al: Hairy cell leukaemia with polyarteritis nodosa. Lancet 1979 (2):280-282

563 Raju SF, Chapman SW, Dreiling B et al: Hairy cell leukemia with the appearance of mixed cryoglobulinemia and vasculitis. Arch Int Med 1984 (144):1300-1302

564 Dorsey JK and Penick GD: The association of hairy cell leukaemia with unusual immunologic disorders. Arch Int Med 1982 (142):902-903

565 Le Pogamp P, Ghandour C and Le Prise PY: Hairy cell leukaemia and polyarteritis nodosa. J Rheumatol 1982 (9):441-442

566 Weh JH, Katz M, Bray B, Rodat O, Degos C and Flandrin G: Lesions ossueses au cours des leucemies a tricholeucocytes. Nouv Pres Med 1979 (8):2253-2254

567 Demanes DJ, Lane N and Beckstead JH: Bone involvement in hairy cell leukaemia. Cancer 1982 (49):1697-1701

568 Embersky BC, Ratain MJ and Golomb HM: Skeletal complications in hairy cell leukaemia: Diagnosis and therapy. J Clin Oncol 1986 (6):1280-1284

569 Linder J, Silberman HR and Croker BP: Amyloidosis complicating hairy cell leukemia Am Clin Path 1982 (78):864-867

570 Bouroncle BA: Unusual presentations and complications of hairy cell leukaemia. Leukemia 1987 (1): 288-293

571 Li CY, Yam LT and Lam KW: Studies of acid phosphatase isoenzymes in human leucocytes. Demonstration of isoenzyme cell specificity. J Histochem Cytochem 1970 (18):901-910

572 Schwarting R, Stein H, Wang CY: Monoclonal antibodies SHCL-1 and SHCL-3 allow the diagnosis of hairy cell leukemia. Blood 1985 (65):974-983

573 Falini B, Palford K, Erber WN et al: Use of a panel of monoclonal antibodies for the diagnosis of hairy cell leukaemia. An immunocytochemical study of 36 cases. Histopathology 1986 (10):671-687

574 Chilosi M and Pizzolo G: Immunophenotypical diagnosis and monitoring of hairy cell leukemia. Leukemia 1990 (4):168-169 (editorial)

575 Thaler J, Dietze O, Faber V et al: Monoclonal antibody B-Ly7: A sensitive marker for detection of minimal residual disease in hairy cell leukemia. Leukemia 1990 (4):170-176

576 Rubin LA, Kurman CC, Fritz ME et al: Soluble interleukin-2 receptors are released from activated human lymphoid cells in vitro. J Immunol 1985 (135):3172-3177

577 Chilosi M, Semenzato G, Cetto G et al: Soluble interleukin-2 receptors in the sera of patients with hairy cell leukemia: relationship with the effect of recombinant alpha-interferon therapy on clinical parameters and natural killer in vitro activity. Blood 1987 (70):1530-1535

578 Pizzolo G, Chilosi, Semenzato G: The soluble interleukin-2 receptor in haematological disorders. Br J Haematol 1987 (67):377-380

579 Semenzato G, Trentin L, Zambellow R et al: Origin of the soluble interleukin-2 receptor in the serum of patients with hairy cell leukemia. Leukemia 1988 (2):788-792

580 Ambrosetti A, Semenzato G, Prior M et al: Serum levels of soluble interleukin-2 receptors in hairy cell leukaemia: a reliable marker of neoplastic bulk. Br J Haematol 1989 (73):181-186

581 Golomb HM: Progress report on chlorambucil therapy in post-splenectomy patients with progressive hairy cell leukemia. Blood 1981 (57):464-467

582 Jansen J and Hermans J: Clinical staging system for hairy cell leukaemia. Blood 1982 (60):571-577

583 Krigel R, Liebes LF, Pelle E and Silber R: Chlorambucil therapy in hairy cell leukemia: effects on lipid composition and lymphocyte subpopulations. Blood 1982 (60): 272-275

584 Porzsolt F, Raghavacher A, Digel W et al: Strategy for the treatment of hairy cell leukemia. Leukemia 1987 (1):334-337

585 Quesada JR, Hersh EM and Gutterman JU: Therapy of hairy cell leukaemia with alpha interferon. Antiviral Research 1984 34: abstract

586 Quesada JR, Reuben J, Manning JT and Hersh EM: Alpha interferon for induction of remission in Hairy Cell Leukaemia. N Engl J Med 1984 (310):15-18

587 Quesada JR, Lepe-Zuniga JL and Gutterman JV: Mid-term observations on the efficacy of alpha-interferon in hairy cell leukemia and status of the interferon system of patients in remission. Leukemia 1987 (1):317-319

588 Worman C, Catovsky D, Cawley JC et al: The UK experience with human lymphoblastic interferon in

HCL: A report of the first 50 cases. Leukemia 1987 (1):320-322
589 Pralle H, Zwingers T, Boedewadt S et al: A prospective multicenter trial with human recombinant alpha 2C interferon in hairy cell leukemia before and after splenectomy. Leukemia 1987 (1):337-340
590 Golomb HM and Ratain MJ: Recent advances in the treatment of hairy cell leukemia. N Engl J Med 1987 (316):870-871 (editorial)
591 Samuels BL, Rosner MC, Giometti CS et al: Action of interferons in hairy cell leukemia. Leukemia 1987 (1):365-369
592 Cheson BD and Martin A: Clinical trials in hairy cell leukaemia. Ann Int Med 1987 (106):871-878
593 Figlin RA: Biotherapy in clinical practice. Semin Haematol 1989 (26 Suppl 3):15-24
594 Golomb HM, Ratain MJ, Fefer A, Johnson J et al: Randomised study of the duration of treatment with interferon alpha-2b in patients with hairy cell leukemia. JNCI 1988 (80):369-373
595 Golomb HM, Fefer A, Golde DW, Ozer H et al: Sequential evaluation of alpha-2b-interferon treatment in 128 patients with hairy cell leukaemia. Semin Oncol 1987 (14 Suppl 2):13-17
596 Ratain MJ, Golomb HM and Bardawil RG: Durability of responses to interferon alfa-2b in advanced hairy cell leukaemia. Blood 1987 (69):872-877
597 Thompson JA, Shields AF, Porter BA and Olsen DO: Magnetic resonance imaging of bone marrow in hairy cell leukaemia: Correlation with clinical response to alpha-interferon. Leukemia 1987 (1):315-316
598 Quesada JR, Talpaz M, Rios A, Kurzroch R and Gutterman JV: Clinical toxicity of interferons in cancer patients - a review. J Clin Oncol 1986 (4):234-243
599 Abrahams PG, McClamrock E and Foon KA: Evening administration of alpha interferon. N Engl J Med 1985 (312):443-444 (letter)
600 Roth MS and Foon KA: Alpha Interferon in the treatment of hematologic malignancies. Am J Med 1986 (81):871-882
601 Roy V and Newland AC: Raynaud's phenomenon and cryoglobulinaemia associated with the use of recombinant human alpha-interferon. Lancet 1988 (i): 944 (letter)
602 Schilsky RL, Davidson HS, Magid D, Dalter S and Golomb HM: Gonadal and sexual functions in male patients with hairy cell leukaemia: lack of adverse effect of recombinant alpha interferon treatment. Cancer Treat Rep 1987 (71):179-181
603 Coci A, Costello A, Pagnucco G, et al: Bone marrow histology in patients with hairy cell leukaemia (HCL) treated by human lymphoblastoid interferon. Haematologica 1987 (72):143-148
604 Dupuy E, Sigaux F, Bryckaert MC et al: Platelet acquired defect in PDGF and beta haemoglobulin content in hairy cell leukaemia: improvement after interferon therapy. Br J Haematol 1987 (65):107-110
605 Heslop HE, Bianchi AC, Cordingley FT et al: Mechanisms of action of alpha-interferon in B lymphoproliferative disorders. Nouv Pres Fr Med 1988 (30):317-319
606 Cordingly FT, Bianchi A, Hoffbrand AV et al: Tumour necrosis factor as an autocrine tumour growth factor for chronic B- cell malignancies. Lancet 1988 (i): 969-971
607 Bianchi AC, Heslop HE, Drexler HG et al: Effects of tumour necrosis factor and alpha interferon on chronic B-cell malignancies. Nouv Rev Fr Hematol 1988 (30):317-319
608 Steis RG, Smith JW II, Urba W and Clark JW: Resistance to recombinant interferon alfa-2a in hairy cell leukemia associated with neutralizing anti-interferon antibodies. N Engl J Med 1988 (318):1409-1413
609 Itri LM, Campion M, Dennin RA, Palleroni AV et al: Incidence and clinical significance of neutralizing antibodies in patients receiving recombinant interferon alfa-2a by intramuscular injection. Cancer 1987 (59 suppl 3):668-674
610 Gauci L: Management of cancer patients receiving interferon alpha-2a. Int J Cancer 1987 (suppl 1):21-30
611 Von Wussaw P, Freund M, Block B and Diedrich H: Clinical significance of anti-1FN-antibody titres during interferon therapy. Lancet 1987 (ii):635-636
612 Spiegel RJ, Spicehandler JR, Jacobs SL and Oden EM: Low incidence of neutralizing factors in patients receiving recombinant alfa-2b interferon (INTRON). Am J Med 1986 (80): 223-228
613 Moormeier JA, Westbrook CA, Ratain MJ and Golomb HM: Interferon Alfa-2b antibodies and clinical resistance in a patient with hairy cell leukaemia. Leuk Lymph 1989 (1):43-45
614 Glaspy JA, Baldwin GC, Robertson BA and Olsen DO: Therapy of neutropenia in hairy cell leukaemia with recombinant human granulocytic colony-stimulating factor. Ann Int Med 1988 (109):789-795
615 Spiers ASD, Parekh SJ and Bishop MB: Hairy cell leukaemia: induction of complete remission with pentostatin (2'deoxycoformycin). J Clin Oncol 1984 (2):1336-1342
616 Spiers ASD, Moore D, Cassileth PA, Harrington DP et al: Remissions in hairy cell leukaemia with

pentostatin (2'-deoxycoformycin). N Engl J Med 1987 (316): 825-830

617 Kraut EH, Bouroncle BA and Grever MR: Low dose deoxycoformycin in the treatment of hairy cell leukaemia. Blood 1986 (68):1119-1122

618 Kraut EH, Bouroncle BA and Grever MR: Pentostatin in the treatment of advanced hairy cell leukaemia. J Clin Oncol 1989 (7):168-172

619 Murphy SB, Sinkule JA and Rivera G: Phase I-II clincal and pharmacodynamic study of the effects of 2'- deoxycoformycin administered by continuous infusion in children with refractory acute lymphoblastic leukaemia. Cancer Treat Symp 1984 (2):55-61

620 Eisenhauer E, Johnston JB, Barr et al: 2'-deoxycoformycin (DCF) in hairy cell leukemia. In: Proceedings of the Fifth NCI/EORTC Symposium on New Drugs in Cancer Treatment. Free University Amsterdam, Netherlands 1986 Abstr No 1208

621 Ho A, Thaler J, Mandelli F et al: Response to Pentostatin in Hairy-Cell Leukemia refractory to interferon- alpha. J Clin Oncol 1989 (7):1533-1538

622 Smyth JF, Paine RM, Jackman AL, Harrap KR et al: The clinical pharmacology of the adenosine deminase inhibitor 2'deoxyco- formycin. Cancer Chemother Pharmacol 1980 (5):93-101

623 Smyth JF and Harrap KR: Adenosine deaminase activity in leukaemia. Br J Cancer 1975 (31):544-549

624 Smyth JF, Prentice HG, Proctor S and Hoffbrand AV: Deoxycoformycin in the treatment of leukaemias and lymphomas. Ann NY Acad Sci 1985 (451):123-128

625 Grever MR, Sian ME, Jacob WF et al: The biochemical and clinical consequences of 2'deoxycoformycin in refractory lymphoproliferative malignancy. Blood 1981 (57): 406-416

626 Seto S, Carvera CJ, Kubota M et al: Mechanism of deoxyadenosine and 2 chlorodeoxyadenosine toxicity to non-dividing human lymphocytes. J Clin Invest 1985 (75):377-383

627 Kefford RF and Fox RM: Deoxycoformycin-induced response in chronic lymphatic leukaemia: Ω deoxyadenosine toxicity in non replicating lymphocytes. Br J Haematol 1982 (50): 627-636

628 Lamballe F, Le Prise P-Y, Le Gall E and David JC: dATP-mediated inhibition of DNA Ligase by 2'-Deoxycoformycin in T and B cell Leukemia. Leukemia 1989 (3): 97-103

629 Urba WJ, Baseler MW, Kopp WC et al: Deoxycoformycin-induced immunosupression in patients with hairy cells. Blood 1989 (73): 38-46

630 Piro LD, Carrera CJ, Carson DA and Beutler E: Lasting remissions in hairy cell leukaemia induced by a single infusion of 2-chlorodeoxyadenosine. N Engl J Med 1990 (322):1117-1121

631 Kim IYZ, Lang CY, Cantoni GL et al: Inactivation of S-adenosylhomocysteine hydrolase by nucleosides. Biochem BioPhys Acta 1985 (829):150-155

632 Golomb HM, Ratain MJ and Moormeier J: What is the choice of treatment for hairy cell leukemia J Clin Oncol 1989 (7):156-158 (editorial)

The Use of Biological Response Modifiers in Acute Myeloid Leukaemia

Peter Reizenstein

Division of Haematology, Karolinska Hospital and Institute, P.O. Box 60500, S-104 01 Stockholm, Sweden

The basis for the use of immunotherapy or biological response modifiers in acute leukaemia is the hypothesis of immune surveillance of leukaemic cells.

Theoretical Basis for Immune Surveillance in Animals and in Man

The major histocompatibility complex, a genetic region encoding the classical class I transplantation antigens HLA-A, B and C, is the cell surface target for cytotoxic T-lymphocytes, but it also protects against natural killer (NK) cells [1]. The class II genes encode the immune response or Ia antigens recognised by T-helper cells, and the class III the complement components. The original immunosurveillance theory was a thymus-based system, and for tumours induced by viruses or ultraviolet radiation this might still be true, but probably not for leukaemias. The main reason is probably that spontaneous tumours are rarely antigenic. However, alteration of the class I antigens associated with the insulin receptor has been found in many human tumours [1] and even in leukaemia [2].

Assuming that an immunosurveillance mechanism uses cytotoxic effectors rather than hypothetical growth inhibiting or differentiating agents, surveillance can be based on the existence of tumour-specific or tumour-associated antigens and mediated by antigen-dependent cytotoxic T-cells or by antibody-dependent complement cytotoxicity. Alternatively, it can be antigen independent and mediated by non-specific cytotoxic mechanisms such as activated natural killer (NK) cells or macrophages. Macrophages and NK-cells recognise biochemical characteristics of malignant cells other than rejection type tumour antigens. NK-cells include a non-MHC restricted cytotoxic T-cell population and a non-T, non-B NK-linkeage.

NK-cells express CD-16 and Leu-19 antigens, but not the T-cell receptor, nor its m-RNA. Thus, NK-cells cannot kill via this receptor. NK-cells do not require previous priming with antigens to be cytotoxic, unlike the CD-4 positive cell, which recognises MHC-I antigens, or the CD-8 expressing cytotoxic T-cell, which recognises MHC-II antigens. However, the LAK-cell population may also contain some activated cytotoxic, possibly MHC unrestricted NK-like T-cells.

A reasonable relationship must be maintained between the tumour volume and the capacity of the effector mechanism [1-5].

In several experimental tumours, tumour-specific antigens have been found. Tumour transplant takes can be prevented or reduced by previous immunisation, and the growth of established tumours slowed down by similar procedures. It is probable that antigen-dependent, T-cell-mediated cytotoxicity plays a part in this immunologic surveillance [2-4]. In addition, some immunoglobulin subclasses, mainly IgG-2, can initiate complement-mediated cytotoxic activity against target cells displaying the corresponding antigens.

Spontaneous tumours in man present a more complex situation. Firstly, there is considerable immunophenotype variability [5], including maturation asynchrony [6] and lineage infidelity [7]. It is not only the expression of tissue-specific or differentiation antigens that varies. Even surface markers as fundamental as insulin receptors or HLA-DR [2] can be absent. While it is certain that so far no tumour-specific antigen has been demonstrated to be regularly present on all tumour cells in all patients for any type of human tumour, it is uncertain whether neo-antigens may occasionally be expressed on some tumour cells in some patients. Differentiation antigens present on melanoma cells and lung cancer cells have been used with some promising results in the prevention of postoperative recurrences.

Many of the tumour-associated antigens originally believed to be tumour specific have been shown to be differentiation antigens. However, even the expression of such antigens is unreliable in malignant cells, which frequently show so-called differentiation asynchrony, or the simultaneous expression of both maturity and immaturity markers, or the absence of both.

Antigen-Independent Cytotoxic Mechanisms

Natural killer cells are largely a laboratory artefact, since they are cytotoxic neither for viable human tumour cells nor for any other viable human cells - with the possible exception of some immature bone marrow cells - nor for many cell lines. In contrast, the activated forms of natural killer cells do show HLA non-restricted cytotoxicity, both for viable human tumour cells and, to a lesser extent, for some normal human cell types. This cytotoxicity is relatively rapid (4-8 hours). If there are specific or non-specific receptors on the target cell surface, these receptors are not yet known, but contact between the effector and the target cell appears to be necessary. Antibodies against several cell surface structures, however, cannot block the cytotoxicity by activated NK-cells [8,9].

NK-cell activation can be achieved in different ways. The lymphokine-activated killer cell, obtained through an approx. 18-hour activation *in vitro* in about 800 IU (Cetus) of IL-2/ml of mononuclear blood cells containing NK-cells, is the best studied [8]. The cytotoxicity displayed by LAK-cells, however, is weaker than that shown by lectin-activated killer cells. In fact, the LAK-cell cytotoxicity can be potentiated by additional antigen activation, with the CD-3 monoclonal antibody [10].

Low doses of cytostatics can also stimulate Lyt 2-cytotoxic T-cells in mice to eradicate some tumours [11]. In human acute myeloid leukaemia with relatively low-dose maintenance chemotherapy, similar conservation of the T-cell mitogen response and the T-helper cell number [12-15].

Macrophage Cytotoxicity

Macrophage cytotoxicity, frequently mediated by lymphotoxin and/or partially homologous tumour necrosis factor, which are internalised via a common receptor and which induce DNA fragmentation, possibly via peroxides and free oxygen radicals, appears to be slower (8-120 hours) than the perforin-mediated cytotoxicity caused by activated NK-cells.

In Vitro Effects of the Cytotoxic Mechanisms

Specific effects against human leukaemic cells have been displayed by monoclonal antibodies against cell surface markers in combination with suitable complement batches [9].

Non-specific cytotoxicity mediated by lymphokine-activated, lectin-activated or antibody-activated natural killer cells has been demonstrated against a number of different cell lines derived from human tumours, but also against a number of different viable human tumour cells.

The fact that NK-cells represent an immunosurveillance mechanism is suggested by the lymphomas in NK-deficient patients, by the ascites regression in ovarian cancer patients with many NK-cells, and by the LAK-cell phenomenon [16].

There are normally about 100 billion circulating T-cells, and 100 billion in the lymph-node paracortical area and the splenic white pulp. The circulating T-cells may be reduced both in number and function in cancer patients [17], and NK-cells from leukaemia patients cannot produce cytotoxic factor and bind to target cells [16]. Although these findings can be secondary to, rather than a cause of the leukaemia, attempts are being made to restore NK-cells in tumour patients. This can be done non-specifically with BCG [14] or more specifically and efficiently with IL-2 [16,20,21]. However, LAK cells seem able to kill only 11-30% of the leukaemic blasts [8,9,16,18,19]. Nonetheless, tumour-infiltrating lymphocytes (Leu-19+, CD-3+ or -) have been claimed to be 50-100 times more potent than LAK-cells in about 90% of the patients [22].

In vivo generation of demonstrable LAK-cells is possible in some, but far from all of the patients given IL-2 intravenously [20,21]. Side effects, mainly in the form of the capillary leak syndrome, can be severe, possibly because circulating IL-2 is non-physiological. Normally, IL-2 has a short plasma half-life and is bound to high, intermediate or low affinity cell surface receptors.

In addition to the attempts to activate LAK-cell precursors and to expand this cell pool *in vivo* with IL-2, there are also speculations that the T-cell pool can be expanded with thymic factors or thymopoietins like isoprenosine.

Target Cell Resistance to Cytotoxic Agents

Major variations in the sensitivity of target cells have been demonstrated. In general, mature, normal human cells are quite resistant, both to complement-mediated toxicity, and to that mediated by activated NK-cells. Immature, normal human cells may be more sensitive and malignantly transformed cells certainly are more sensitive. However, even within the malignant cell population there are usually some resistant cells. Even when activation and confrontation conditions are apparently optimal, only a minority of many human leukaemic cell populations are killed. This is true both for lymphokine, lectin and antibody-activated cells, as well as for complement-mediated cytotoxicity [8,9].

Combining Several Cytotoxic Agents

Leukaemic cells can apparently be cross-resistant to cytotoxicity mediated by killer cells and by complement. This cross-resistance is only partial, however, since some of the cells surviving confrontation with LAK-cells are still sensitive to complement-mediated cytotoxicity, although the opposite is not true. Cells surviving complement-mediated cytotoxicity are also resistant to LAK-cells [8,9].

As mentioned, it is also possible to increase LAK-cell cytotoxicity by additionally stimulating the cells with CD-3 antibody [10]. Studies of the possibility to further combine these modes by prolonged IL-2 stimulation, by using tumour infiltrating cells, or by exposure to certain lymphotoxins like tumour necrosis factor, are in progress.

The sad fact is that no combination of specific or non-specific cytotoxic agents so far has been able to reproducibly kill a majority of the leukaemic cells. What actually happens to the clonogenic leukemic cells is of course unknown. Unless the clonogenic cells are preferentially killed, treatment with these combinations of cytotoxic agents may therefore well be compared to the partial resection of a tumour, which may have a palliative, but certainly not a curative effect.

In Vivo Effects of Biological Response Modifiers on Immunological Parameters in Mice

Many studies show that immunomodifiers can affect the delayed hypersensitivity reaction, the lymphocyte subpopulations, and certain macrophage and natural killer cell activities in mice. This is likewise true of thymus factors and thymomimetic agents like levamisol and isoprenosine. It is also true of bacterial products like BCG, as well as of immunoglobulins and immunoglobulin fractions like tuftsine. Many synthetic agents such as low-dose cytostatics, zinc, or bestatine can stimulate different components of the immune system in relatively well-defined ways [23-25].

The term immunocompetence is generally poorly defined. It may relate both to delayed hypersensitivity reactions, to immunoglobulin synthesis, to T-cell proliferation or cytotoxicity, to various macrophage functions, to NK-cell function, and to T-helper/T-suppressor cell ratios. In some of these respects, aged animals as well as tumour-bearing animals show reduced immunocompetence, which can partially be restored by some of the immunomodifiers mentioned above.

Effects of Biological Response Modifiers on Laboratory Parameters in Man

Relatively few studies are available on healthy controls. In patients with mammary carcinoma, radiotherapy leads to a longstanding decrease in the T-helper/T-suppressor ratio, which has, however, not been demonstrated to increase the rate of infectious disease in these patients [19].
In patients with acute myeloid leukaemia in complete remission, relatively low-dose cytostatic maintenance chemotherapy leads initially to an *increase* in the T-helper/T-suppressor ratio [13]. This can be compared to similar findings by Dray [11] in animals with low doses of cytostatics. However, prolonged treatment eventually leads to a decrease in the T-helper/T-suppressor cell ratio. Also the NK-cell activity is decreased in these patients, as is the macrophage release of colony-stimulating activity. If the biological response modifier BCG is given together with maintenance chemotherapy, the decrease in colony-stimulating factor production and NK-cell activity can be prevented [14,15].
While it is thus obvious, both in animals and in patients, that biological response modifiers can in fact affect certain instruments in the immunological orchestra, it is far from clear whether these effects improve the final symphony. There are two reasons for this. One is that systematic monitoring of patients treated with immunomodifiers has been relatively rare. The other is that it has been, and still partially is, quite uncertain, which, if any, of the parameters mentioned really is related to an immunosurveillance of the tumour and to the clinical outcome in the patients. However, recent results suggest that antigen-independent cytotoxicity mediated by activated NK-cells and possibly macrophages and cytotoxic T-cells are plausible candidates for the effector mechanism. It has been shown, in fact, that infusions of interleukin-2, which can activate NK-cells and cytotoxic T-cells, can lead to partial tumour regressions. Similar data are available for so-called adoptive immunotherapy, i.e., infusion of lymphokine-activated killer cells prepared *in vitro*.

Minimal Residual Disease

At present there are no specific methods to distinguish patients with acute myeloid leukaemia in complete remission who are really cured from those who still have minimal residual disease. Tentative calculations based on allogeneic and autologous transplant data, together with assumptions about the remaining tumour volume when complete remission is achieved, suggest that one million leukaemic cells or less, and even fewer clonogenic cells suffice to cause a relapse [26]. Since this number is close to what can be detected considering the number of cells in a bone marrow aspirate, it is difficult to see how immunological, cytochemical or morphological characteristics of individual malignant cells could help in the diagnosis of minimal residual disease [26]. The technique of break point cluster region studies, however, may be an exception to this rule.

Non-Specific, Systemic Signs

The biological response to minimal residual tumours can be observed. Although less pronounced, the biological response to malignant tumours resembles the inflammatory reaction. The first initiator is unknown but the first mediator is probably the macrophage which triggers a whole cascade of reactions in a network with many feedback loops. Macrophage-colony stimulating factor (M-CSF) is produced first and switches on granulocyte-CSF, GM-CSF, etc. A leukocytosis results, leading to protease liberation and activation of the coagulation cascade. Interleukin-1 is produced and activates the hepatic production of acute phase reactants like fibrinogen and ferritin, which prevent damage from liberated proteases. This biological response seems to be sensitive to a

surprisingly small tumour volume and it can be monitored.
For instance, the fibrinogen in the serum leads to an erythrocyte sedimentation rate increase in acute myeloid leukaemia, in Hodgkin's disease, and in ovarian carcinoma. If it remains high in complete remission, this is an indication of minimal residual disease and is seen mainly in those patients who are later found to relapse [26]. Similar indicators of the presence of minimal residual disease could be the serum ferritin value [26] or other non-specific acute phase reactants, a deregulation of lymphocyte subpopulations, and signs of an inflammatory reaction.
The biological response can be activated in more than one way. Hormonal activation may play a part, in addition to cytokine activation. Lymphocytes and bone marrow cells have receptors for glucocorticoids, growth hormone, and prolactin, which may activate the c-myc gene in these cells. Transmitter substances may also play a role, and lymphocytes also have receptors for muscarinic acetylcholine and nicotinic acid [27].
IL-1 may, together with M-CSF, TNF and endotoxin-like substances, initiate the acute phase host response. It stimulates endothelial cells to produce platelet activating factor, and this response can be inhibited by cyclooxygenase inhibitors [28,29]. IL-1 can auto-induce IL-1 gene expression in an amplification loop [30].
There are also some indications that the amplification involved in the studies of the break point cluster region can be a sensitive, and of course much more specific sign of minimal residual leukaemia. However, even with the sensitivity increase afforded by the amplification, at least one cell that has undergone leukaemic transformation must be obtained in the sample, which would not always be the case if the cell numbers just calculated were correct.

Clinical Effect

Interferon, the only immunomodulator to have found a place in routine treatment of, e.g., hairy cell leukaemia and possibly chronic myelocytic leukaemia, blocks expression both of growth factor regulating oncogenes like c-myc and of growth factor receptors like those for transferrin and insulin. Conversely, it can be a differentiation inducer for, e.g., erythroleukaemia cells.
It is likely that the antitumour effect of interferon is mediated by its anti-growth activity rather than by immunomodulation [30]. 2.5 million units of interferon alpha three times weekly for one year will reduce splenomegaly and the white blood cell count in hairy cell leukaemia, but hairy cells remain, the survival benefit is not yet proven, toxicity is considerable and splenectomy should remain the first choice [31]. The reason for the sensitivity of hairy cells is a partial autocrine loop where the tumour cells both produce and express receptors for B-cell growth factor.
In chronic myelocytic leukaemia, 3-8 million units daily of interferon alpha leads to 71% of haematologic remissions and an annual mortality of only 8% as compared to 25% after chemotherapy. The Philadelphia Chromosome could be suppressed in 39% of the patients [31], and the three-year survival was 76%.
Responses are also frequent in non-Hodgkin's lymphoma, Kaposi's sarcoma, where a partial autocrine loop based on basic fibroblast growth factor and IL-1-beta may be the explanation, essential thrombocythaemia and IgA myeloma.

Tumour Necrosis Factor has 30% homology with lymphotoxin, the receptors of which it shares. It synergises with interferon in growth inhibition and antigen expression induction, and it has several other effects. It is still very toxic and no clinical results in leukaemia were found.

Interleukin-2 stimulated NK-cells (LAK-cells) used for passive immunotherapy induced a response in 31% and a complete response in 8% of Rosenberg's 106 tumour patients, among others also lymphomas. Severe side effects have been discussed above [30,31].
I have not yet been able to find IL-2 results in human leukaemia. However, it is very likely that the so-called graft versus leukaemia effect, essential for the clinical result of allogeneic bone marrow transplants, is mediated by LAK-like cells. A combination of IL-2 treatment and autologous marrow transplants in

leukaemia is therefore recommended. It could improve the autologous transplant results to what is seen in allogeneic transplants, without the risk of chronic GVH-disease, and it could achieve a reasonable LAK effector cell to target cell ratio, which is far too low in the earlier studies of advanced tumours with large tumour cell masses.

Platelet-Derived Growth Factor, partially homologous with a protein product of the v-sis gene, is functional in wound healing. Antagonists now exist, for instance interferon [30], and should be tested in attempts to prevent the bone marrow fibrosis complicating essential thrombocythaemia and polycythaemia vera.

Bestatin has been claimed in one study to prolong remission in elderly patients with acute myeloid leukaemia [32].

Growth Factors. Recombinant versions are now available of growth factors for numerous cell types. IL-1 and IL-2 have been discussed. IL-3 is multi-CSF or M-CSF or burst-promoting activity. IL-4 is the B-cell growth factor that activates macrophages and that, together with IL-5, induces the immunoglobulin production switch. IL-6 is also a B-cell and plasmacyte growth factor.
GM-CSF and G-CSF have some use in shortening the leukopaenic phase (but not necessarily the septicaemic one) after marrow transplants and chemotherapy. However, many leukaemic blasts have receptors for and respond to GM-CSF, and also to G-CSF and IL-3, both by colony formation and by DNA-synthesis. Biological therapy to patients with residual acute leukaemia has to be used with caution. These factors may possibly have a place in the treatment of cyclic neutropaenia and aplastic anaemia refractory to antithymocyte globulin. G-CSF may have fewer side effects than GM-CSF.

Conclusion

It is traditional to conclude almost all papers about immunotherapy in an optimistic fashion suggesting that further studies will in fact open the door for immunotherapy of acute leukaemia into clinical routine practice. There is some justification for this optimism, but in man it consists only of four sets of data. The most important is the graft versus leukaemia reaction. The second is the finding that discontinuation of cyclosporine treatment in patients with chronic myelocytic leukaemia after an allogeneic transplant can restore their Philadelphia negativity. Hypothetically, the third is the so-called 4S-neuroblastomas in the newborn, which disappear spontaneously as the babies' immune defense develops, and also the high frequency of neuroblastoma in newborn babies dying of unrelated causes and examined post mortem. This frequency is much higher than that of clinically manifest neuroblastoma, which could possibly suggest immunosurveillance, although other explanations exist. The fourth is the contradictory empirical clinical trials. Here, two recent long-term follow-up studies of non-Hodgkin's lymphoma [33] and acute myeloid leukaemia [34], both of which showed an effect of BCG-immunotherapy, would appear to support the findings suggesting that immunotherapy does have an effect. So would the finding [35] that fewer patients with acute lymphoblastic leukaemia relapse after chemo-immunotherapy than after chemotherapy alone. Mathé has listed 11 tumours where at least one controlled study suggests that immunotherapy can be effective [32]. In one leukaemia study where no effect was found on survival, there was nevertheless one on second remissions [36].
In addition to this, there is experimental data on which an elaborate theoretical structure has been built. Man is usually proud of his theoretical and educational capacities. If they are compared to those of a chicken, this is justified, but if they are compared to the complexity of biological systems, I am not so sure. Still, the vast majority of our treatment methods, all the way from salicylic acid via digitalis, vitamin B-12, and cytostatic agents to immunotherapy, were based on coincidence, chance, or incorrect hypotheses. We can be humble enough to realise that we understand but a small fraction of the biological response to and defense against disease. If we are lucky enough, however, to stumble onto anything that can improve the quality of care to our patients, we should keep our eyes open so that we can recognise it and use it.

REFERENCES

1 Linsk RL and Goodenow RS: Immunologic and non-immunologic roles of the major histocompatibility complex in tumorigenesis. Cancer Rev 1986 (6):40

2 Öst Å, Christensson B, Andersson R, Hast R, Lagerlöf B, Reizenstein P, Trowbridge S and Biberfeld P: Immune phenotype heterogeneity in AML. Scand J Haematol 1985 (34):293

3 Olsson L, Mathé G and Reizenstein P: The biological and immunologic response to tumors. In: Karrer N (ed) Clinical Chemotherapy Vol. 3. Antineoplastic Chemotherapy. Thieme Stratton, New York 1984 p 308

4 Reizenstein P, Olsson L and Mathé G: Immunomodulation and cancer therapy. In: Ray PK (ed) Immunobiology of Transplantation, Cancer and Pregnancy. Pergamon Press, Oxford 1983 p 241

5 Minowada J, Mathé G, Barcos M, Ginsbourg M, Preisler H, Canon C and Reizenstein P: Cytological and immunological study of 139 patients with acute leukemia. Med Oncol and Tumor Pharmacother 1984 (1):3

6 Reizenstein P, Öst Å, Skoog L, Christensson B, Biberfeld P and Lagerlöf B: Maturation asynchrony in leukemic cells. An abnormal combination of normal cell markers. Anticancer Res 1985 (5):361

7 Reizenstein P, Beksac M, Biberfeld P, Christensson B, Lagerlöf B, Laurén L, Öst Å and Porwit A: Leukemic myeloblasts expressing lymphoid markers. Acta Haematol 1985 (74):148

8 Vasilopoulos G, Sjögren AM and Reizenstein P: Cytotoxic effects on viable human leukemic cells by combinations of lymphokine activated killer cells and monoclonal antibodies. Leukemia Res 1989 (13):87

9 Beksac M, Porwit A, Hast R, Biberfeld P and Reizenstein P: Cytotoxicity of monoclonal antibodies against individual immunophenotyped human leukemic cells. Cancer Immunol Immunother 1985 (19):231

10 Reizenstein P and Vasilopoulos G: Effect of CD3 antibodies on cytotoxicity against leukemic cells resistant to activated killer cells. Submitted to Leukemia Res, Aug 1988

11 Dray S and Mokyr B: Cyclophosphamide and melphalan as immunopotentiating agent in cancer therapy. Med Oncol and Tumour Pharmacother 1989 (6):77

12 Miale T, Stenke L, Penchansky M, Lehtinen T and Reizenstein P: The role of macrophages in phagocytosis and mixed leukocyte reactivity in human acute myeloid leukemia. Immunological Communications 1979 (8):279

13 Arends-Merino A, Giscombe R, Ogier C, Reizenstein P, Sjögren AM and Wasserman J: Modifying the biological response in acute myeloid leukemia. II. Effect of BCG and leukemic cells on lymphocyte response to mitogens, and on helper and suppressor activity. Cancer Immunol Immunother 1982 (14):32

14 Reizenstein P, Andersson B and Beran M: Possible mechanisms of immunotherapy action in acute non-lymphatic leukemia: Macrophage production of colony-stimulating activity. Recent Results in Cancer Research 1982 (80):64

15 Arends-Merino A, Sjögren AM and Reizenstein P: Modifying the biological response to acute myeloid leukemia. I. BCG, allogenic leukemic cells and spontaneous cytotoxicity. Anticancer Res 1983 (3):239

16 Lotzova E: Cytotoxicity and clinical application of activated NK cells. Med Oncol and Tumor Pharmacother 1989 (6):93

17 Hadden JW and Hadden EM: Therapy of secondary T-cell immunodeficiencies with biological substances and drugs. Med Oncol and Tumor Pharmacother 1989 (6):11

18 Fierro MT, Liao XS, Lusso P, Bonferroni M, Matera L, Cesano A, Lista P, Arione R, Forni G and Foa R: In vitro and in vivo susceptibility of human leukemic cells to lymphokine activated killer activity. Leukemia 1988 (1):50

19 Reizenstein P, Ogier C, Blomgren H, Petrini B and Wasserman J: Cells responsible for tumor surveillance in man; effects of radiotherapy, chemotherapy, and biological response modifiers. In: Ray PK (ed) Advances in Immunity and Cancer Therapy. Springer Verlag, New York 1985 p 1

20 Hank J, Kohler P, Weil-Hillman G, Rosenthal N, Moore K, Storer B, Minkoff D, Bradshaw J, Bechhofer R and Sondel P: In vivo induction of the lymphokine-activated killer phenomenon: Interleukin 2-dependent human non-major histocompatibility complex-restricted cytotoxicity generated in vivo during administration of human recombinant interleukin 2. Cancer Res 1988 (48):1965

21 Thompson JA, Lee DJ, Lindgren CG, Benz LA, Collins C, Levitt D and Fefer A: Influence of dose and duration of infusion of interleukin-2 on toxicity and immunomodulation. J Clin Oncol 1988 (4):669

22 Whiteside TL: Cytolytic antitumor effector cells identified in cultures of tumour infiltrating lymphocytes. Cancer Immunol Immunother 1988 (26):1

23 Reizenstein P, Mathé G, Vriz N and Lomme L: Nonspecific immunomodulators in oncology and hematology. In: Oldham RK (ed) Principles of Cancer Biotherapy. Raven Press Ltd, New York 1987 p 163

24 Mathé G, Blazsek I, Gil-Delgado MA, Canon C, Misset JL, Gaget H and Reizenstein P: The effect of zinc on normal and neoplastic T-lymphocyte proliferation. Med Oncol and Tumor Pharmacother 1985 (3):203

25 Reizenstein P, Andreasen R, Biberfeld P, Canon C, Hast R, Lagerlöf B, Olsson L and Öst Å: Biological response to acute leukemia. I. Tumor-associated antigens and antigen-independent tumor surveillance. Cancer Treatment Symp 1985 (1):101

26 Reizenstein P: The monitoring of minimal residual disease in patients with malignant tumors. In: Reizenstein P, Mathé G, Dicato (eds) Managing Minimal Residual Malignancy in Man. Pergamon Press, Oxford 1988 p 5

27 Berczi I: The influence of pituitary hormones and neurotransmitters on the immune system. EOS, J Immunol Immunopharmacol 1988 (3):186

28 Stenke L, Lindgren L, Laurén L and Reizenstein P: Leukotrienes in bone marrow: Abnormal lipoxygenase activity in CML (in Swedish). Abstract, Sc and Soc Hematol, Stockholm 1986 (17)
29 Stenke L, Reizenstein P and Lindgren JÅ: Increased leukotriene C4 synthase activity in acute and chronic myelogenous leukemia. Abstract. Int Soc Hematol, Milan 1988 (22)
30 Dupere SL, O'Connor TE and Oldham RK: Lymphokines/cytokines: Biotherapeutic applications. EOS, J Immunol Immunopharmacol 1988 (8):201
31 Platzer E, Gramatzki M, Kalden JR and Roelinghoff M: Clinical trials with cytokines; a review. EOS, J Immunol Immunopharmacol 1988 (8):216
32 Mathé G: Bestatin compared to other pharmacologic immunoregulator or modulator agents. Horizons on antibiotic research. In: Proceedings of the symposium dedicated to the late professor Hamao Umozawa. Tokyo 1987 p 44
33 Hoerni B, Ravand A, Eghbal H, Hoerni-Simon G: Adjuvant therapy by BCG of non-Hodgkin's malignant lymphoma in a controlled trial. An update. Brit J Haematol 1989 (71):161
34 Reizenstein P and Laurén L: Immunotherapy of acute myeloid leukemia - a fifteen-year follow up. Submitted to Br J Haematol
35 Komada Y, Azuma E, Yamamoto H, Tanaka S, Shimizu K, Kamiya H, Sakurai M and Izawa T: Discontinuing chemoimmunotherapy in childhood acute lymphoblastic leukemia. Biomed and Pharmacother 1988 (42):597
36 Hayat M, Jehn N, Willemze R, Haanen C, Zittoun R, Monconduit M, Lowenberg B, Stryckmans P, Peetermans M, De Cataldo F: A randomized comparison of maintenance treatment with androgens, immunotherapy, and chemotherapy in adult acute myelogenous leukemia. A leukemia-lymphoma group trial of the EORTC. Cancer 1986 (58):617

Biological Characteristics of Acute Myeloblastic Leukaemia Contributing to Management Strategy

E.A. McCulloch

The Ontario Cancer Institute and the University of Toronto, 500 Sherbourne Street, Toronto, Canada M4X 1K9

Introduction

Malignant tumours are cellular clones [1], each maintained by a minority population consisting of stem cells, capable of renewing themselves or entering into terminal divisions; these divisions are limited in number and finish with cells that are proliferatively inert [2]. The kinetics of clonal expansion are determined by the balance between self-renewal, the process that leads to an increase in clonogenic cells, and determination, the event that limits growth by the initiation of terminal divisions. The goals of therapy may be considered in the light of this cellular model. Control of malignant growth might be achieved by altering the balance so that determination was favoured. Cure, the extinction of the malignant clone, might occur if the pressures towards terminal divisions were sufficiently strong. A direct cytotoxic attack on stem cells would have the same effect if the last of the crucial stem cell population were eliminated. Successful treatment might require both; dose-response curves for chemotherapeutic agents are often negative exponentials; it follows that to achieve cure by cytoreduction alone requires doses that reduce tumour stem cell numbers well below levels where only one viable cell would be expected to survive. However, if treatment regimens could be devised that were not only cytotoxic but also decreased self-renewal, a few surviving stem cells might become extinct by passing through determination.

It is the purpose of this chapter to review some of the biological properties of the clonal haemopathies generally and Acute Myeloblastic Leukaemia (AML) in particular [3]. The implications of clonal origin and expansion will be considered, together with regulatory mechanisms as these effect the balance between stem cell growth and differentiation. Attention will be given to certain growth factors, active on myelopoietic cells. Cell culture studies of the blast population in AML will be summarised. Specifically, evidence will be presented that some chemotherapeutic agents, in addition to their general capacity for cell kill, may have some selective toxicity for cells that are in the process of self-renewal. Certain growth factors can be shown to increase or decrease blast stem cell self-renewal and concomitantly to alter drug sensitivity.

The view is advanced that a research priority exists to develop novel therapeutic strategies based on the biology of leukaemic populations. Particularly, attention might be directed to the question whether the interactions between growth factors or other biological response modifiers and chemotherapeutic drugs observed in culture also occur *in vivo*; if this proves to be the case, therapists may have enhanced opportunities for controlling or eliminating malignant cells.

The Clonal Haemopathies

Clonal Analysis

Several methods are available for detecting members of normal cellular clones *in vivo*. Chromosome markers have long been used for this purpose [4]; early studies with radiation-induced markers in mice showed that haemopoietic stem cells were capable of differentiation along several lineages, but that the distribution of lineages within clones varied with time [5]; very similar results have been obtained recently using cells marked by the random integration of retroviruses [6-10]. Abnormal chromosome markers have been used extensively in the study of leukaemic clones. The Philadelphia Chromosome provided the first evidence both for the clonal nature of a leukaemia (Chronic Myeloblastic Leukaemia, CML) and the pluripotent nature of its cell of origin [11]. An ingenious combination of chromosome analysis and radioautography with radioiron provided early evidence for extensive differentiation capacity in AML [12]. Karyotypic analysis has been a mainstay in the analysis of heterogeneity among patients with AML; several non-random karyotypic patterns have been identified and associated with clinical outcome [13 and Freireich, EJ, in this monograph]. However, the most extensive studies of abnormal haemopoietic clones have been done by Fialkow and his colleagues, using alleles for the x-linked gene for the enzyme Glucose-6-Phosphate Dehydrogenase (G6PD) [14].

X-linked Clonal Markers

These methods depend on x-inactivation, the process by which one X chromosome becomes inactive early in embryogenesis. As a consequence, females are genetic mosaics, with one X chromosome functional in some cells and the other X chromosome in the remainder. If different alleles, with products that can be distinguished, are present on the X chromosomes, the mosaicism can be detected. In the case of G6PD, alleles specify isoenzymes that can be separated electrophoretically. In normal female heterozygotes, cells containing each of the enzymatic forms are present at approximately equal frequencies. Clones, however, contain only one isoenzyme, that which was present in the cell of origin. Thus, against a background of two isoenzymes, the cells of a clone can be detected by the presence of only one form of the protein. The technique is easily applied to haemopoietic cells since these can be obtained in quantity and safely. Isoenzyme distributions in each haemopoietic lineage can then be compared to normal somatic cells, usually fibroblasts. Recently, molecular techniques have been used for clonal analysis. One of these is based on sex-linked restriction fragment length polymorphism (RFLP); as the methylation patterns are different in the active and inactive chromosomes, these RFLPs can be applied to clonal analysis of cells from female patients in the same way as G6PD isoenzymes are assessed [15].

Abnormal Haemopoietic Clones

The G6PD method readily confirmed the chromosome findings for CML and extended the work to considerations of pathogenesis [16-18]. In addition, Polycythemia Vera (P-vera) [19], Ideopathic Myelofibrosis (IMF) [20] and at least one case of aplastic anaemia [21] have been shown to be clonal expansions from pluripotent stem cells. The malignant populations in AML patients are also clones; however, there has been controversy about the differentiation stage of the cell of origin. G6PD studies in some patients showed that their malignant clones contained only blast cells and granulopoietic progenitors while in others, multilineage differentiation was observed [22,23]. A possible interpretation of the findings is that leukaemic transformation is heterogeneous in respect to target. In some patients the event might occur in granulopoiesis-committed progenitor cells; in others, as in the diseases enumerated above, pluripotent stem cells might be the original transformants. Deduction of the properties of an ancestor from the cellular composition of its clonal descendants provides only a minimum estimate of potential for differentiation since some lineages may not be expressed or detected. Thus, it remains possible that all cases of AML begin in pluripotent stem cells.

Biological Properties

Consideration of the biological properties of such diverse diseases as AML and IMF discloses certain common features. Firstly, all, or almost all, are derived from pluripotent stem cells; these, because of their self-renewal capacity, are the normal source of clones, and can serve the same function after transformation. Secondly, abnormal clones become dominant; co-existing normal populations may be absent, or, if present, may only be demonstrated by sensitive cell culture methods [24]. Dominance may be achieved because transformed stem cells have a proliferative advantage; for example, such stem cells may have lost the capacity to enter into a G_0 state. A third general property of abnormal clones may also contribute to dominance. Interactions occur between abnormal clones and accompanying normal populations. These may lead to suppression of normal haemopoiesis, and even to the extinction of normal stem cells. Interactions with transformants may also stimulate marrow stroma, leading to the fibrosis that is characteristic of IMF and other haemopathies (CML). Finally, abnormal haemopoietic clones are genetically unstable and often show progression. Blast transformation in CML is an example of this phenomenon. Taken together, these properties are sufficiently important for the behaviour of the clones that it is reasonable to abandon the practice of considering some phenotypes to be leukaemic and others not. Rather, it may be helpful to consider all diseases that share the properties described above as a single class of clonal haemopathies [25]. The distribution of cells within each abnormal clone is then the basis for the diagnosis of recognised clinical entities.

Remission

Acute leukaemias are remarkable in their responses to chemotherapy. Widely-disseminated and aggressive cancers become undetectable following successful treatment and normal haemopoiesis resumes. The disease remains, however, since, with very few exceptions, malignant cells reappear. If the mechanisms responsible for remission and relapse were known, it might be possible to extend the period of time in remission and increase the number of patients cured of their disease.

It is widely held that cytotoxic chemotherapeutic drugs induce remission by killing a very high proportion of leukaemic stem cells. Then, normal co-existing populations emerge, restoring haemopoiesis. An alternative, attractive mechanism has been proposed; differentiation in culture has been reported in leukaemic cell lines or the blasts of some patients with leukaemia following exposure to agents such as dimethylsulphoxide (DMSO) or retinoic acid [26-32]. Recent clinical trials support the view that retinoic acid may be active against leukaemic or preleukaemic cells *in vivo* [33,34]. If differentiation could be achieved regularly in leukaemia, a physiological remission might be obtained. Regrettably, normal differentiation is seldom observed when AML blasts, rather than cell lines, are exposed to inducing agents in culture.

The observations of apparently normal granulocytes and erythropoietic precursors found in AML clones in relapse [15,22,23] suggest a further possibility; that apparently normal cells characteristic of remission might represent the continuing differentiation capacity of pluripotent leukaemic stem cells. Experience with CML provides a precedent. In relapse, CML clones contain predominantly granulopoietic elements, although erythropoiesis and platelet formation continue. When CML is treated with conservative chemotherapy, cytoreduction is associated with a more normal representation of the lineages within malignant clones. In each patient, the disease remains clonal. Polyclonal, presumably normal, haemopoietic cells are seen only when aggressive chemotherapy is used [35]. In contrast, studies of AML in remission usually show polyclonal patterns. However, in a substantial minority of patients (20-30%) the abnormal clone persists, although the clinical state is remission [15,36].

The observations of clonal remissions support a model of haemopoiesis that considers that AML pluripotent stem cells may not only be capable of originating the normal myelopoietic lineages (and, indeed, at least B lymphopoiesis [37]) but also have the capacity to give rise to blast cells (Figure 1). Chemotherapy might destroy the self-renewing blast population; if no normal stem cells persisted, or, if present, failed to grow, functional granulopoietic, erythropoietic and megakaryocytic elements might derive from a transformed pluripotent stem cell. Relapse

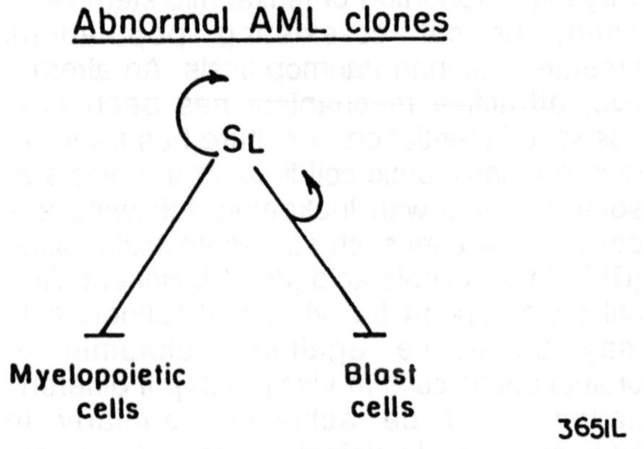

Fig. 1. A diagram of an abnormal AML clone. A leukaemia pluripotent stem cell(SL) is shown capable of self-renewal and differentiation along myelopoietic pathways. In addition, the stem cell is pictured giving rise to a novel lineage of blast cells; the blast cells of origin have the stem cell property of self-renewal; therefore, the blast lineage can be maintained independently of its pluripotent ancestor. If the blasts are eliminated by therapy but the leukaemic stem cell remains, a clonal remission can be observed; relapse will occur when the pluripotent stem cell again gives rise to one or more blast stem cells. Reprinted from [232], by permission of the publisher

would occur if that stem cell exhibited its capacity to give rise to new blast stem cells. If the probability of that event were small, clonal remission might be long-lasting.

Support for the view that relapse might be the re-emergence of blast cells as a new subclone comes from recent studies of the ras oncogene in AML. Using the polymerase chain reaction [38] to enhance the sensitivity of detection, mutated N-ras was detected in 14 of 52 samples from AML patients. In four of these instances, where mutated N-ras was present in initial samples, it could no longer be found in specimens obtained at relapse after an intervening remission [39]. Since studies with clonal markers almost always show that the same abnormal clone is present at presentation and relapse, it is reasonable to consider that the blast populations in these four instances belonged to the same clones at both examinations but that the blast genotypes changed. This interpretation is consistent with the model shown in Figure 1, since the model includes the capacity of leukaemic pluripotent stem cells to generate self-maintaining blast lineages.

Regulation

Clonal Heterogeneity

Analysis of haemopoietic clones may cast light on mechanisms regulating their expansion. Such analysis regularly shows clone-to-clone variation much greater than could be explained on the basis of heterogeneity in the stem cells of origin; it follows that clonal expansion is not rigidly controlled. Several models have been proposed to explain the findings. Firstly, examination of new clonogenic cells in spleen colonies *in vivo* [40,41] showed a gamma distribution, a form that is generated by random events occurring with fixed probabilities. For the example of spleen colonies, a stochastic model was proposed based on the stem cell properties of self-renewal and determination. The former was considered to be a "birth" probability since it is the mechanism that generates new stem cells; it follows that the latter, determination, acts as a "death" probability since it subtracts stem cells from the growing population as they enter into terminal divisions. For each stem cell about to divide, the "birth" and "death" probabilities sum to unity since no other fate is available. Variation is generated because of the random nature of the alternative stem cell fates [42]. Similar analytic techniques have been applied to colonies in culture and the stochastic concept extended to them [43,44].

Neither lax control nor a stochastic model implies the absence of regulation. For the latter, mechanisms are postulated that determine the probabilities of "birth" and "death"; the orderly behaviour of a polyclonal population may be considered to be the outcome of averaging many heterogeneous clones. Alternatively, inductive mechanisms have been proposed. A popular concept was advanced on the basis of morphological examination of spleen colonies. Early in their growth these were found to contain predominantly cells of a single lineage; only later were cells detected along other myelopoietic pathways. It was proposed that marrow and spleen contained discrete microenvironments, each with the capacity to induce differentiation along a line specified by the microenvironment [45]. Support for this model was not obtained when early progenitors, rather than morphologically differentiated cells, were used to analyse the differentiation patterns in spleen colonies [46].

Regardless of the mechanism underlying their generation, clonal heterogeneity must be considered in interpreting the results of cellular analysis in patients with clonal haemopathies. Since the haemopoietic populations in these individuals are clonal, variation is to be expected on the same basis as that seen when distributions are determined of cells in colonies *in vivo* or in culture. If the mechanism for generating patient-to-patient differences is clonal expansion, it is unlikely that the cellular phenotype at a point in time will be related to disease mechanisms or correlated with clinical outcome. If the cellular pattern in a given patient is not consistent with time, clonal expansion should be considered to be its source, unless there are compelling counter arguments.

An example is provided by analysis of the marrow content of granulopoietic and erythropoietic progenitors at different points in time in patients with AML [47]. The distribution of both progenitor classes among the populations conformed to the gamma form of the binomial distribution expected on the basis of the stochastic model. Treatment resulted in cytoreduction; with recovery, the malignant clones re-expanded. At a second observation, gamma distributions were observed again, although with different medians. However, the values from each patient had re-assorted in the distributions with no correlation between the first and second observations. Thus, the cellular composition of each malignant clone was not consistent with time, indicating that the details of the phenotype might well be attributed to random events during clonal expansion.

Receptors, Ligands and Signal Transduction

Soluble factors are known to be potent regulators of haemopoiesis and have been used to construct models of regulation. For example, erythropoietin has long been accepted as a hormone essential for the maintenance of normal erythropoiesis [48]. It has been proposed that such hormones might "instruct" cells to follow one or other lineage [49]. A more comprehensive insight may be provided by new knowledge of cellular receptors, their ligands and the mechanism by which ligand-receptor binding signals the nucleus.

Receptor-ligand interactions occur at both the cell surface and the nucleus; both are important in haemopoiesis. Several growth factor receptors have been found on the cell surface [50-62]; following binding to ligand, signal transduction mechanisms [63-65] lead to the initiation of nuclear events. These may include changes in the transcription of certain growth-regulated oncogenes [66-70]. Recent experiments using antisense to c-myb have provided strong evidence that this gene is important in early cell proliferation in haematopoietic cells, with effects on both granulopoiesis and erythropoiesis [71]. It is reasonable to expect that similar direct evidence will be forthcoming for the roles of other growth-regulated oncogenes.

A second family of nuclear receptors is also important in haemopoietic regulation [72,73]. Their ligands include vitamin D, cortico--steroids and thyroid hormones [74-77]. Nuclear receptors appear to act by binding to ligand, then, after translocation to the nucleus, they interact with regulatory stretches of DNA [73]. Recently, it has been shown that the differentiation-inducer, retinoic acid (RA), has two very similar nuclear receptors [78-81]. The alpha receptor, but not the beta receptor, is expressed in myelogenous leukaemia cells [82,83].

Genetic Regulation

The receptor-ligand dependent regulatory system provides a way for cells to sense their environment and react to it. It requires both external signals, often provided by growth factors or stromal elements, and internal mechanisms governing cell behaviour. These two aspects of regulation are explicit in the genetically-determined stem cell defects found in mice with mutations in the W and Sl loci. Genetically anaemic mice of genotype W/W^v have defective stem cells, unable to form macroscopic spleen colonies [84]; however, marrow from W/W^v mice is able to regenerate committed progenitors on transplantation and even occasionally to reconstitute haemopoiesis in recipient animals [85]. It appears likely, then, that the W locus encodes information that regulates early stem cell behaviour; since proliferative capacity, but not differentiation, appears to be affected by mutation, the gene may act on stem cell self-renewal.

Mice of genotype Sl/Sl^d are also anaemic because of a defect in stem cell function; however, in these animals the stem cells are normal; the lesion affects the capacity of marrow and spleen stromal cells to support haemopoietic cell growth and differentiation [86]. Indeed, physiological complementation is possible, since the anaemia of W/W^v mice can be cured by transplantation with marrow from Sl/Sl^d donors. Thus, the W locus contains a gene affecting self-renewal mechanisms intrinsic to stem cells, while the Sl gene controls an extrinsic factor necessary for their function.

Recently, two groups have mapped the proto-oncogene c-kit to the W locus [87,88]. C-kit encodes a gene product with the properties of a transmembrane receptor, with a tyrosine kinase internal domain and extensive homology with the receptors for CSF-1 and Platelet-Derived Growth Factor (PDGF) [89,90]. Both groups of investigators included in their descriptions of the linkage between c-kit and the W locus the hypothesis that the ligand for this receptor might be the product of a gene in the Sl locus. Since physiological studies with Sl/Sl^d animals show that the affected gene product does not circulate [91], it follows that the putative ligand will usually be cell-associated. Thus, short-range regulatory mechanisms, such as those mediated by marrow or splenic stromal cells, may use ligand-receptor interactions similar to those identified for secreted factors. Indeed, some growth factors, identified by their capacity to stimulate differentiation in culture, may act physiologically while remaining bound to the membranes of producing cells [92,93].

It is evident that the behaviour of haemopoietic stem cells is the result of many factors interacting in the regulatory network linking outside factors to intrinsic functions. It is probable that no single determinant is responsible for the balance between stem cell renewal and determination; rather, each cell follows one or other course as a consequence of the melded influences coming from a regulatory milieu. Many growth factors and receptors have been shown to be highly homologous to oncogenes or proto-oncogenes [94], observations that extend the concept of genetic regulation. In this context, one may consider that a genetically-determined regulator may not act directly to settle the outcome of each cell division but rather contribute to a milieu that sets the probabilities of stem cells undergoing self-renewal or entering into a specific differentiation pathway. From this prospective, new molecular information is consistent with the stochastic model of stem regulation while providing concrete mechanisms by which both the environment and growth factors can play effective roles.

Myelopoietic Growth Factors

Most known growth factors active on myelopoietic cells are derived from activated lymphocytes, mononuclear cells and fibroblasts, all components of the haemopoietic environment [95,96]. With the exception of erythropoietin, growth factors were identified originally by their capacity to promote or support differentiation during colony-formation in cell culture. In these culture systems, growth factor effects were usually obtained using whole cells or culture media conditioned by cells. As a consequence, definitions of factors were often descriptive, although improved with more extensive factor purification. Now, molecular clones have been obtained for many factors and recombinant proteins are available [97]. Some difficulties have been resolved as factors, thought to be different on the basis of their effects in cultures, proved to be identical molecules or different only in the extent of their glycosylation. Not unexpectedly, the availability of cloned reagents has disclosed other complexities, particularly as interactions between factors were explored.

Directly-Acting Factors

When the activities of growth factors are determined in culture, it is a recurrent concern whether the observed effects are the consequences of direct action of factor on target cell (ligand-binding); alternatively, the mechanism may be indirect, mediated through a second cell population which responds by producing one or more directly-acting factors. Molecular clones are available for five factors where evidence exists for direct and important action on myelopoiesis. Two of these, IL-3 and GM-CSF, have multilineage effects; the others, G-CSF, CSF-1 and erythropoietin are predominantly lineage restricted.

IL-3 [53,98,99] is essential for the growth and differentiation of the most primitive cells that can be detected in culture. In addition, it has effects on many cell lines, and will promote the differentiation of mature progenitors. Its effects, therefore, are seen throughout the myelopoietic lineages. GM-CSF [96,100-102] was first described as a factor that could stimulate in culture colonies of granulocytes, macrophages or both lineages together. When recombinant GM-CSF became available, some stimulation of erythropoietic differentiation was observed, indicating an action on a precursor with potential for differentiation along at least three pathways [99,100]. The multilineage effects of GM-CSF are not as obvious as those of IL-3, although this hormone has been shown to increase differentiated leukocyte function [103-105] as well as to stimulate proliferation. Lineage-restricted factors include Erythropoietin, the earliest recognised haemopoietic growth factor; it acts directly on committed precursors of erythropoiesis and appears to be essential for haemoglobinisation [48,106]. CSF-1 also acts directly, stimulating only macrophages and monocytes [107,108]. The receptor for CSF-1 has been cloned [109] and shown to be the c-fms oncogene [52]. G-CSF is also a cloned growth factor with activity restricted to granulopoiesis [110-113].

Cooperative Factors

It is becoming increasingly evident that growth factors often act in concert. In addition to causing the secretion of additional factors from populations co-existing with their targets, factors may act directly on target cells with other factors, giving synergistic, additive or even antagonistic effects. The finding of cooperation has also shown that factors may act on cells of both the myelopoietic and lymphoid components of haemopoiesis. For example, IL-1 was originally described as a factor required for T lymphocyte activation, has been shown to be identical with haemopoietin-1 [114,115], identified by its capacity to act synergistically with CSF-1 to stimulate early stem cells [116]. IL-1 has also been shown to stimulate the production of GM-CSF and G-CSF by fibroblasts or endothelial cells [117,118]. IL-4 and IL-5 were first described as factors acting on lymphocytes; indeed, there was some confusion about their terminology [119]. Both are now known to act synergistically or to cooperate with other factors on committed myelopoietic progenitors. IL-4 [120-123] has its most prominent myelopoietic action on mast cells or basophil production, while IL-5 [124] increases eosinophil numbers. IL-6, originally described as an interferon [125] with effects on a wide variety of lymphoid cells and cell lines, has been shown to act synergistically with IL-3 and GM-CSF on haemopoietic stem cells [126-128]. Indeed, only for IL-2, described first as a T-cell growth factor (TCGF) [129], does there still appear to be specificity for lymphocyte production; even in this case, IL-2-stimulated T-cells produce other haemopoietic factors and increase the cytotoxic effects of monocytes [130]. Thus, in general, the activities of growth factors do not coincide with the standard lineage diagrams used to describe haemopoiesis. In fact, their activity is not restricted to haemopoietic populations; recently it has been shown that G-CSF and GM-CSF can stimulate migration and proliferation in human endothelial cells cultured from umbilical veins [131].

Myelopoietic Growth Factors In Vivo

The myelopoietic growth factors have been discussed above in the context of their effects in culture. Before molecular technology was available, it was feasible only to ascribe activity *in vivo* to erythropoietin. Now, with the availability of cloned genes and recombinant proteins, three lines of evidence have emerged bearing on their roles in intact animals.

Firstly, transgenic mice [132] were engineered with the GM-CSF gene introduced under the control of a promotor and enhancer in the LTR of the Moloney Murine Leukaemia Virus [133]. The transgenic animals had a high constitutive expression of GM-CSF with elevated levels of the protein in serum and urine resulting in extensive accumulations of macrophages in the abdominal and pleural cavities. The transgenic mice were born blind because of ocular damage associated with accumulation of macrophages. Their survival was shortened, with death associated with a wasting illness. GM-CSF and IL-3 have both been transferred to bone marrow stem cells by retroviruses and these stem cells used to reconstitute recipient mice. In both instances extensive lethal myeloproliferation was observed [134,135]. Thus, large and unregulated production of IL-3 or GM-CSF leads to a massive fatal non-clonal proliferation of macrophages and granulocytes. It will be important to see if similar results are obtained when genes for lineage-restricted factors are tested as transgenes or after transfer to stem cells.

Secondly, recombinant growth factors have been administered experimentally to animals and tested in man in clinical trials.

Both GM-CSF and G-CSF increased granulopoiesis in nonhuman primates [136,137] and, as expected from its activities in culture, GM-CSF also caused reticulocytosis. Both factors were also able to improve the speed of recovery of neutrophils following chemotherapy [138,137]. IL-3 has little activity by itself in monkeys; however, animals have a much greater response to GM-CSF if they have been pretreated with IL-3, as might be expected by the major activity of IL-3 on very early stem cells [139].

Erythropoietin has been shown to be effective in increasing haemoglobin and red cell levels in patients with uraemia [140]. Both GM-CSF and G-CSF [141,105] have been tested in man; both showed the expected improvement in granulopoiesis. G-CSF reduced the toxic effects of chemotherapy given for carcinoma [142]. GM-CSF administration was clinically beneficial in myelodysplastic syndrome. Adverse effects were slight, but included fever, and thrombosis at the site of injection. Where blasts were present in the marrow, their numbers increased, sometimes requiring chemotherapy [143]. In patients with AIDS, GM-CSF increased neutrophil counts but did not affect the course of the disease [144]. In all of these trials, clear dose-response relationships were observed, providing strong evidence that the effects of the factors as seen in culture were indeed reproduced *in vivo*.

Thirdly, the effects of growth factors with specificity for human cells have been studied in a system where these cells proliferate following transplantation into mice. The recipient animals carried mutations in three loci, nude (nu), beige (bg) and xid (xid); after 400cGy of radiation, transferred marrow cells could be detected and identified as human by the detection of satellite DNA sequences after amplification with PCR. Some growth factors (IL-3 and GM-CSF) are species specific while others (CSF-1 and G-CSF) are active across species boundaries. However, in nu/bg/xid irradiated mice, human marrow cells grew regardless of whether or not recipients were continuously infused with rGM-CSF. Indeed, colonies requiring human GM-CSF for growth were obtained from animals that had been transplanted with human cells but had not received the species-specific growth factor [145].

The experiments with transgenic mice or animals transplanted with stem cells constitutively expressing high levels of GM-CSF or IL-3 show that massive amounts of these factors can produce lethal, although not neoplastic, proliferation of macrophages and granulocytes. The experiments with primates and the clinical trials are evidence that pharmacological doses of growth factor are well tolerated and may have clinically beneficial effects. However, the growth of human GM-CSF-dependent cells in mice without human growth factor makes it necessary to consider the physiological role of these regulators. It remains possible that most or all of the factors now available as recombinant proteins function normally to resist infection or react to foreign material. Their action may not be necessary for establishment or maintenance of haemopoiesis. If this proves to be the case, their role is not diminished, nor is their therapeutic potential lessened; however, a need emerges to identify yet other environmentally-derived mechanisms for haemopoietic regulation. The putative factor encoded by genes in the Sl locus, and binding to the product of W locus genes, described earlier, are obvious candidates.

Blast Cells of AML

Regulatory mechanisms affecting haemopoiesis in general and the myelopoietic growth factors in particular are important in considering the biology of the clonal haemopathies since freshly-obtained leukaemic cells have been shown to retain responsiveness to growth factors. The challenge is to recognise those properties or control elements that may exploited in management.

The blast cells of AML provide a useful way of meeting this challenge. The model of AML depicted in Figure 1 indicated that the blast cells may be considered as a separate lineage within abnormal clones, maintained by stem cells derived from leukaemic pluripotent stem cells prior to determination [146,147]. This population may safely be obtained from patients and examined using cellular or molecular techniques in the laboratory; conclusions or hypotheses based on such experiments may be tested clinically by seeking correlations between laboratory measurements and clinical parameters or even through clinical trials.

Blast Cells in Culture

Culture methods provide a way in which blast cell self-renewing and terminal differentiation processes can be assessed with some degree of independence. Blast cells can be obtained from marrow or peripheral blood. The latter is the source of choice since blood of AML patients contains many fewer myelopoietic or lymphoid progenitors co-existing with the blast cells. Almost pure blast populations can be prepared by simple separation procedures designed to remove normal leukocytes and T cell progenitors [148]. Clonogenic cells can then be detected specifically, using a culture assay in which the cells are immobilised in methylcellulose, usually in the presence of one or more growth factors [149]. Counting colonies developing in this procedure yields a plating efficiency in methylcellulose, PE_{mc}. Blast colonies can also be recovered readily from methylcellulose; their phenotypic characteristics are similar to those of the blasts cells found in the patients from whom the samples were obtained. The cells can also be resuspended and replated. In about 70% of cases, secondary colonies can be grown [150]; their enumeration gives a secondary plating efficiency, PE_2. However, PE_2 values are usually less than one percent, and evidence is available that most of the non-clonogenic cells in colonies are the outcomes of terminal divisions [151]. Further, attempts to replate secondary colonies are seldom successful. These observations are interpreted to mean that most divisions during colony formation in methylcellulose are post-deterministic and that the culture conditions are not favourable for self-renewal. Nonetheless, the observation of any secondary plating efficiency is important; the finding provided the first evidence that clonogenic blast cells have the stem-cell-defining property of self-renewal. PE_2 was also the first blast property determined in culture with a clinical correlation. As might be anticipated from the role of self-renewal in clonal expansion, high values of PE_2 have been shown, in several separate series, to be associated with a low probability of successful remission induction [150-154].

AML blasts will also proliferate in suspension. Using ^{3}HTdR incorporation into DNA to assess growth, it was possible to show requirements for soluble growth factors as supplied by media from leukocytes grown in the presence of PHA (PHA-LCM) and for high cell density, as well as marked patient-to-patient variation [155,156]. However, the method only became sufficiently flexible when the development of the blast colony assay described above made it possible to monitor changes in clonogenic cells in suspension [157]. It was then shown that blast stem cells from many patients increased in suspension. For these populations, subculture was often possible; cells could be maintained in exponential growth for weeks or even months. Rarely, the blasts became established as cell lines, preserving most of the biological properties observed when the cells were first examined [158,159]. Growth patterns in suspension varied from patient to patient. In some instances, clonogenic cell number was maintained or declined. Adherent cells were also observed in some cultures; these often had the morphology of macrophages and showed increased amounts of the macrophage-associated antigen MO2 on their surfaces [160]. These adherent cells were never seen to divide; their generation was considered to be a manifestation of terminal divisions in blast populations. The most important conclusion from the study was that changes in clonogenic cell number reflected their self-renewal capacity rather than recruitment from a more primitive precursor. A numerical value can be determined, the plating efficiency after suspension (PE_S). Evidence was also provided that cell-cell contact was essential for growth of clonogenic cells. Daily examination of the cultures showed that growth was usually associated with the formation of large loose cell aggregates; these did not form if methylcellulose was added to the cultures and growth of clonogenic cells was also inhibited. Thus, it may be that in the clonogenic assay methylcellulose prevents a cell-cell interaction that supports blast cell self-renewal.

The Balance between Self-Renewal and Differentiation

The methylcellulose assay for clonogenic blast cells and the suspension method complement each other in experiments designed to estimate the balance between blast stem cell renewal and terminal divisions analogous to differentiation. PE_{mc} in the clonogenic assay reflects principally terminal divisions. In contrast, when plating efficiency is measured after 7 days in suspension (PE_S), it is not correlated to the primary plating efficiency, but rather reflects self-renewal. The suspension culture also allows for the enumeration of adherent cells; their number is the outcome of terminal divisions. The number of non-adherent cells can also be determined. During suspension culture clonogenic cells have doubling times varying from 3 to 9 days; this contrasts with 5 to 8-hour values for the DNA synthesis times of clonogenic blasts [161], values that suggest generation times for blast stem cells of less than 12 hours. Such a discrepancy between doubling time and generation time is characteristic of cultures where a proportion of the cells are lost regularly from the proliferating population. Thus, many of the non-adherent cells are also the consequence of terminal rather than self-renewal divisions, a conclusion supported by the values of PE_S, which rarely approach 10%. However, PE_S and total nucleated cells can be multiplied, to give the number of clonogenic cells recovered after suspension culture. This is then a self-renewal associated value. In summary, the two assays give three values that estimate terminal divisions, the outcome of the "death probability"; these are PE_{mc}, adherent cell number, and, perhaps less reliably, non-adherent cell number. Two values, PE_S and clonogenic cell recovery after suspension, reflect self-renewal or the "birth" probability.

In practice it is possible to use an experimental protocol that separates exposure of cells to various experimental conditions from "read out" procedures that reflect responses to those conditions. The protocol depends on using media conditioned by the continuous bladder carcinoma cell line 5637 (5637-CM) [162], to provide a constant and nearly maximum stimulation of AML blasts. In the first step, the population under test, either directly obtained from patients, recovered after cryopreservation or maintained as a stable strain or line, is exposed to 5637-CM for 2-3 days, in order to establish exponential growth and constant conditions. In the second step the cells are then either plated in methylcellulose or cultured in suspension under experimental conditions. Third, the "read-out" is obtained: 1) by counting colonies in the methylcellulose dishes; 2) by harvesting the suspension cultures and counting adherent and non-adherent cells; and 3) by plating the non-adherent cells from the suspension cultures in methylcellulose with 5637-CM in order to measure PE_S and, from it and the non-adherent cell count, to determine clonogenic cell recovery.

A graphic display is a valuable aid to considering data emerging from such a protocol. Regrettably, the scales of the parameters are different, making it inconvenient to use such well-known techniques as histograms. Star diagrams overcome the difficulty since they permit the display of multiple parameters with different scales [163]. The diagrams consist of axes, radiating from a central point. Each axis is scaled for one of the parameters measured experimentally. Values are plotted on each axis at the scaled distance from the central point; the points on each axis are joined to form a multi-sided figure. The "death"-related values are plotted on axes to the right and up; the "birth"-related values are assigned axes to the left and down. Thus, a star predominantly to the right and up shows a population growing under conditions that favoured differentiation while a star to the left and down reflects predominantly self-renewal events. Star diagrams for different conditions can be compared, either directly, as matrices or by superimposition. Then, inspection alone provides a sense of how the experimental conditions have affected the balance between self-renewal and determination for the blast population under test. Examples of the use of star diagrams are given in Figures 2 and 3.

Leukaemic Cells and Growth Factors

Leukaemic Cell Lines

Observations on leukaemic cell lines have led to the hope that growth factors might reduce or eliminate cell proliferation by the induction of differentiation [164,32]. Several myelopoietic growth factors have been shown to increase the number of differentiated cells in myelopoietic lines. Prominent among them is G-CSF, whose effects on WEHI-3 cells have been examined extensively [110,111,165,166]. Recently, a factor termed Leukaemia Inhibitory Factor (LIF) has been isolated from Krebs II ascites cells and cloned from a cDNA library made from a murine T lymphocyte cell line, LB3 [167]. This induces differentiation in the ML-1 myeloid leukaemia cell line but not in WEHI-3 cells; however, unlike G-CSF it has not been reported to stimulate any of the normal haemopoietic lineages. The possibility might be entertained that the activity of LIF was only inhibitory, particularly when it was found to maintain embryonic stem cells in their undifferentiated state in culture [168,169]. However, molecular clones were isolated for the interleukin that stimulates human DA cells to proliferate and shown to be identical with LIF clones [170]; it follows that the response following this ligand-receptor interaction is determined by many factors rather than only by the structural information in the ligand and that the outcomes of these interactions may be diverse.

Freshly Obtained AML Blast Cells

Growth factors have been studied extensively using AML blast cells as targets. Il-3 [171,172], GM-CSF [171,173-175], G-CSF [171,175,176] and CSF-1 [177,178] have been shown to be stimulators. Both Tumour Growth Factor beta [179] and Tumour Necrosis Factor [180] inhibit blast cell colony formation. As with stimulatory factors, the effects of these peptides varied from patient to patient and seldom was the inhibition very marked. Synergistic effects have also been seen, notably between GM-CSF and G-CSF [181] or IL-6 [182]. These studies all serve to emphasise the importance of attempting to distinguish between self-renewal and terminal divisions; further, since many growth factors are derived from lymphocytes, monocytes or endothelial cells, it is anticipated that they will be presented to targets in combination. Therefore, studies of their interactions are required.

The protocol for studies of blast cells in culture, described earlier, can be used to examine the effects of growth factors both singly and in combination. IL-3, GM-CSF, G-CSF and CSF-1 were tested on blasts by exposing cells as single agents or combinations of two agents both in suspension and in methylcellulose as determined by the protocol [183]. The experimental data was presented as star diagrams; The "death"-related values, adherent cell number and PE_{mc} were plotted on axes to the right and up; the "birth"-related values, PE_S and clonogenic cell recovery assigned axes to the left and

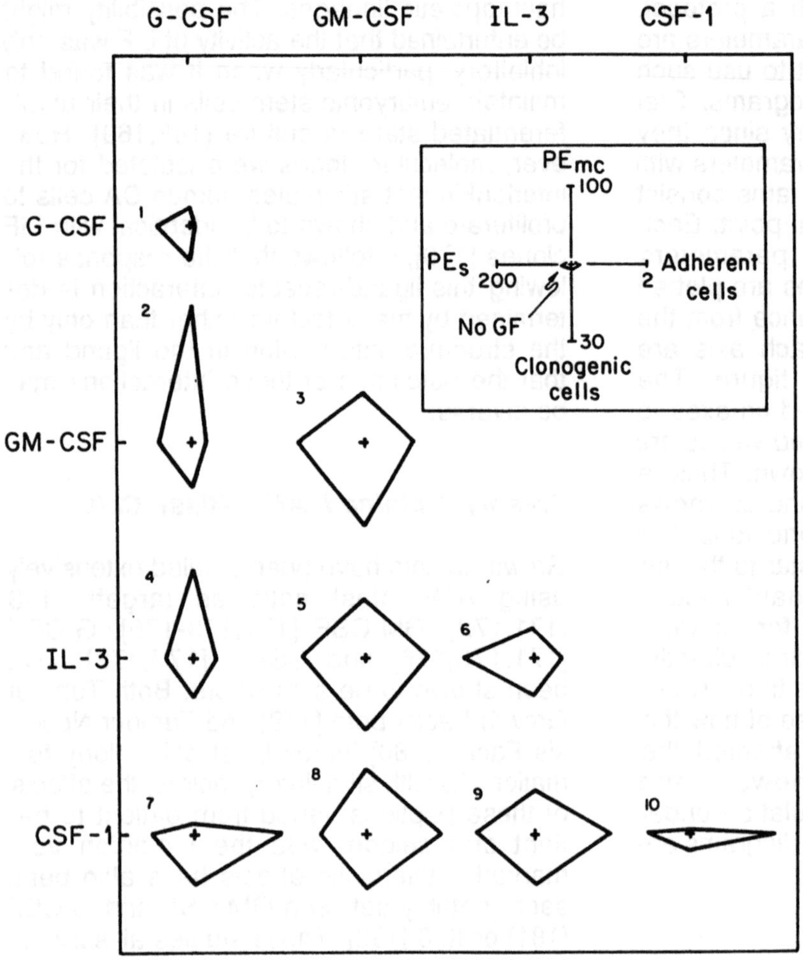

Fig. 2. Star diagrams depicting the responses of a single blast population of IL3, GM-CSF, G-CSF and CSF-1, alone or in combination. The diagrams are arranged as a matrix, with a star diagram in each box. The insert at the top right corner of the figure shows the scales and axes of the star, together with the response of the population when no factors were added to the cultures. For explanation, see text.
Reproduced from reference [231] by permission of the publisher

down. This arrangement of axes follows the convention that a star predominantly to the right and up shows a population growing under conditions that favour differentiation, while a star to the left and down reflects predominantly self-renewal events.

The star diagrams are shown as a matrix in Figure 2, with factor designations shown at the top and on the left. Star diagrams along the diagonal (cells 1, 3, 6 and 10) are drawn from data for each factor tested alone. The remaining diagrams are data for factors in combination, as indicated by the matrix labels. The cell at the top-right of the figure shows the scaled axes used to construct the star diagram together with the data obtained when no factor was added to the cultures. In Figure 2 this insert shows that the cells under test had little or no spontaneous growth; the blast cells under test responded to all of the culture conditions. G-CSF had only modest activity and this was principally stimulation of self-renewal, as seen by a small star to the left and down in respect to the central point. The star diagram from GM-CSF alone (Figure 2, cell 3) showed that both self-renewal and differentiation increased similarly in response to this factor. Next in the diagonal of the Figure 2 matrix, the star diagram of IL-3 shows that this factor favoured renewal divisions, although some adherent cells were also formed. The star diagram for CSF-1 is the last in the diagonal; it has the triangular shape, with apex down, indicating that colonies did not form in methylcellulose (PE_{mc}) in response to this factor. However, in suspension, the "death" probability emerged strongly, as seen by adherent cell formation, although some "birth"-related events were also detected.

The effects of combining all factors with one another are shown in the remaining star diagrams of Figure 2. Interactions between factors are most evident at the left and bottom of the matrix. Cells 2, 4 and 7, on the left side, contain stars for G-CSF combined with GM-CSF, Il-3 and CSF-1. The changes in the star diagrams for each combination are evident by comparison with the diagram in cell 1 for G-CSF alone. GM-CSF and IL-3 had qualitatively similar synergistic effects when combined with G-CSF, both increasing the "death" probability as seen as a shift of the star upwards, as PE_{mc} became greater. The addition of CSF-1 to G-CSF increased the "death" probability by promoting the generation of adherent cells. Similar although less marked CSF-1 effects are seen in the star diagrams on cells 8 and 9 at the bottom of the matrix, representing the combination of CSF-1 with GM-CSF and IL-3, respectively. Little interaction was seen when GM-CSF and IL-3 were combined. The star diagram for this combination seen in cell 5 is not different from that in the cell above it (cell 3), for GM-CSF alone.

Figure 2 contains the data for blasts from only a single patient. Variation in response is seen regularly. In other examples, G-CSF increased the "death" probability while IL-3 favoured the "birth" probability. However, the general pattern seen in Figure 2 was also observed in other instances studied in equivalent detail. IL-3, GM-CSF and G-CSF stimulated both self-renewal and differentiation, although to varying degrees [171]. CSF-1 often did not increase colony formation, but activity could be detected using suspension assays [177]. The effects of CSF-1 are more consistent than those of the other factors, since differentiation is usually favoured.

When the four factors are combined in pairs, the pattern of Figure 2 is seen regularly. The increase in the "death" probability associated with CSF-1 persists and may be amplified when CSF-1 is combined with any of the other four hormones. The normally early-acting factors, IL-3 and GM-CSF, are synergistic in combination with the late-acting G-CSF and CSF-1 [181], but, when used together, only the response to the most active factor is observed.

Mechanisms

The requirement of some cell lines and most blast cells for growth factors raises the issue of their role in the neoplastic state. Specifically, are autocrine or paracrine mechanisms operative [184]? First, the experiments described earlier, where factor-overproduction *in vivo* was achieved by inserting genes for growth factors into the germline or the genomes of stem cells [132,134,168], show that high levels of these factors by themselves do not result in leukaemia. However, transfection of IL-3 or GM-CSF into factor-dependent cell lines renders them both secretors of the factors and capable of malignant growth following transplantation [185,186]. Moreover, many leukaemic cell lines grow independently of added factor and, for murine cells, regularly give rise to leukaemias in recipient animals.

Blast cells from patients have been examined extensively for evidence of autocrine or paracrine mechanisms. Factor expression at the RNA level has been demonstrated in up to 50% of blast populations [187-190]. Secretion of biologically active growth factors is much less common. Further, many populations that express genes for growth factors continue to respond to the hormones and very few are autonomous in culture. Nor is it evident that autocrine mechanisms are essential for the establishment of permanent cell lines.

Indirect evidence exists that CSF-1 has autocrine activity. About half of AML blasts were positive for CSF-1 expression by Northern analysis; of these only one secreted bioactive factor. However, the expression-positive clones were found to renew themselves significantly less well than expression-negative populations [191]. This observation is consistent with the findings described earlier, showing that exogenous CSF-1 regularly increased the "death" probability for sensitive blast populations; although CSF-1 protein has yet to be found in most expression-positive populations, studies with the fms gene, known to encode the receptor for CSF-1 [52], are consistent with the view that CSF-1 expression reduces cell growth by ligand receptor interactions. Only fms expression-positive clones responded to CSF-1, as expected since the fms gene encodes the CSF-

1 receptor [52]. Most CSF-1 expression-positive clones were also fms expression positive. Regrettably, too few CSF-1-positive, fms-negative examples were identified to test whether cells with this phenotype had different growth characteristics than the commoner fms-positive type, although a trend towards better growth was seen in CSF-1 expression-positive clones when fms was not expressed. Taken together, these data support the view that CSF-1 acts directly to inhibit blast growth by binding with its receptor, and that such interaction may take place intracellularly. Such a mechanism might be considered autocrine inhibition of growth.

Lineage Infidelity

Information about the responses of blast cells to growth factors may contribute to the ongoing discussion of the biological nature of leukaemia. The model of AML clones shown in Figure 1 has provided a conceptual basis for much of the discussion in this chapter. However, the model is not widely accepted. Indeed, many investigators consider that leukaemic blast cells represent the proliferation of early progenitors whose differentiation has been blocked. Strong support for this view comes from studies of cell lines; as described earlier, many of these respond to chemicals (DMSO or retinoic acid) or growth factors (G-CSF or LIF) by the production of morphologically differentiated cells. The model in Figure 1 was developed in the context of the cellular composition of AML clones and supported by the findings that blast cells behaved in culture like an independent lineage. However, relevant information can also be obtained from the phenotypes of blast cells. A blocked differentiation model would predict that each blast cell population would express markers characteristic of a normal lineage and differentiation stage (lineage fidelity); in contrast, if blasts are a novel lineage, their phenotypes might be unusual. The first prediction appeared to be fulfilled in early descriptions of immunophenotypes, particularly in B lymphocytic leukaemias and lymphomas [192,193]. As more reagents were used, marked heterogeneity was found in leukaemic cells. In ALL, lymphoid markers were found in abnormal combinations, which were considered to be evidence for asynchronous development of malignant clones from very early progenitors [194]. Friend cells, considered to be erythroleukaemic, were shown to express markers of granulopoiesis [195]; cells of the human K562 line, also often described as an erythroleukaemia, were seen to express spontaneously erythropoietic and granulopoietic markers on single cells [196]. Using histochemical or immunologically-detected markers, several groups found markers usually associated with different lineages together on single leukaemic blasts directly obtained from patients [197-201]. This immunophenotypic lineage infidelity was considered as evidence of abnormal gene expression in leukaemia and not easily reconciled with the concept of blocked differentiation and lineage fidelity. The immunophenotypic data for infidelity was soon supported by molecular evidence; rearrangements of immunoglobulin and T cell receptor genes, events essential to lymphoid differentiation, were found in blast populations considered on morphological and immunophenotypic grounds to be AML [202-206].

An explanation that might accommodate the data without entirely discarding the concept of lineage fidelity was introduced by Greaves [207]. He accepted the view that leukaemic transformation usually occurs in pluripotent stem cells, but suggested that such cells might have latitude in expression of lineage-associated genes; such cells might express transiently genes for one lineage before becoming committed at determination irreversibly to a different differentiation pathway (Lineage promiscuity). Leukaemic transformation occurring in such cells might then "immortalise" the "promiscuous" predeterministic phenotype.

The issue might be resolved if the phenotypes of pluripotent stem cells were known. Then, one might see if these differed from those of leukaemic blast cells either qualitatively or in the extent of their heterogeneity. Recently, a cell purification procedure has been published based on both negative and positive cell sorting for immunologically-defined markers [208]. The procedure yielded a small population of homogeneous cells; good evidence was presented that each of these was able to give rise to a spleen colony, repopulate a thymus or a Whitlock-Witte long term lymphoid cell culture. Thus, the population obtained after purification consisted almost entirely of pluripotent stem cells. The separation procedure also gave phenotypic information about the cells. They were null for lineage markers. It follows that differentiation is a positive event leading to the appearance of lineage- or stage-specific markers rather than selection of some markers from a large array already present. This general view is compatible with the molecular events that are required for B or T cell differentiation; these also are positive, consisting of molecular re-arrangements. This concept of differentiation is not easily reconciled with an interpretation of the diverse marker phenotypes on leukaemic blasts as the continuing expression of primitive phenotypes, expressed promiscuously and made permanent by transformation.

Highly purified murine stem cells respond to IL-3 and GM-CSF by colony formation in culture [209]. This observation is consistent with the activity of these factors on very primitive cells. However, the considerations about differentiation given above make it unlikely that receptors for late-acting factors, such as G-CSF or CSF-1, are also expressed on primitive cells. Yet such receptors and the biological responses associated with ligand binding are found on AML blast cells. They are also variable from population to population. Thus, the growth factor-related phenotypes of blast cells are unlikely to resemble those of primitive precursors which are expected to be more homogeneous and without expression of lineage-associated markers. While neither this, nor the conclusions drawn from any of the data are conclusive in support of any model of leukaemic blast cells, together the immunophenotypic, molecular and growth factor characteristics of blast cells are highly consistent with the view that genes, normally expressed in an orderly fashion in differentiation, are turned on or off in abnormal sequences and combinations in these malignant cells. If, as proposed, the AML blasts belong to a novel lineage, differentiation programmes in that lineage may be assembled abnormally from normal components. Recently, molecular support for the concept that abnormal gene expression may change differentiation programmes has come from experiments where v-raf insertion was shown to convert B-lineage to macrophage differentiation [205].

Biology and Chemotherapy

A remarkable feature of acute leukaemia in general and AML in particular is the response to chemotherapy with complete remission (see earlier). Induction and maintenance or remission have been studied extensively in multi-institutional randomised clinical trials such as those conducted by Cancer and Leukaemia Group B in the USA [210] and the Medical Research Council in the United Kingdom [Rees, this volume]. Major improvements have not been seen in recent trials. Similar evidence, indicating that remission induction and duration of survival are not strongly dependent on drug regimen, was obtained in four sequential historically controlled trials at a single Institution (The Princess Margaret Hospital/Ontario Cancer Institute), where combinations of active drugs or a single agent, cytosine arabinoside (ara-C) [211] led to survival and remission outcomes that were not significantly different [63,212,213]. In these series, patient characteristics, like details of chemotherapy regimen, were shown to be less important contributors to outcome than biological parameters of the disease [152,153]. Nonetheless, treatment is crucial since in its absence remissions are not seen and very few patients survive a year after diagnosis. The interaction between chemotherapy, the malignant clone and the human host is, therefore, an important issue.

A very useful model was introduced by Bruce and his collaborators [214]. They related the cytotoxic actions of agents to the cell cycle parameters of their targets. Particularly they noted that some, such as ionising radiation, were active at cells throughout the cycle or in a resting (G_0) state. Others showed cycle specificity, either acting only during DNA synthesis or requiring proliferation to be lethal. Since normal haemopoietic stem cells are often in G_0 while tumour cells are in active cell cycle, drugs with S-phase or cycle specificity are able to destroy tumour cells while sparing normal cells. This model remains a useful explanation of how chemotherapy reduces the size of a malignant clone while leaving normal cells with intact growth capacity. Attempts have been made to extend the model to explain variation in response of leukaemic cells to chemotherapy, based on ^{3}HTdR labelling studies [215]. Low levels of labelled cells were taken to indicate that leukaemic cells were in G_0 and changes in labelling indices were considered evidence for their recruitment into active cell cycle [216]. With the development of the cell culture assays for normal and leukaemic stem cells, it became apparent that the populations have great functional heterogeneity in respect to their proliferative capacity, with many cells incapable of division because of differentiation or its analogue in leukaemia. Kinetic experiments using ^{3}HTdR radioautography would not have the resolution to distinguish between such cells and G_0 cells; it is possible, therefore, that the interpretation of the kinetic studies as indicating the presence of resting leukaemic cells was erroneous because of the large number of proliferatively-inert cells in the populations. This view is consistent with studies in which the proliferative status of AML blasts was examined, using the capacity of high specific-activity ^{3}HTdR to kill cells by internal irradiation ("suicide") to measure percentage of clonogenic cells in the S-phase of the cycle. By this technique a high proportion of clonogenic AML blast cells were shown to be killed specifically by brief exposure of ^{3}HTdR, indicating that all the blast stem cells are in active cell cycle [217]. It follows that the model of Bruce and his collaborators may be valid for comparisons of normal and leukaemic cells, the case for which it was proposed, but its extension to putative cycle differences within leukaemic populations may not be justified.

Drug Sensitivity in Suspension and Methylcellulose Compared

From the foregoing it is apparent that the heterogeneity of leukaemic cell populations must be considered in any approach to the mechanism of response to chemotherapy. Cell kill models are often based on negative exponential dose response curves, relating drug exposure to cell kill; curves of this form are obtained regularly under experimental conditions [218,219]. Such curves would be hard to accept as explanations of the elimination of blasts if it were necessary to inactivate all blast cells. However, if only stem cells rather than all cells must be eliminated in order to destroy blast populations, the requirement for cell kill might be reduced sufficiently to be credible [220]. A further refinement of the target has emerged from experiments where dose-response curves were constructed for blast stem cells exposed to drug either in suspension or in methylcellulose.
Comparisons of exponential survival curves obtained using the two methods fell into three patterns [221,222]. For adriamycin both procedures yielded curves with the same slope, expressed as the drug concentration required to reduce survival to 10% of control (D10) [223,224]. In contrast, cytosine arabinoside (ara-C) was more toxic when tested in suspension than in methylcellulose. The third pattern was observed with 5-azacytidine (5-aza) or 5-deoxyazacytidine; D10 values for these agents were greater when determined using the clonogenic assay in methylcellulose than when measured in suspension.
The proposal was advanced that the differences observed between the two assays may be explained as a differential toxicity in suspension or in methylcellulose depending on the probability of either stem cell renewal or determination; thus, where conditions favoured self-renewal (that is, in suspension) ara-C was more toxic and 5-aza less toxic. In contrast, where terminal divisions were favoured (that is, in methylcellulose), the reverse was seen with 5-aza more toxic than ara-C.
All three drugs act on DNA; the anthracyclines intercalate in DNA and may be cytotoxic by inhibiting preribosomal RNA synthesis; there is no known specificity for particular sequences in DNA [225]. In contrast, ara-C is a cytidine analogue that is converted enzymatically to ara-CTP and then incorporated into DNA [226]. 5-Aza is also a cytidine analogue, processed by different enzymes prior to incorporation into both RNA and DNA. It is considered to have functional specificity

based on nitrogen substituted for carbon in the 5 position of the cytidine ring. This carbon is the site of methylation of DNA and the 5-substituted base cannot accept methyl groups. Hypomethylation following 5-aza treatment has been shown to alter gene expression [227] and to affect differentiation [228]. The observed effects of 5-aza on self-renewal might be explained if it were integrated more efficiently into DNA bearing information related to self-renewal than into DNA generally [221]. By analogy a similar suggestion may be made for ara-C. The suggestion implies that specific genes exist whose activity determines the balance between self-renewal and determination. Regardless of the mechanisms, the results of comparing survival curves in suspension and methylcellulose suggest that, in addition to their general cytotoxicity, some chemotherapeutic drugs might have some specificity for cell cycles leading to terminal cells on the one hand or new stem cells on the other.

Clinical Correlations

Measuring in culture the sensitivity of pathogens to antibiotics has undoubted clinical value. It has long been a goal to devise an analogous culture test for chemotherapeutic agents, based on their capacity to destroy the capacity of stem cells to form colonies in culture. Studies by Salmon and his associates were pioneering efforts in this direction [229]. Unfortunately, experience since Salmon's first proposals has not established a reliable correlation between drug sensitivity measured with clonogenic assays and outcome. In AML ara-C or adriamycin D10 values measured in methylcellulose were not regularly associated with response to chemotherapy regimens that included both agents [152].

This negative result might be attributed to the use of the wrong test. D10 measured in suspension might be more useful, if, as suggested, the suspension assay is a sensitive way of detecting the inhibition of self-renewal. Indeed, for both ara-C and 5-aza, a significant association was found between sensitivity in suspension and successful response to chemotherapy [223,230,231]. The patients used in these studies were treated with a single agent, high dose ara-C [211]; it was reasonable, therefore, to find that the ara-C sensitivity of the self-renewal function was an attribute contributing to successful therapy. No such argument can be made for the association between 5-aza sensitivity and response to treatment with ara-C. Rather, it might be postulated that the self-renewal function varies in its sensitivity to agents that are incorporated into DNA, a view consistent with the hypothesis that there are self-renewal specific genes. Further, that clones with "sensitive" renewal machinery respond to chemotherapy, while those with "resistant" systems fail. The data support the suggestion that each AML patient has an intrinsically-determined response to commonly-used treatment regimens, provided these regimens contain active drugs, a view that is consistent with the clinical observations that response in AML is not strongly associated with any specific drug regimen. From this point of view, sensitivity in suspension is associated with response because it helps to identify those patients with chemotherapy-sensitive self-renewal mechanisms.

Growth Factors and Chemosensitivity

Two postulates have emerged from the cell culture studies of AML blasts. Firstly, that an operational distinction can be made between self-renewal and terminal divisions by combining or comparing assays in suspension and in methylcellulose. Secondly, that certain drugs are more toxic for cells in renewal divisions than cells that are dividing terminally. The first postulate was the basis for considering that growth factors influence the balance between self-renewal and differentiation. The second postulate is the basis for considering that self-renewal of stem cells may be the appropriate target for chemotherapy. Together, these considerations lead to the suggestion that the sensitivity of blast cells in culture could be altered using growth factors; specifically, changing the "birth" and "death" probabilities of blast cells in culture should lead to alterations in drug sensitivity.

A test of the prediction is presented in Figure 3; the figure contains data from experiments on two stable AML lines in culture (OCI/AML1 and OCI/AML2) [159]. The cells were chosen

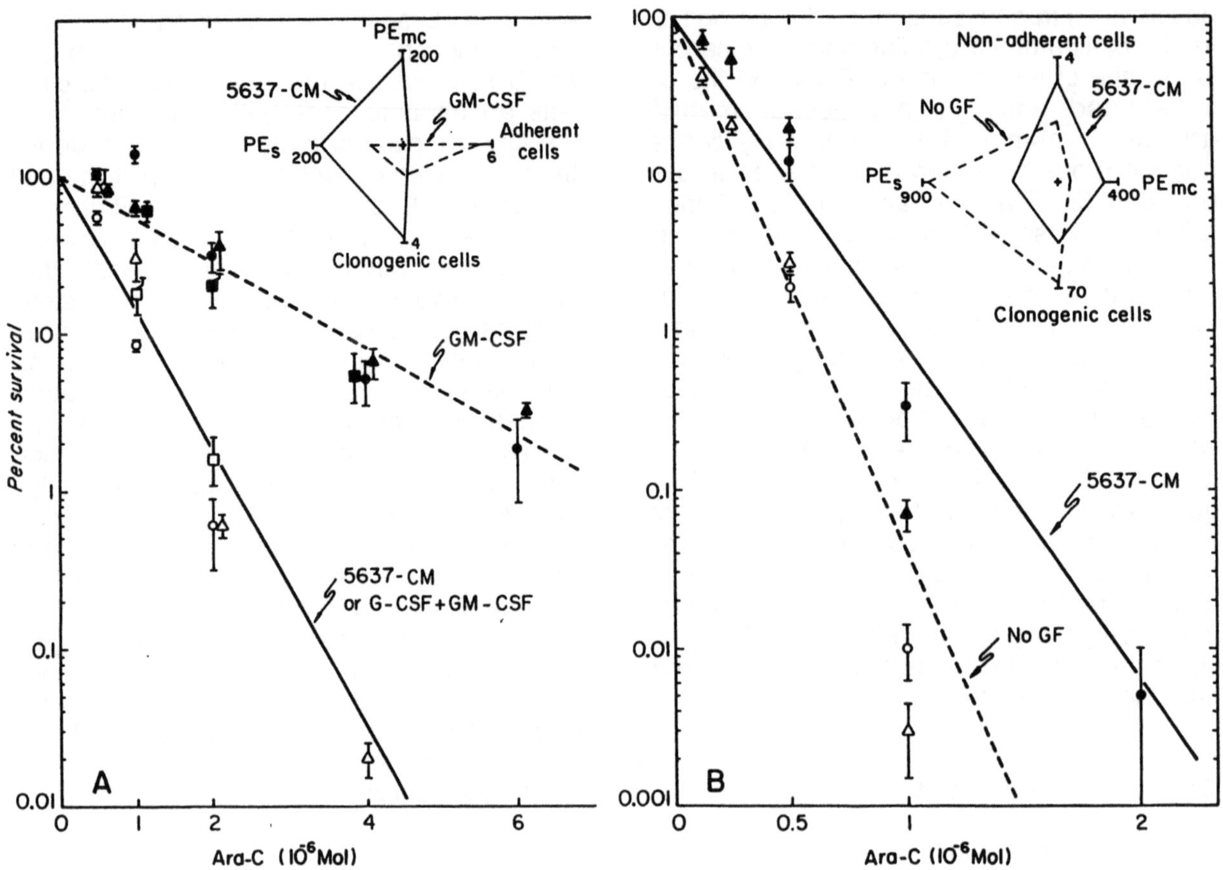

Fig. 3. Simple negative exponential survival curves [223] for recovery of clonogenic cells from suspension cultures of OCI/AML1 (panel A) and OCI/AML2 (panel B) exposed to increasing concentrations of ara-C under different growth conditions. For OCI/AML1 (A), survival curves obtained in the presence of 5637-CM are shown as open symbols and with GM-CSF as closed symbols; additional experimental points obtained with GM-CSF or GM-CSF and G-CSF are shown as closed and open squares, respectively. For OCI/AML2 (B), open symbols represent curves obtained in cultures without added growth factors and closed symbols for curves obtained in the presence of 5637-CM. In each instance, replicate experiments are shown as triangles or circles. For each panel, two superimposed star diagrams are included; scales for each axis are shown in the figure: for panel A, the up axis is PE_{mc} (colonies/10^4 cells), the down axis is clonogenic cell recovery (x 10^4/ml), the right horizontal axis is adherent cell number (x 10^4/culture), the left horizontal axis is PE_s (colonies/10^4 cells). For panel B, the up axis is non-adherent cell number (x 10^6/ml) after suspension culture, the down axis is clonogenic cell recovery (x 10^4/ml), the right horizontal axis is PE_{mc} (colonies/3 x 10^3 cells) and left horizontal axis is PE_s (colonies/3 x 10^3 cells). The axes in both panels have been chosen so that a movement to the left and down indicates a shift towards "birth" probabilities and a movement to the right and up a shift towards "death" probabilities. Reprinted from [159], by permission of the publisher

on the basis of their responses to growth factors. OCI/AML1 is factor dependent; its growth requires 5637-CM, known to contain at least GM-CSF, G-CSF, IL-1 and IL-6. Exposure of OCI/AML1 to recombinant GM-CSF in suspension results in the production of adherent cells incapable of further division [173]. OCI/AML2 cells grow in the absence of added factor but their growth pattern changes on exposure to growth factors. The inserts at the upper right hand corners of the panels of Figure 3 contain star diagrams indicating the responses of the cells to varying conditions. For panel A, the star diagram shows a comparison between the growth of OCI/AML1 in 5637-CM or GM-CSF; however, the results with a combination of G-CSF and GM-CSF were very similar. For panel B the star diagrams were for OCI/AML2 growing with or without added factor 5637-CM. Since adherent cells were found in suspension cultures of OCI/AML1 but not in cultures of OCI/AML2, different axes were chosen to construct stars for these populations. In each instance the axes were chosen so that a star predominantly to the left and down is an indication that "birth" is favoured, while a star to the right and up signals increased "death" probability (see caption for Figure 3 for details). The ara-C survival curves in Figure 3 were then obtained for exponentially growing cells using the growth conditions specified in the figure for each curve.

For OCI/AML1, (Panel A) 5637-CM favoured self-renewal, as evident from a star showing high values for the "birth"-related parameters PE_S and clonogenic cell recovery; in contrast, the star diagram for cells grown in GM-CSF shows the generation of adherent cells and decreases in the "birth"-related functions. The survival curves show that OCI/AML1 blasts were more sensitive to ara-C in 5637-CM or a combination of G-CSF and GM-CSF than in GM-CSF. This change is compatible with the prediction that a shift in the balance between "birth" and "death" probabilities to favour "birth" would lead to increased ara-C sensitivity.

The results for OCI/AML2 (Panel B) also agree with the prediction, but provide a contrast. For these cells growth without added factor was dominated by self-renewal, as evident from the star diagram, showing high values for the "birth"-related parameters PE_S and clonogenic cell recovery. When cultured with 5637-CM, the star moved towards parameters indicating "death". The cells were more sensitive to ara-C without added factors than in the presence of the differentiation-inducing influences of the factors in 5637-CM.

Cells freshly obtained from two AML patients were also examined for changes in ara-C D10 values under different growth conditions. For these examples the results were also consistent with the prediction relating ara-C sensitivity to "birth" and ara-C resistance to "death" probabilities. No association was found between ara-C sensitivity and other parameters, such as intrinsic sensitivity or the extent of growth stimulation. Further examples need to be tested and agents other than growth factors should be examined for their interactions with drugs. Studies are also needed to see if these culture effects occur *in vivo*. If, as postulated, the chemosensitivity of self-renewal is important in obtaining favourable responses, growth factors or other biological response modifiers provide a potential tool for improving the therapeutic effectiveness of drugs. The use of such approaches will depend on detailed measurements of biological responses in individual patients.

Conclusion

The major theme of this review is that biological properties of leukaemic cells provide potent levers for therapists to exploit in management. The review was written at a time when the revolution in molecular biology had begun to have a major impact on models of normal and leukaemic growth and differentiation. It is now possible to consider in concrete terms a genetically-controlled system which regulates both the internal economy of cells and their relations with their environment, including their neighbours. The mechanism depends on ligand-receptor interactions based on genetically-determined binding sites. However, the signals that follow receptor binding are complex; their effects are modified and influenced by many cellular factors in addition to the specificity of binding sites. Further, each cell may experience, perhaps simultaneously, several binding events, some of which will use similar biochemical mechanisms to carry their messages. Thus, the cellular milieu is a complex of signals, which, together, may set probabilities rather than acting in a highly deterministic fashion.

It is not sufficient to consider single cells as units in the problem of the control of leukaemia. The heterogeneity of the cell populations is also highly significant. Stem cells, a small minority of the population, may be essential; their replication is not exact. Indeed, the change that is introduced during the expansion of single cells to clones is recognised as differentiation.

Malignant transformation affects not only the genetically-controlled mechanisms of regulation. Cell organisation is also changed. Normal polyclonal haemopoiesis is replaced, in the haemopathies, by clonal proliferation and dominance. Thus, the long-accepted view that fully-developed leukaemia requires multiple steps is a natural match for a picture of populations with the many regulatory mechanisms, changes in several of which might be required for the leukaemic phenotype. It is a goal to see which changes are necessary and sufficient for normal cells to become malignant and which are secondary. The cellular and molecular techniques are now available to approach such fundamental questions. In doing so, it should not be forgotten that secondary events may still provide targets for therapeutic manipulation. For example, autocrine mechanisms may not often be essential for leukaemic growth; but growth factors may still be very useful in treatment of the disease. The challenge is to take advantage of the great technological capacity that has been developed; yet technology by itself may not suffice. It may be that a special requirement now exists for radical thought if new biologically-based management strategies are to be successful.

Acknowledgements

This contribution was supported by grants from the Medical Research Council of Canada and the National Cancer Institute of Canada. The author is grateful to Dr. Mark Minden for his critical reading of the manuscript.

REFERENCES

1 Fialkow PJ: Clonal origin of human tumors. Biochim Biophys Acta 1976 (456):283-321

2 Buick RN, McCulloch EA: The role of stem cells in normal and malignant tissue. In: Boynton AL and Leffert HL (eds) Control of Animal Cell Proliferation. Academic Press, Orlando 1985 pp 25-57

3 McCulloch EA: Normal stem cells and the clonal hemopathies. In: Cronkite EP, Dainiak N, McCaffrey RP, Palek J and Quesenberry PJ (eds) Progress in Clinical and Biological Research. Hematopoietic Stem Cell Physiology. Alan R Liss Inc, New York 1985 pp 21-38

4 Nowell PC: The clonal evolution of tumor cell populations. Science 1976 (194):23-28

5 Barnes DWH, Ford CE, Gray SM, Loutit JF: Spontaneous and induced changes in cell populations in heavily irradiated mice. In: Bugher J, Coursaget J and Loutit JF (eds) Progress in Nuclear Energy: Proceedings 2nd International Conference on Peaceful Uses of Atomic Energy. Pergamon Press, London 1959 pp 10-16

6 Williams DA, Lemischka IR, Nathan DG, Mulligan RC: Introduction of new genetic material into pluripotent hematopoietic stem cells of the mouse. Nature (London) 1984 (310):476-480

7 Lemischka IR, Raulet D, Mulligan RC: Developmental potential and dynamic behaviour of hematopoietic stem cells. Cell 1986 (45):917-927

8 Dzierzak EA, Papayannopouli T, Mulligan RC: Lineage-specific expression of a human beta-globin gene in murine bone marrow transplant recipients reconstituted with retrovirus-transduced cells. Nature 1988 (331):35-41

9 Joyner A, Keller G, Phillips RA, Bernstein A: Retrovirus mediated transfer of a bacterial gene into mouse hematopoietic progenitor cells. Nature 1983 (305):556-558

10 Dick JE, Magli MC, Huszar D, Phillips RA, Bernstein A: Introduction of a selectable gene into primitive stem cells capable of long-term reconstitution of the hematopoietic system of W/W_v mice. Cell 1985 (42):71-79

11 Nowell PC, DA Hungerford: Chromosome studies in human leukemia. II Chronic granulocytic leukemia. JNCI 1961 (27):1013-1035

12 Blackstock AM, Garson OM: Direct evidence for involvement of erythroid cells in acute myeloblastic leukemia. Lancet 1974 (2):1178-1179

13 Rowley JD: Chromosomes in leukemia and lymphoma. In: Freireich EJ and Hersh EM (eds) Seminars in Hematology - Leukemia and Lymphoma. Grune and Stratton, New York 1978 pp 258-276

14 Fialkow PJ: Cell lineages in hematopoietic neoplasia studied with glucose-6-phosphate dehydrogenase cell markers. J Cell Physiol (Suppl 1) Alan Liss New York 1982

15 Fearon ER, Burke PJ, Schiffer CA, Zehnbauer BA, Vogelstein B: Differentiation of leukemic cells to polymorphonuclear leukocytes in patients with acute nonlymphocytic leukemia. N Engl J Med 1986 (315):15-24

16 Fialkow PJ, Gartler SM, Yoshida A: Clonal origin of chronic myelocytic leukemia in man. Proc Natl Acad Sci USA 1967 (58): 1468-1471

17 Fialkow PJ, Jacobson RJ, Papayannopoulou T: Chronic myelocytic leukemia: clonal origin in a stem cell common to the granulocyte, erythrocyte, platelet and macrophage/monocyte. Am J Med 1977 (63):125-131

18 Fialkow PJ, Martin PJ, Najfeld V, Jacobson RJ, Hansen JA: Evidence for a multistep pathogenesis of chronic myelogenous leukemia. Blood 1981 (56):773-781

19 Adamson JW, Fialkow PJ, Murphy S, Prchal JE, Steinmann L: Polycythemia vera: stem cell and probable clonal origin of the disease. N Engl J Med 1976 (295):913-916

20 Jacobson RJ, Salo A, Fialkow PJ: Agnogenic myeloid metaplasia: a clonal proliferation of hematopoietic stem cells with secondary myelofibrosis. Blood 1978 (51):189-194

21 Abkowitz JL, Fialkow PJ, Niebrugge DJ, Rasskind WH, Adamson JA: Pancytopenia as a clonal disorder of a multipotent hematopoietic stem cell. J Clin Invest 1984 (73):258-261

22 Fialkow PJ, Singer JW, Adamson JW, Vaidya K, Dow LW, Ochs J, Moohr JW: Acute nonlymphocytic leukemia: heterogeneity of stem cell origin. Blood 1981 (57):1068-1073

23 Fialkow PJ, Singer JW, Raskind WH, Adamson JW, Jacobson RJ, Bernstein DI, Dow LD, Najfeld, V, Veith R: Clonal development, stem-cell differentiation and clinical remissions in acute nonlymphocytic leukemia. N Engl J Med 1987 (317):468-473

24 Prchal JF, Adamson JW, Murphy S, Steinman L, Fialkow PJ: Polycythemia vera: The in vitro response of normal and abnormal stem cell lines to erythropoietin. J Clin Invest 1978 (61):1044-1047

25 McCulloch EA, Till JE: Stem cells in normal early haemopoiesis and certain clonal haemopathies. In: Hoffbrandt AV, Brain MC and Hirsch J (eds) Recent Advances in Haematology. Churchill-Livingston, London-New York 1977 pp 85-110

26 Friend C, Scher W, Holland JG, Sato T: Hgb synthesis in murine virus-induced leukemic cells in vitro: stimulation of erythroid differentiation by DMSO. Proc Natl Acad Sci USA 1971 (68):378-382

27 TR Breitman, Collins SJ, Keene BR: Terminal differentiation of human promyelocytic leukemia cells in primary culture in response to retinoic acid. Blood 1981 (57):1000-1004

28 Lawrence JH, Conner K, Kelly MA, Haussler MR, Wallace P, Bagby GC, Jr: cis-Retinoic acid stimulates the clonal growth of some myeloid leukemia cells in vitro. Blood 1987 (69):302-307

29 Collins SJ, Ruscetii FW, Gallagher RE, Gallo RC : Terminal differentiation of human promyelocytic leukemia cells induced by dimethylsulphoxide and other polar compounds. Proc Natl Acad Sci USA 1978 (75):2458-2462

30 Collins SJ, Ruscetti FW, Gallagher RE, Gallo RC: Normal functional characteristics of cultured human promyelocytic leukemia cells (HL-60) after induction of differentiation by dimethylsulphoxide. J Exp Med 1979 (149):969-974

31 Breitman TR, Selonick SE, Collins SJ: Induction of differentiation of the human promyelocytic leukemia cell line (HL-60) by retinoic acid. Proc Natl Acad Sci USA 1980 (77):2936-2940

32 Sachs L: The molecular control of blood cell development. Science 1987 (238):1374-1379

33 Meng-er H, Yu-chen Y, Shu-rong C, Jin-ren C, Jia-Xiang L, Lin Z, Long-jun G, Zhen-yi W: Use of all-trans retinoic acid in the treatment of acute promyelocytic leukemia. Blood 1988 (27):567-572

34 Hoffman SJ, Robinson WA: Use of differentiation-inducing agents in the myelodysplastic syndrome and acute non-lymphocytic leukemia. Am J Hemat 1988 (28):124-127

35 Singer JW, Arlin ZA, V Najfeld, Adamson JA, Kempin SJ, Clarkson BD, Fialkow PJ: Restoration of nonclonal hematopoiesis in chronic myelogenous leukemia following a therapy-induced loss of the PH^1 chromosome. Blood 1980 (56):356-360

36 Jacobson RJ, Temple MJ, Singer JW, Powell J, Fialkow PJ: A clonal complete remission in a patient with acute myeloblastic leukemia originating in a multipotent stem cell. N Engl J Med 1984 (310):1513-1517

37 Raskind WH, Jacobson R, Murphy S, Adamson JW, Fialkow PJ: Evidence for the involvement of B lymphoid cells in polycythemia vera and essential thrombocythemia. J Clin Invest 1985 (75):1388-1390

38 Saiki R, Gelfand D, Stoffel S, Scharf S, Higuchi R, Horn G, Mullis K, Erlich H: Primer-directed amplification of DNA with a thermostable DNA polymerase. Science 1987 (239):487-491

39 Farr CJ, Saiki RK, Erlich HA, McCormick F, Marshall CJ: Analysis of ras gene mutations in acute myeloid leukemia by polymerase chain reaction and oligonucleotide probes. Proc Natl Acad Sci USA 1988 (85):1629-1633

40 Siminovitch L, McCulloch EA, Till JE: The distribution of colony-forming cells among spleen colonies. J Cell Comp Physiol 1963 (62):327-336

41 Korn AP, Henkelman RM, Ottensmeyer FP, Till JE: Investigations of a stochastic model of haemopoiesis. Exp Hemat 1973 (35b):1-14

42 Till JE, McCulloch EA, Siminovitch L: A stochastic model of stem cell proliferation, based on the growth of spleen colony forming cells. Proc Natl Acad Sci USA 1964 (51):29-36

43 Nakahata T, Gross AJ, Ogawa M: A stochastic model of self-renewal and commitment to differentiation of the primitive hemopoietic stem cells in culture. J Cell Physiol 1982 (113):455-458

44 Kobayashi T, Nakahata T: Stochastic model of mast cell proliferation in culture of murine peritoneal cells. J Cell Physiol 1989 (138):24-28

45 Trentin JJ: Influence of hematopoietic organ stroma (hematopoietic inductive microenvironments) on stem cell differentiation. In: Gordon AS (ed) Regulation of Hematopoiesis. Appleton, Century and Croft, New York 1970 pp 161-186

46 Gregory CJ, Henkelman RM: Relationships between early hemopoietic progenitor cells determined by correlation analysis of their numbers in individual spleen colonies. In: Baum SJ and Ledney GD (eds) Experimental Hematology Today. Springer-Verlag, New York, Heidelberg 1977 pp 93-101

47 Lan S, McCulloch EA, Till JE: Cytodifferentiation in the acute myeloblastic leukemias of man. JNCI 1978 (60):265-269

48 Goldwasser E: Erythropoietin and its mode of action. Blood Cells 1984 (10):147-162

49 Goldwasser E: Erythropoietin and the differentiation of red blood cells. Fed Proc 1976 (34):2285-2292

50 Park LS, Friend D, Gillis S, Urdal DL: Characterization of the cell surface receptor for a multi-lineage colony stimulating factor (CSF-2 alpha). J Biol Chem 1986 (261):205-210

51 Sorenson P, Farber NM, Kyrstal G: Identification of the interleukin-3 receptor using an iodinatable, cleavable, photo-reactive cross-linking agent. J Biol Chem 1986 (261):9094-9097

52 Sherr CJ, Rettenmier CW, Sacca R, Roussel MF, Look AT, Stanley ER: The c-fms proto-oncogene product is related to the receptor for the mononuclear phagocyte growth factor, CSF-1. Cell 1985 (41):665-676

53 Mufson RA, Gesner TG, Turner K, Norton C, Yang Y-C, Clark S: Characterization of IL-3 receptors on human acute myelogenous leukemia cell line KG-1. Blood 1987 (70 suppl 1)118a

54 Avalos BR, Hedzat C, Baldwin GC, Golde DW, Gason JC, DiPersio JF: Biological activities of human G-CSF and characterization of the human G-CSF receptor. Blood 1987 (70 suppl 1) 165a

55 Kelleher CA, Wong GG, Clark SC, Schendel PF, Minden MD, McCulloch EA: Binding of iodinated recombinant human GM-CSF to the blast cells of acute myeloblastic leukemia. Leukemia 1988 (2):211-215

56 Gasson JC, Kaufman SE, Weisbart RH, Tomonaga M, Golde DW: High-affinity binding of granulocyte-macrophage colony-stimulating factor to normal and leukemic human myeloid cells. Proc Natl Acad Sci USA 1986 (83):669-673

57 Fraser JK, Lin F-K, Berridge MV: Expression and modulation of specific high affinity binding sites for erythropoeitin on the human erythroleukemic cell line K562. Blood 1988 (71):104-109

58 DiPersio J, Billing P, Kaufman S, Eghtesady P, Williams RE, Gasson JC: Characterization of the human granulocyte-macrophage colony-stimulating factor receptor. J Biol Chem 1988 (263):1834-1841

59 Park LS, Friend D, Gillis S, Urdal DL: Characterization of the cell surface receptor for human granulocyte/macrophage colony-stimulating factor receptor. J Exp Med 1986 (164):251-262

60 Dower SK, Kronheim SR, Hopp TP, Cantrell M, Deely M, Gillis S, Henney CS, Urdal DI: The cell surface receptors for Interleukin-1 alpha and interleukin-1 beta are identical. Nature 1986 (324):266-268

61 Sawada K, Krantz SB, Sawyer ST, Civin CI: Quantitation of specific binding of erythropoietin to human erythroid colony-forming cells. J Cell Physiol 1988 (137):337-345

62 Sawyer ST, Krantz SB, Luna J: Identification of the receptor for erythropoietin by cross-linking to Friend virus-infected erythroid cells. Proc Natl Acad Sci USA 1987 (84):3690-3694

63 Gilman AG: G proteins: transducers of receptor-generated signals. Ann Rev Biochem 1987 (56):615-649

64 Majerus PW, Connolly TM, Deckmyn H, Ross TS, Bross TE, Ishii H, Bansal VS, Wilson DB: The metabolism of phosphoinositide-derived messenger molecules. Science 1987 (234):1519-1526

65 Sibley DR, Benovic JL, Caron MG, Lefkowitz RJ: Regulation of transmembrane signalling by receptor phosphorylation. Cell 1987 (48):913-922

66 Kelly K, Cochran B, Stiles CD, Leder P: Cell-specific growth regulation of the c-myc gene by lymphocyte mitogens and platelet-derived growth factor. Cell 1983 (35):603-610

67 Greenberg ME, Ziff EB: Stimulation of 3T3 cells induces transcription of c-fos proto-oncogene. Nature 1984 (311):433-438

68 Thompson CB, Challoner PB, Neiman PE, Groudine M: Expression of the c-myb proto-oncogene during cellular proliferation. Nature 1986 (319):374-380

69 Reich NE, Levine AJ : Growth regulation of a cellular tumor antigen p^{53} in non-transformed cells. Nature 1984 (308):199-201

70 Ryder K, Lau LF, Nathans D: A gene activated by growth factors is related to the oncogene v-jun. Proc Natl Acad Sci USA 1988 (85):1487-1491

71 Gewirtz AM, Calabretta B: A c-myb antisense oligonucleotide inhibits normal human hematopoiesis in vitro. Science 1988 (242):1303-1306

72 Minghetti PP, Norman AW: 1,25$(OH)_2$-vitamin D_3 receptors: gene regulation and genetic circuitry. FASEB Journal 1988 (2):3043-3053

73 Beato M: Gene regulation by steroid hormones. Cell 1989 (56):335-344

74 Arriza JL, Weinberger C, Cereli G, Glaser TM, Handelin BL, Housman DE: Cloning of human mineralocorticoid receptor complementary DNA: structural and functional kinship with the glucocorticoid receptor. Science 1987 (238):268-275

75 Meisfeld R, Okret S, Wilstrom A-C, Wrange O, Gustafsson J-A, Yamamoto KR: Characterization of a steroid hormone receptor gene and mRNA in wild-type and mutant cells. Nature 1984 (312):779-781

76 Sap J, Munoz A, Damm K, Goldberg Y, Ghysdael J, Leutz A, Beug H, Vennstrom B: The c-erb-A protein is a high-affinity receptor for thyroid hormone. Nature 1986 (324):635-640

77 Weinberger C, Thompson C, Ong ES, Lebo R, Gruol DJ, Evans RM: The c-erb-A gene encodes a thyroid hormone receptor. Nature 1986 (324):641-646

78 Giguere V, Ong ES, Segui P, Evans RM: Identification of a receptor for the morphogen retinoic acid. Nature 1987 (330):624-629

79 Petkovitch M, Brand NJ, Krust A, Chambon P: A human retinoic acid receptor which belongs to the family of nuclear receptors. Nature 1987 (330):444-450

80 Brand N, Petkovich M, Krust A, Chambon P, de The H, Marchinol A, Tiollais P, Dejean A: Identification of a second human retinoic acid receptor. Nature 1988 (332):850-853

81 Benbrook D, Lernhardt E, Pfahl M: A new retinoic acid receptor identified from a hepatocellular carcinoma. Nature 1988 (333):669-672

82 de The H, Marchio A, Tiollais P, Dejean A: Differential expression and ligand regulation of the retinoic acid receptor alpha and beta genes. Embo J 1989 (8):429-433

83 Wang C, Curtis JE, Minden MD, McCulloch EA: Expression of a retinoic acid receptor gene in myeloid leukemia cells. Leukemia 1989 (3):264-269

84 McCulloch EA, Siminovitch L, Till JE: Spleen colony formation in anemic mice of genotype W/W^{v}. Science 1964 (144):844-846

85 Sutherland DJA, Till JE, McCulloch EA: A kinetic study of the genetic control of hemopoietic progenitor cells assayed in culture and in vivo. J Cell Physiol 1970 (75):267-274

86 McCulloch EA, Russell ES, Siminovitch L, Till JE, Bernstein SE: The cellular basis of the genetically determined hemopoietic defect in anemic mice of genotype S1/S1^{d}. Blood 1965 (26):399-410

87 Geissler EN, Ryan MA, Housman DE: The dominant white-spotting (W) locus of the mouse encodes the c-kit proto-oncogene. Cell 1988 (55):185-192

88 Chabot B, Stephenson DA, Chapman VM, Besner P, Bernstein A: The proto-oncogene c-kit encoding a transmembrane tyrosine kinase receptor maps to the mouse W locus. Nature 1988 (335):88-89

89 Yarden Y, Kuang W-J, Yang-Feng T, Coussens L, Mumenitsu S, Dull, TJ, Chen E, Schlesinger J, Francke U, Ullrich A: Human proto-oncogene c- kit: a new cell surface receptor tyrosine kinase for an unidentified ligand. Embo J 1987 (6):3341-3351

90 Qiu F, Ray P, Brown K, Barker PE, Jhanwar S, Ruddle FH, Besner P: Primary structure of c-kit: relationship with the CSF-1/PDGF receptor kinase family - oncogenic activation of v-kit involves deletion of extracellular domain and C terminus. Embo J 1988 (7):1003-1011

91 Bernstein SE: Tissue transplantation as an analytic and therapeutic tool in hereditary anemias. Am J Surg 1970 (119):448-451

92 Gordon MY, Riley GP, Watt SM, Greaves MF: Compartmentalization of a haemopoietic growth factor (GM-CSF) by glycosaminoglycans in bone marrow microenvironment. Nature 1987 (326):403-405

93 Roberts R, Gallagher J, Spooner E, Allen TD, Bloomfield F, Dexter TM: Heparin sulphate bound growth factors: a mechanism for stromal cell mediated haemopoiesis. Nature 1988 (332):332-378

94 Marshall CJ: Oncogenes and growth control 1987. Cell 1987 (49):723-725

95 Metcalf D: The Hemopoietic Colony-Stimulating Factors. Elsvier, Amsterdam 1984

96 Metcalf D: The molecular biology and functions of the granulocyte-macrophage colony-stimulating factors. Blood 1986 (67):257-267

97 Clark SC, Kamen R: The human hematopoietic colony-stimulating factors. Science 1987 (236):1229-1237

98 Fung MC, Hapel AJ, Ymer S, Cohen DR, Johnson RM, Campbell HD, Young IG: Molecular cloning of cDNA for murine interleukin-3. Nature 1984 (307):233-237

99 Messner HA, Yamasak K, Jamal N, Minden MD, Wong GG, Clark SC: Growth of human hemopoietic colonies in response to recombinant gibbon interleukin-3: comparison with human recombinant granulocyte-macrophage colony-stimulating factor (GM-CSF). Proc Natl Acad Sci USA 1987 (84):1-5

100 Sieff CA, Emerson SG, Donahue RE, Nathan DG, Wang EA, Wong GG, Clark SC: Human recombinant granulocyte-macrophage colony-stimulating factor: a multilineage hematoprotein. Science 1985 (230):1171-1173

101 Gough NM, Gough J, Metcalf D, Kelso A, Grail D, Nicola N, Burgess AW, Dunn AR: Molecular cloning of cDNA encoding a murine hematopoietic growth regulator, granulocyte-macrophage colony stimulating factor. Nature 1984 (309):763-767

102 Stanley E, Metcalf D, Sobieszczuk P, Gough NM, Dunn AR: The structure and expression of the murine gene encoding granulocyte-macrophage stimulating factor: evidence for utilization of alternative promotors. Embo J 1985 (4):2569-2573

103 Weisbart RH, Kwan L, Golde DW, Gasson JC: Human GM-CSF primes neutrophils for enhanced oxidative metabolism in response to major physiological chemoattractants. Blood 1987 (69):18-21

104 Weisbart RH, Golde DW, Clark SC, Wong GG, Gasson J: Human granulocyte-macrophage colony-stimulating factor is a neutrophil activator. Nature 1985 (314):361-363
105 Yuo A, Kitagawa S, Okabe T, Urabe A, Komatsu Y, Itoh S, Takaku F: Recombinant human granulocyte colony-stimulating factor repairs the abnormalities of neutrophils in patients with myelodysplastic syndromes and chronic myelogenous leukemia. Blood 1987 (70):404-411
106 Lin FK, Suggu S, Lin CH, Browne JK, Smalling R, Egrie JC, Chen KK, Fox GM, Martin F, Stabinsky Z, Badrawi SM, Lai PH, Goldwasser E: Cloning and expression of the human erythropoietin gene. Proc Natl Acad Sci USA 1985 (82):7580-7584
107 Stanley ER, Guilbert LJ, Tushinski RJ, Bartelmez SH: CSF-1: a mononuclear phagocyte lineage-specific hemopoietic growth factor. Cell Biochem 1983 (21):151-159
108 Das SK, Stanley ER: Structure-funtion studies of a colony stimulating factor (CSF-1). J Biol Chem 1982 (257):13679-13684
109 Wong GG, Temple PA, Leary A, Witek-Giannotti JS, Yang Y, Ciarletta AB, Chung M, Murtha P, Kritz R, Kaufman RJ, Ferenz CR, Sibley BS, Turner KJ, Hewick RM, Clark SC, Yanai N, Yokota H, Yamada M: Human CSF-1: Molecular cloning and expression of 4-kb cDNA encoding the human urinary protein. Science 1987 (235):1504-1508
110 Nicola NA, Metcalf D, Matsumo M, Johnston GR: Purification of a factor inducing differentiation in murine myelomonocytic leukemia cells. Identification as granulocyte-colony-stimulating factor. J Biol Chem 1983 (258):9017-9023
111 Souza LM, Boone TC, Gabrilove J, Lai PH, Zsebo KM, Murdock DC, Chazin VR, Bruszewski J, Lu H, Chen KK, Barendt J, Platzer E, Moore MAS, Mertelsmann R, Welte K: Recombinant human granulocyte colony-stimulating factor: effects on normal and leukemic myeloid cells. Science 1986 (232):61-65
112 Nagata S, Tsuchiya M, Asano S, Kaziro Y, Yamazaki T, Yamamoto O, Hirata Y, Kubota, N, Oheda M, Nomura,H, Ono M: Molecular cloning and expression of cDNA for human granulocyte colony-stimulating factor. Nature 1986 (319):415-417
113 Nagata S, Tsuchiya T, Asano S, Yamamoto O, Hirata Y, Kubota N, Yasmazaki T: The chromosome gene structure and two mRNAs for human granulocyte colony-stimulating factor. Embo J 1986 (5):575-581
114 Jubinsky PT, Stanley ER: Purification of hemopoietin 1: A multilineage hemopoietic growth factor. Proc Natl Acad Sci USA 1985 (82):2764-2768
115 Bartelmez SH, Stanley ER: Synergism between hemopoietic growth factors (HGFs) detected by their effects on cells bearing receptors for a lineage specific HGF: assay of hemopoietin-1. J Cell Physiol 1985 (122):370-378
116 Mochizuki DY, Eisenman JR, Conlon PJ, Larsen AD, Tushinski RJ: Interleukin-1 regulates hematopoietic activity, a role previously ascribed to hemopoietin-1. Proc Natl Acad Sci 1987 (84):5267-5271
117 Zucali JR, Dinarello CA, Oblon DJ, Gross MA, Anderson L, Weiner RS: Interleukin 1 stimulates fibroblasts to produce granulocyte-macrophage colony stimulating activity (GM-CSA) and prostoglandin E2 (PGE2). J Clin Invest 1986 (77):1857-1863
118 Broudy VC, Kaushansky K, Harlan JM, Adamson JW: Interleukin-1 stimulates human endothelial cells to produce granulocyte-macrophage colony-stimulating factor and granulocyte colony-stimulating factor. J Immunol 1987 (139):464-468
119 Warren DJ, Moore MAS: Synergism among interleukin-1, interleukin-3 and interleukin-5 in the production of eosinophils from primitive hemopoietic stem cells. J Immunol 1988 (140):94-99
120 Lee F, Yokota T, Otsuka T, Meyerson P, Villaret D, Coffman R, Mosman T, Rennick D, Roehm N, Smith C, Zlotnick A, Arai K-I: Isolation and characterization of a mouse interleukin cDNA clone that expresses BSF-1 activities and T cell and mast cell stimulating activities. Proc Natl Acad Sci USA 1986 (83):2061-2065
121 O'Garra A, Warren DJ, Holman M, Popham AM, Sanderson CJ, Klaus GBB: Interleukin 4 (B-cell growth factorII/eosinophil differentiation factor) is a mitogen and differentiation factor for preactivated murine B lymphocytes. Proc Natl Acad Sci USA 1986 (83):5228-5232
122 Rennick D, Yang G, Muller-Sieburg C, Smith C, Arai N, Takabe Y, Gemmell L: Interleukin 4 (B-cell stimulatory factor 1) can enhance or anatagonize the factor dependent growth of hemopoietic progenitor cells. Proc Natl Acad Sci USA 1987 (84):6889-6893
123 Hamaguchi Y, Kanakura Y, Fujita J, Takeda S, Nakano T, Tarui S, Honjo T, Kitamura Y: Interleukin 4 as an essential factor for in vitro clonal growth of murine connective tissue-type mast cells. J Exp Med 1987 (165):268-273
124 Campbell HD, Tucker WQJ, Hort Y, Martinson ME, Mayo G, Clutterbuck EJ, Sanderson CJ, Young

IG: Molecular cloning, nucleotide sequence, and expression of the gene encoding human eosinophil differentiation factor (interleukin 5). Proc Natl Acad Sci USA 1987 (84):6629-6633

125 Garman RD, Jacobs KA, Clark SC, Raulet DH: B-cell-stimulatory factor 2 (beta 2 interferon) functions as a second signal for interleukin 2 production by mature murine T cells. Proc Natl Acad Sci USA 1987 (84):7629-7633

126 Ikebuchi K, Wong GG, Clark SC, Ihle JN, Hirai Y, Ogawa M: Interleukin 6 enhancement of interleukin 3-dependent proliferation of multipotential hemopoietic progenitors. Proc Natl Acad Sci USA 1987 (84):9035-9039

127 Ogawa M, Clark SC: Synergistic interaction between interleukin-6 and interleukin-3 in support of stem cell proliferation in culture. Blood Cells 1988 (14):329-337

128 Caracciolo D, Clark SC, Rovera G: Human interleukin-6 supports granulocytic differentiation of hemopoietic progenitor cells and acts synergistically with GM-CSF. Blood 1989 (73):666-670

129 Morgan DA, Ruscetti FW, Gallo RC: Selective in vitro growth of T lymphocytes from normal human bone marrow. Science 1976 (193):1002-1008

130 Makovsky M, Loveland B, North M, Sherto GL, Gao L, Ward P, Fiers W: Recombinant interleukin-2 directly augments the cytotoxicity of human monocytes. Nature 1987 (325):262-265

131 Bussolino F, Wang MJ, Defilipi P, Turrini F, Sanovio F, Edgell C-JS, Aglietti M, Arese P, Mantovani A: Granulocyte- and granulocyte-macrophage-colony stimulating factors induce human endothelial cells to migrate and proliferate. Nature 1989 (337):471-473

132 Brinster RL, Chen HV, Trumbauer ME, Yagle MK, Palmiter RD: Factors effecting the efficiency of introducing foreign DNA into mice by microinjecting eggs. Proc Natl Acad Sci USA 1985 (82):4438-4442

133 Lang RA, Metcalf D, Cuthbertson RA, Lyons I, Stanley, E, Kelso A, Kannourakis G, Williamson DJ, Klintworth GK, Gonda TJ, Dunn, AR: Transgenic mice expressing a hemopoietic growth factor (GM-CSF) develop accumulations of macrophages, blindness and a fatal syndrome of tissue damage. Cell 1987 (51):675-686

134 Johnson GR, Gonda TJ, Metcalf D, Hariharan IK, Cory S: A lethal myeloproliferative syndrome in mice transplanted with bone marrow cells infected with a retrovirus expressing granulocyte-macrophage colony stimulating factor. Embo J 1989 (8):335-341

135 Chang JM, Metcalf D, Lang RA, Gonda TJ, Johnson GR: Non-neoplastic hemopoietic myeloproliferative syndrome induced by dysregulated Multi-CSF (IL-3) expression. Blood 1989 (73):1487-1497

136 Donahue RE, Wang EA, Stone DK, Kamen R, Wong GG, Sehgal PK, Nathan DG, Clark SC: Stimulation of haematopoiesis in primates by continuous infusion of recombinant GM-CSF. Nature 1986 (321):872-875

137 Welte K, Bonilla MA, Gillo AP, Boone TC, Potter GK, Gabrilove JL, Moore MAS, O'Reilly RJ, Souza LM: Recombinant human granulocyte colony-stimulating factor: effects on hematopoiesis in normal and cyclophosphamide-treated primates. J Exp Med 1987 (165):941-948

138 Monroy RL, Skelly RR, Taylor P, Dubois A, Donnahue RE, Macvittie TJ: Recovery of severe hematopoietic suppression using recombinant human granulocyte-macrophage colony-stimulating factor. Exp Hematol 1988 (16):344-348

139 Donahue RE, Seehra J, Metzger M, Lefebvre D, Rock B, Carbone S, Nathan DG, Garnick M, Sehgal PK, Laston D, Lavallie E, McCoy J, Schendel PF, Norton C, Turner K, Yang Y, Clark SC: Human Il-3 and GM-CSF act synergistically in stimulating hematopoiesis in primates. Science 1988 (241):1820-1823

140 Eschbach JW, Egrie JC, Downing MR, Browne JK, Adamson JW: Correction of the anemia of end-stage renal disease with recombinant human erythropoietin. N Engl J Med 1987 (316):73-78

141 Vadhan-Raj S, Keating M, LeMaistre A, Hittleman WN, McCredie K, Trujillo JM, Broxmeyer HE, Henney C, Gutterman JU: Effects of recombinant human granulocyte-macrophage colony-stimulating factor in patients with myelodysplastic syndromes. N Engl J Med 1987 (25):1545-1552

142 Gabrilove J, Jakubowsk A, Sher H, Sternberg C, Wong G, Grous J, Yagoda A, Fain K, Moore MAS, Clarkson B, Oettegen HF, Alton K, Welte K, Sousa L: Effect of granulocyte colony-stimulating factor on neutropenia and associated morbidity due to chemotherapy for transition cell carcinoma of the urothelium. N Engl J Med 1988 (318):1414-1422

143 Ganser A, Volkers B, Greher J, Ottmann OG, Walther F, Becker R, Bergmann L, Schutz G, Hoelzer D: Recombinant human granulocyte-macrophage colony-stimulating factor in patients with myelodysplastic syndromes - a phase I/II trial. Blood 1989 (73):31-37

144 Groopman JE, Mitysyasu RT, Deleo MJ, Oette DH, Golde DW: Effect of recombinant human

granulocyte-macrophage colony-stimulating factor on myelopoiesis in the acquired immunodeficiency syndrome. N Engl J Med 1987 (317):593-598
145 Kamel-Reid S, Dick JE: Engraftment of immune-deficient mice with human hematopoietic stem cells. Nature 1988 (242):1706-1709
146 McCulloch EA: Stem cells in normal and leukemic hemopoiesis (Henry Stratton Lecture 1982). Blood 1983 (62):1-13
147 Griffin JD, Lowenberg B: Clonogenic cells in acute myeloblastic leukemia. Blood 1986 (68):1185-1195
148 Minden MD, Buick RN, McCulloch EA: Separation of blast cell and T-lymphocyte progenitors in the blood of patients with acute myeloblastic leukemia. Blood 1979 (54):186-195
149 Buick RN, Till JE, McCulloch EA: Colony assay for proliferative blast cells circulating in myeloblastic leukaemia. Lancet 1977 (1):862-863
150 Buick RN, Minden MD, McCulloch EA: Self-renewal in culture of proliferative blast progenitor cells in acute myeloblastic leukemia. Blood 1979 (54):95-104
151 McCulloch EA, Till JE: Blast cells in acute myeloblastic leukemia: A model. Blood Cells 1981 (7):63-77
152 McCulloch EA, Curtis JE, Messner HA, Senn JS, Germanson TP: The contribution of blast cell properties to outcome variation in acute myeloblastic leukemia (AML). Blood 1982 (59):601-608
153 Curtis JE, Messner HA, Hasselback R, Elhakim TM, McCulloch EA: Contributions of host- and disease-related attributes to the outcome of patients with acute myelogeneous leukemia (AML). J Clin Oncol 1984 (2):253-259
154 Nara N, Nagata SK, Yamashita Y, Murohashi I, Adachi Y: Relationship between in in vitro sensitivity to cytosine arabinoside of blast progenitors and the outcome of treatment in acute myeloblastic leukemia. Br J Haematol 1988 (70):187-191
155 Aye MT, Niho Y, Till JE, McCulloch EA: Studies of leukemic cell populations in culture. Blood 1974 (44):205-219
156 McCulloch EA, Till JE: Interacting cell populations in cultures of leukocytes from normal or leukemic peripheral blood. Blood 1977 (49):269-280
157 Nara N, McCulloch EA: The proliferation in suspension of the progenitors of the blast cells in acute myeloblastic leukemia. Blood 1985 (65):1484-1493
158 Lange B, Valierie M, Santoli D, Caracciola D, Mavillo F, Gemperlein I, Griffin C, Emanuel B, Nowell P, Rovera G: Growth factor requirements of childhood acute leukemia: establishment of GM-CSF-dependent cell lines. Blood 1897 (70):192-199
159 Miyauchi J, Kelleher CA, Wang C, Minkin S, McCulloch EA: Growth factors influence the sensitivity of leukemic stem cells to cytosine arabinoside in culture. Blood, 1989 (73):1272-1278
160 Langley GR, Smith LJ, McCulloch EA: Adherent cells in cultures of blast progenitors in acute myeloblastic leukemia. Leukemia Res 1986 (10):953-959
161 Minden MD, Major P, Wu A, Kufe DW: Generation time of leukemic blast progenitor cells. Cell Tissue Kinet 1981 (16):577-582
162 Hoang T, McCulloch EA: Production of leukemic blast growth factor by a human bladder carcinoma cell line. Blood 1985 (66):748-751
163 Chambers JM, Cleveland WS, Kleiner B, Tukey PA: Graphical Methods for Data Analysis. Duxbury Press, Boston 1983
164 Sachs L: Control of normal cell differentiation in the phenotypic reversion of malignancy in myeloid leukemia. Nature 1978 (274):535-539
165 Nicola NA, Metcalf D: Binding of the differentiation-inducer, granulocyte-colony-stimulating factor, to responsive but not unresponsive leukemic cell lines. Proc Natl Acad Sci USA 1984 (81):3765-3769
166 Griffin JD, Sullivan R, Beveridge RP, Lacom P, Schlossman SF: Induction of proliferation of purified human myeloid progenitor cells. A rapid assay for granulocyte colony-stimulating factors. Blood 1984 (63):904-911
167 Gearing DP, Gough NM, King JA, Hilton DJ, Nicola NA, Simpson RJ, Nice EC, Kelso A, Metcalf D: Molecular cloning and expression of cDNA encoding a murine myeloid leukaemia inhibitory factor (LIF). Embo J 1987 (6):3995-4002
168 Williams RL, Hilton DJ, Pease S, Wilson TA, Stewart CL, Gearing DP, Wagner EF, Metcalf D, Nicola NA, Gough NM: Myeloid leukaemia inhibitory factory maintains developmental potential of embryonic stem cells. Nature 1988 (336):684-687
169 Smith AG, Heath JK, Donaldson DD, Wong GG, Moreau J, Stahl M, Rogers D: Inhibition of pluripotential embryonic stem cell differentiation by purified polypeptides. Nature 1988 (336):688-690
170 Moreau J-F, Donaldson DD, Bennet F, Witek-Gianotti J, Clark SC, Wong GG: Leukaemia inhibitory factor is identical to the myeloid growth factor human interleukin for DA cells. Nature 1988 (336):690-692

171 Miyauchi J, Kelleher C, Yang Y-C, Wong GC, Clark SC, Minden MD, Minkin S, McCulloch EA: The effects of three recombinant growth factors, IL-3, GM-CSF and G-CSF, on the blast cells of acute myeloblastic leukemia maintained in short term suspension culture. Blood 1987 (70):657-663

172 Delwel R, Dorssers L, Touw I, Wagemaker ER, Lowenberg B: Human recombinant multilineage colony stimulating factor (Interleukin-3): stimulator of acute myelocytic leukemia progenitor cells in vitro. Blood 1987 (70):333-336

173 Hoang T, Nara N, Wong G, Clark S, Minden MD, McCulloch EA: The effects of recombinant GM-CSF on the blast cells of acute myeloblastic leukemia. Blood 1986 (67):313-316

174 Griffin JD, Young D, Herrman F, Wiper D, Wagner K, Sabbath DK: Effects of recombinant GM-CSF on the proliferation of clonogenic cells in acute myeloblastic leukemia. Blood 1986 (67):1448-1453

175 Vellenga E, Young DC, Wagner K, Wiper D, Otapovicz D, Griffin JD: The effects of GM-CSF and G-CSF in promoting growth of clonogenic cells in acute myeloblastic leukemia. Blood 1987 (69):1771-1776

176 Nara N, Murohashi I, Suzuki T, Yamashita Y, Maruyama Y, Aoki N, Tanikawa S: Effects of recombinant human granulocyte colony-stimulating factor (G-CSF) on blast progenitors from acute myeloblastic leukaemia patients. Br J Cancer 1987 (56):49-51

177 Miyauchi J, Wang C, Kelleher CA, Wong GG, Clark SC, Minden MD, McCulloch EA: The effects of recombinant CSF-1 on the blast cells of acute myeloblastic leukemia in suspension culture. J Cell Physiol 1988 (135):55-62

178 Suzuki T, Nagata K, Murohashi I, Nara N: Effect or recombinant human CSF-1 on the proliferation of leukemic blast progenitors in AML patients. Leukemia 1988 (2):358-362

179 Tessier T, Hoang T: Transforming growth factor beta inhibits proliferation of the blast cells of acute myeloblastic leukemia. Blood 1988 (72):159-164

180 Beran M, McCredie KB, Keating MJ, Gutterman JU: Antileukemic effect of recombinant tumor necrosis factor alpha in vitro and its modulation by alpha and gamma interferons. Blood 1988 (72):728-738

181 Kelleher C, Miyauchi J, Wong G, Clark S, Minden MD, McCulloch EA: Synergism between recombinant growth factors, GM-CSF and G-CSF, acting on the blast cells of acute myeloblastic leukemia. Blood 1987 (69): 1498-1503

182 Hoang T, Haman A, Goncalves O, Wong GG, Clark SC: Interleukin-6 enhances growth factor-dependent proliferation of the blast cells of acute myeloblastic leukemia. Blood 1988 (72):823-826

183 Miyauchi J, Kelleher CA, Wong GG, Yang Y-C, Clark SC, Minkin S, Minden MD, McCulloch EA: The effects of combinations of the recombinant growth factors GM-CSF, G-CSF, IL-3 and CSF-1 on leukemic blast cells in suspension culture. Leukemia 1988 (2):382-387

184 Sporn MB, Roberts AB: Autocrine growth factors and cancer. Nature 1985 (313):745-747

185 Lang RA, Metcalf D, Gough NM, Dunn AR, Gonda TJ: Expression of a hematopoietic growth factor cDNA in a factor-dependent cell line results in autonomous growth and tumorigenicity. Cell 1985 (43):531-542

186 Hapel AJ, Vande Woude G, Campbell HD, Young IG, Robbins T: Generation of an autocrine leukemia using a retroviral expression vector carrying the interleukin-3 gene. Lymphokine Res 1986 (5):249-254

187 Young DC, Griffin JD: Autocrine secretion of GM-CSF in acute myeloblastic leukemia. Blood 1986 (68):1178-1181

188 Young DC, Wagner K, Griffin JD: Constitutive expression of the granulocyte-macrophage colony-stimulating factor gene in acute myeloblastic leukemia. J Clin Invest 1987 (79):100-106

189 Cheng GYM, Kelleher CA, Miyauchi J, Wang C, Wong G, Clark S, McCulloch EA, Minden MD: Structure and expression of genes of GM-CSF and G-CSF in blast cells from patients with Acute Myeloblastic Leukemia. Blood 987 (71):204-208

190 Young DC, Demetri GD, Ernst TJ, Cannistra SA, Griffin JD: In vitro expression of colony-stimulating factor genes in human acute myeloblastic leukemia cells. Exp Hematol 1988 (16):378-382

191 Wang C, Kelleher CA, Cheng GYM, Miyauchi J, Wong GG, Clark SC, Minden MD, McCulloch EA: Expression of the CSF-1 gene in the blast cells of acute myeloblastic leukemia: Association with reduced growth capacity. J Cell Physiol 1988 (135):133-138

192 Greaves MF: "Target" cells, cellular phenotypes, and lineage fidelity in human leukaemia. J Cell Physiol 1982 (111 Suppl 1):113-125

193 Seligmann M, Vogler LB, Preud'Homme JL, Guglielmi P, Brouet JC: Immunological phenotypes of human leukemias of the B-cell lineage. Blood Cells 1981 (7):237-246

194 Hurwitz CA, Loken MR, Graham ML, Karp JE, Borowitz MJ, Pullen DJ, Civin CI: Asynchronous antigen expression in B lineage acute lymphoblastic leukemia. Blood 1988 (72):299-307
195 Fioritoni G, Bertolini L, Revoltella R: Cytochemical characteristics of leukopoietic differentiation in murine erythroleukemic (Friend) cells. Cancer Res 1980 (40):866-872
196 Marie JP, Izaguirre CA, Civin CI, Mirro J, McCulloch EA: The presence within single K-562 cells of erythropoietic and granulopoietic differentiation markers. Blood 1981 (58):708-711
197 McCulloch EA, Smith LJ, Minden MD: Normal and malignant haemopoietic clones in man. Cancer Surv 1982 (1):279-298
198 Smith LJ, Curtis JE, Messner HA, Senn JS, Furthmayr H, McCulloch EA: Lineage infidelity in acute leukemia. Blood 1983 (61):1138-1145
199 Mirro J, Antoun GR, Zipf TF, Melvin S, Stass S: The E rosette-associated antigen of T cells can be identified on blasts from patients with acute myeloblastic leukemia. Blood 1985 (65):363-367
200 Neame PB, Soamboonsrup P, Browman G, Barr, RD, Saeed N, Chan, BB, Berger A, Wilso, WEC, Walker IR, McBride JA: Simultaneous sequential expression of lymphoid and myeloid phenotypes in acute leukemia. Blood 1985 (65):142-148
201 Lanham G, Bollum FJ, Williams DL, Stass SA: Simultaneous occurrence of terminal deoxynucleotidyl transferase and myeloperoxidase in individual leukemic blasts. Blood 1984 (64):318-320
202 Cheng GYM, Minden MD, Toyonaga B, Mak TW, McCulloch EA: T-cell receptor and immunoglobulin gene rearrangements in acute myeloblastic leukemia. J Exp Med 1986 (65):894-901
203 Norton JD, Campana D, Hoffbrand AV, Janossy G, Coustan-Smith E, Jan H, Yaxley JC, Prentice HG: Rearrangement of immunoglobulin and T cell antigen receptor genes in acute myeloblastic leukemia with lymphoid- associated markers. Leukemia 1987 (1):757-761
204 Ackland SP, Westbrook CA, Diaz MO, Le Beau MM, Rowley JD: Evidence favoring lineage fidelity in Acute Nonlymphocytic Leukemia: absence of immunoglobulin gene rearrangements in FAB types M4 and M5. Blood 1987 (69):87-89
205 Klinken SP, Alexander WS, Adams JM: Hemopoietic lineage switch: v-raf oncogene converts Emu-transgenic B cells into macrophages. Cell 1988 (53):857-867
206 Gerhartz HH, Bartram CR, Raghavachar A, Schmetzer H, Clemm C, Wilmanns W, Thiel E: Spontaneous Epsein-Barr transformed B cell line sharing the identical immunoglobulin gene rearrangement with acute myeloid leukemia. Blood 1989 (73):684-687
207 Greaves MF, Chan LC, Furley AJW, Watt SM, Molgaard HV: Lineage promiscuity in hemopoietic differentiation and leukemia. Blood 1986 (67):1-11
208 Spangrude GJ, Heimfeld S, Weissman IL: Purification and characterization of murine hemopoietic stem cells. Science 1988 (241):58-62
209 Muller-Sieburg CE, Townsend K, Weissman IL, Rennick D: Proliferation and differentiation of highly enriched mouse hematopoietic stem cells and progenitor cells in response to defined growth factors. J Exp Med 1988 (167):1825-1840
210 Preisler H, Davis RB, Kirshner J, Dupre E, Richards F,III, Hoagland C, Kopel, S, Levy RN, Carey R, Schulman P, Gottlieb AJ, McIntyre OR (Cancer and Leukemia Group B): Comparison of three remission induction regimens and two postinduction strategies for the treatment of acute nonlymphoblastic leukemia: a Cancer and Leukemia Group B study. Blood 1987 (69):1441-1449
211 Curtis JE, Messner HA, Minden MD, Minkin S, McCulloch EA: High dose cytosine arabinoside in the treatment of acute myeloblastic leukemia: Contributions to outcome of clinical and laboratory attributes. J Clin Oncol 1987 (5):532-543
212 Curtis JE, Till JE, Messner HA, Sousan P, McCulloch EA: Comparison of outcomes and prognostic factors for two groups of patients with acute myeloblastic leukemia. Leuk Res 1979 (3):409-416
213 McCulloch EA, Kelleher CA, Miyauchi J, Wang C, Cheng GYN, Minden MD, Curtis JE : Heterogeneity in acute myeloblastic leukemia. Leukemia Supplement 1988 (2):38S-49S
214 Bruce WR, Valeriote FA : Normal and malignant stem cells and chemotherapy. In: The Proliferation and Spread of Neoplastic Cells. M.D. Anderson Annual Symposium on Fundamental Cancer Research. Williams and Wilkins Co, Baltimore 1967 pp 409-420
215 Saunders EF, Lampkin BC, Mauer AM: Variation of proliferative activity in leukemic cell populations of patients with acute leukemia. J Clin Invest (46):1356-1363
216 Saunders EF, Mauer EM: Re-entry of non-dividing cells into a proliferative phase in acute childhood leukemia. J Clin Invest 1969 (48):1299-1305
217 Minden MD, Till JE, McCulloch EA: Proliferative state of blast cell progenitor in acute myeloblastic leukemia. Blood 1978 (52):592-600

218 Niho Y, Till JE, McCulloch EA: Effect of arabinosyl cytosine on granulopoietic colony formation by marrow cells from leukemic and non-leukemic patients. Exp Hematol 1976 (4):63-69

219 Buick RN, Messner HA, Till JE, McCulloch EA: Cytotoxicity of adriamycin and daunorubicin for normal and leukemic progenitor cells of man. JNCI 1979 (63):249-255

220 McCulloch EA: Experimental approaches to outcome prediction in acute myeloblastic leukemia. In: Hofman V, Berens ME and Martz G (eds) Predictive Tests for Hematological Malignancies. Recent Results in Cancer Research. Springer-Verlag, Heidelberg 1984 pp 76-92

221 Motoji T, Hoang T, Tritchler D, McCulloch EA: The effect of 5-azacytidine and its analogues on blast cell renewal in acute myeloblastic leukemia. Blood 1985 (65):894-901

222 Wang C, McCulloch EA: The sensitivity to 5-azacytidine of blast progenitors in acute myeloblastic leukemia. Blood 1987 (69):553-559

223 Nara N, Curtis JE, Senn JS, Tritchler DL, McCulloch EA: The sensitivity to cytosine arabinoside of the blast progenitors of acute myeloblastic leukemia. Blood 1986 (67):762-769

224 Nara N, Yamashita Y, Murohashi I, Tanikawa S, Imai Y, Aoki N: The effects on leukemic clonogenic cells in murine myeloid leukemia of 1-beta-D-Arabinofuranosylcytosine and the anthracyclines adriamycin, daunomycin, aclacinomycin and 4'-epidoxorubicin. Cancer Res 1987 (47):2376-2379

225 Myers CE: Anthracyclines. In: Chabner BA (ed) Pharmacological Principles of Cancer Treatment. WB Saunders Co, Philadelphia 1982 pp 416-434

226 Chabner BA: Cytosine arabinoside. In: Chabner BA (ed) Pharmacological Principles of Cancer Treatment. WB Saunders Co, Philadelphia 1982 pp 387-401

227 Riggs AD, PA Jones: 5-methylcytosine, gene regulation and cancer. Adv Cancer Res 1983 (40):1-25

228 Taylor SM, Jones PA: Multiple new phenotypes induced in 10 1/2 and 3T3 cells treated with 5-azacytidine. Cell 1979 (7):771-779

229 Salmon SE, Hamburger AW, Soehnlen B, Drurie BGM, Alberts DS, Moon TE: Quantitation of differential sensitivity of human tumor stem cells to chemotherapeutic drugs. N Engl J Med 1978 (298):1321-1327

230 Wang C, Curtis JE, Senn JS, Tritchler DL, McCulloch EA: Response to 5-azacytidine of leukemic blast cells in suspension: a biological parameter associated with response to chemotherapy. Leukemia 1987 (1):753-756

231 McCulloch EA, Minden MD, Miyauchi J, Kelleher CA, Wang C: Stem cell renewal and differentiation in acute myeloblastic leukemia. J Cell Sci 1989 (10 Suppl):1-15

232 McCulloch EA: The blast cells of acute myeloblastic leukemia. In: McCulloch EA (ed) Clinics in Hematology. Saunders, London 1984 pp 503-515

Bone Marrow Transplantation

Alberto M. Marmont

Scientific Consultant, Bone Marrow Transplantation Centre, Ospedale San Martino, Genoa and Istituto Nazionale per la Ricerca sul Cancro (IST), Genoa, Italy
Councillor of the International Bone Marrow Transplant Registry

Introduction

The ablation of pathological bone marrow by means of myelosuppressive "conditioning" regimens, with the purpose of eradicating disease-perpetuating clonogenic cells, be they leukaemic, congenitally altered or merely irreversibly insufficient, must be followed by the administration of an allogeneic or syngeneic bone marrow suspension containing a number of haemopoietic stem cells (HSC) adequate to ensure engraftment and subsequent reconstitution. Autologous bone marrow transplantation (AutoBMT) is closely similar to the allogeneic/syngeneic procedure (AlloBMT) in the treatment of leukaemia and other malignancies, while being obviously out of the question for the treatment of marrow aplasia, inborn errors and others, in which HSCs must come from a healthy donor. Immune problems (donor availability, graft-versus-host disease, GvHD) and scarcely elucidated but undisputably favourable effects (graft-versus-leukaemia, GvL) dominate the allogeneic setting, while in the autologous one elimination of the residual leukaemic clonogenic cells in the remission marrow is a major problem. However, the utilisation of peripheral HSCs is gradually becoming a procedure of major importance, especially when they are collected in the overshoot waves associated with haemopoietic reconstitution following myelosuppressive chemotherapy [1-5], where contamination with residual leukaemic cells is even less than in the marrow [6]. The successful utilisation of non-clonal HSCs, grown in and harvested from long-term cultures of marrows of patients with acute myeloid leukaemia (AML), has also been reported [7].

Although Allo- and Auto-marrow transplants are biologically distinct procedures, to contrast them would amount to making a "false debate" [8]. Each of them has its well-defined preferential or even specific indications, but there are certain areas, such as the acute leukaemias, in which a considerable degree of overlap has developed.

Increasing Use of BMT

The history of AlloBMT has been rightly defined as "courageous and dramatic" [9], and has been reviewed elsewhere [10,11]. While prior to July, 1980, 72% of the transplants were performed for non-malignant diseases, after that date 77% were for patients with malignancies, primarily leukaemias [12]. Of the 1713 AlloBMTs reported to the International Bone Marrow Transplant Registry (IBMTR) during 1988, more than 84% were for haematological malignancies, and 75% for leukaemia [13].

The cumulative number of AlloBMTs worldwide has been estimated at 20,000, performed by 200 teams. By the end of 1988 there were 8578 patients transplanted by 179 teams registered in the IBMTR database [13], and as of June 30, 1989, there have been little less than 1000 (Fig. 1); by the same date the EMBT had registered and evaluated data of 3563 AlloBMTs, of which 2086 patients with leukaemia [14]. Many of these data are superimposable, since they are generally

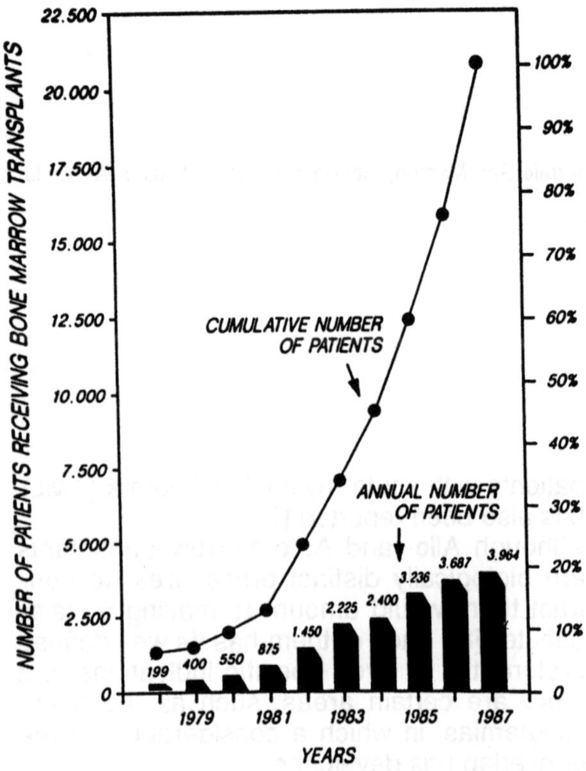

Fig. 1. Number of patients worldwide receiving AlloBMT up to 1987. From: Bortin MM and Rimm AA: Increasing utilization of bone marrow transplantation. II. Results of 1985-1987 survey. Transplantation 1989 (48):453-458

supplied to both Registries. To all of these, the fundamental clinical studies from Seattle must still be added [15,16]. Finally, the origination of national study groups such as GEGMO (France), GITMO (Italy) [17], NORDIC (Scandinavian countries) and others must be mentioned.

This impressive development is reflected in an equally impressive number of articles and in a series of monographs, symposia proceedings and review articles. Leaving aside the less recent literature, AlloBMT has been the object of 6 monographs and monographic journal issues [18-24], 4 UCLA [25-27] and 15 EBMT meeting proceedings, of which only the last 4 will be indicated [28], other symposia [29] and a number of review articles [30-34]. Finally, a specific journal, Bone Marrow Transplantation, is being published since 1986. AutoBMT has a shorter history, but is developing an equally impressive list of monographs [35,36], symposia proceedings and reviews [37-39]. Very rapid progress, new drugs and procedures, and the resulting changes of philosophies and attitudes, all contribute to making the whole field of BMT extremely variable. An attempt to adhere to essentials will be made in this section, which will start with some aspects that both types of BMT have in common.

Bone Marrow Seeding and Reconstitution

Since it is difficult to determine the number of HSCs, allogeneic and/or autologous, that are infused into the recipient's venous system, all nucleated cells are counted. An efficient reconstitution after AlloBMT is generally obtained with inocula containing $3x10^8$ nucleated cells per kg of the recipient's weight; however, all of them have a finite survival, and only HSCs are capable of regenerating haemopoiesis. For AutoBMT, doses of over $50x10^4$/kg of body weight of CFU-GMs have been ascertained to ensure complete engraftment [5,6]; however, other types of more undifferentiated, non-committed progenitors have been shown to be capable of reconstitution [40].

Although the haematologist/oncologist's main concern is with the clinical outcome of transplantation, it is quite unthinkable to pass over the first steps of marrow reseeding and transplantation haemopoiesis. The following brief survey includes both types of BMT, with special emphasis on some aspects of allogeneic haemopoiesis.

HSCs circulate throughout the organism, but are specifically recognised and bound by the marrow microenvironment [41], also in virtue of their adhesive properties and interactions with different stromal cells [42,43]. Endothelial galactosyl receptors [44-46] and a heparan sulphate component of the extracellular matrix [47] provide anchorage sites for the HSCs, which subsequently migrate to the haemopoietic space, probably by means of a "reverse" transendothelial passage [41,48]. Inhibitory glycoproteins, called restrictins, preferentially inhibit HSC accumulation in non-medullary environments [49].

Animal marrow transplantation studies demonstrated that reconstitution can occur from one (monoclonal) or small numbers (oligoclonal) of HSCs [50-51]. Monoclonal reconstitution in man was demonstrated in some cases of AML after chemotherapy [52]. Two important studies addressed this question after AlloBMT employing clonal analysis using restriction fragment length polymorphisms (RFLP) on the X-chromosome. Although marrow reconstitution was found generally to be a polyclonal event [53], there was also evidence in some cases for monoclonal haemopoiesis [54], thus confirming the enormous proliferative capability of HSCs.
Cellular interactions [55,56], specific inductive microenvironments [57,58] and a number of growth factors [59-61] are all of primary importance for the development and regulation of HSC growth and development. The origin of stromal cells is complex because of its heterogeneity [62]. Endothelial cells become of donor origin [63], although a subpopulation of recipient origin has been identified. While fibroblast and fat cell progenitors may be transplantable following the injection of large numbers of cells, the weight of evidence is against colonisation of recipient marrows by infused F-CFUs [62].
The dynamics of marrow macrophages after BMT are also complex. In the first 2-3 weeks after BMT, there is a marked wave of recipient macrophages, which engulf all sorts of cellular debris and morphologically intact cells [64,65]. Subsequently, the mononuclear-macrophage system's stem cells, which are extremely versatile [66], take over and eventually produce pulmonary macrophages [67], hepatic macrophages [68] (Kuppfer's cells), cutaneous Langerhans cells [69] and, leaving aside other somewhat disputed cells, osteoclasts [70]. This last remarkable effect is at the origin of the cure of infantile malignant osteopetrosis (Albers-Schoenberg's disease) by means of AlloBMT [71].
Erythropoiesis is normoblastic, although, in some patients who receive methotrexate (MTX) for GvHD prophylaxis, a transient but not striking megaloblastosis may be observed in the first 2-3 days after administration. Erythroblastic islets, most probably representing CFU-Es *in vivo*, are found in supravital observations on carefully spread preparations [64,65]. These islets are intensively reticulocytopoietic [41,64,65]; however, in some cases of major ABO incompatibility, erythroid aplasia takes place, superimposable to classical pure red cell aplasia (PRCA) [72]. Granulocytopoiesis generally precedes megakaryocytopoiesis, in the same way as neutrophils precede platelets in the circulation. Progenitor and precursor cells all appear, but some degree of loss of haemopoietic potential is generally detectable [73,74]. An exhaustive review of the reconstruction of the haemopoietic and immune systems after marrow transplantation has been published recently [75].
While most of these aspects can be found after both types of BMT, there may be marked differences in peripheral kinetics. In AlloBMT, the mean time to greater than 500 neutrophils/mm^3 is little over 2 weeks, and for 20-30x10^9/l platelets about 3 weeks. In AutoBMT, these measurements may be much more variable, depending on whether relatively intact or heavily pretreated marrow was harvested. In addition, bone marrow purging (see later) may severely affect HSCs in general, and more specifically those of patients having previously undergone prolonged and aggressive CT. Conversely, the speed of reconstitution can be considerable stepped up by the utilisation of haemopoietins.

Collection, Processing and Infusion of Marrow

Bone marrow harvesting is performed in the operating room under sterile conditions. In most cases general anaesthesia is used, but epidural anaesthesia may be possible in special situations. The posterior pelvis is mostly utilised.
Special hardened steel needles are employed, and through puncture sites in the skin a "rose" of about 5-10 aspirations is performed. No more than 2-4 ml of medullary blood must be aspirated to avoid dilution. The aspirate is expelled into a heparinised beaker, and, after filtration, into a second; then to a standard blood transfer pack. Subsequently, the harvested marrow suspension may be infused directly into the patient, or transferred to the laboratory for spe-

cial procedures (AlloBMT: T-cell depletion, red cell removal for major ABO incompatibility; AutoBMT: purging and/or cryopreservation). "Back-up" marrows indicate a fraction of the aspirated marrow that remains untreated when purging or other procedures are performed. It may rescue the patient in case of the no-engraftment/rejection syndrome.
Although this whole procedure has not changed perceptively over the last 20 years [76], the proposal of surgical procurement has not met with success [77]. Cadaveric marrow has attracted attention, but even after TCD [78] its utilisation remains dubious.
Donor complications are extremely rare [79,80] and severe ones even rarer (0.8%) [80]; this is particularly remarkable in the autologous setting, in which the donors are patients. More powerful analgesics to alleviate donors' pain have been suggested [81]. Autologous blood transfusions should be employed in healthy, allogeneic/syngeneic donors. The use of erythropoietin might be considered in this situation (see later).

Supportive Therapy

Supportive therapy with blood products after BMT is practically superimposable in both the allogeneic and the autologous setting, and does not differ from state-of-the-art supportive therapy after aggressive, myelosuppressive CT. While leucocyte transfusions are rarely performed, the regular infusion of platelet concentrates, preferably from single donors, is mandatory. Red cell requirements vary considerably depending on the haematocrit level one wishes to maintain and, in AlloBMT, ABO matching. The ABO mismatch is not a barrier for successful engraftment [82] but, in the case of major incompatibility, prevention of haemolysis must be ensured by means of appropriate procedures, including plasmapheresis [83], the use of immunoabsorbent columns to decrease the isohaemagglutinin titer and removal of the incompatible erythrocytes from the donor marrow *ex vivo* with the IBM 2991 [84]. In such cases, the red cell requirements are almost invariably greater, especially in a situation of post-BMT pure red cell aplasia (PRCA). In rare cases of minor ABO incompatibility, a "late" immunohaemolytic anaemia may develop, which can be quite severe; it is thought to be the consequence of donor B memory lymphocytes expanding post-BMT and reacting against the recipient's erythrocytes. In a study performed on 337 patients having received AlloBMT in Genoa, the red cell transfusion requirements were more than double in the case of major ABO incompatibility. In a recent Seattle study, platelet transfusion independence was most significantly affected by the development of acute GvHD, which is often associated with graft failure [85], and the drug used for GvHD prophylaxis [86].

Haemopoietic Growth Factors

The introduction of recombinant human haemopoietins, or haemopoietic growth factors (HGFs), consequent to the molecular cloning of cDNAs encoding their amino-acid sequence, has already brought and is still bringing considerable advantages in the treatment both of some specific haemopoietic disorders and of the marrow insufficiency following CT and both types of BMT. Besides discussions in former sections, excellent review articles on the clinical utilisation of HGFs have appeared recently [87-92]. In general, while IL-3 and GM-CSF stimulate a broad range of progenitors, G-CSF, M-CSF and Ep are lineage restricted and stimulate more mature granulocyte, monocyte and erythroid progenitor cells.
Maybe also because of the comparative ease of the administration of erythrocytes, recombinant erythropoietin (rHuEp) has not been seriously considered in the setting of BMT. Perhaps its indications are greater in the anaemia of prolonged CT [93], although its use in AutoBMT could be beneficial, similarly to what was found for autologous blood transfusion [94].
GM-CSF has been utilised in the setting of BMT in 3 main directions. Firstly, it has been administered in AutoBMT for lymphoid malignancies, where it was followed by a significantly quicker granulocytic recovery [95-96], thus decreasing the number of febrile episodes and infectious complications due to

granulocytopenia. A significantly less marked effect was found in another clinical study [97], in which, however, the marrows had been treated with 4-hydroxyperoxycyclophosphamide (4HC), an alkylating agent that eliminates residual malignant cells but also the majority of early myeloid progenitors, which are the target of GM-CSF.

The situation is more complex in AML, since myeloid blasts have been shown to be capable of aberrant haemopoietin production, reflecting autocrine growth stimulation. The activation of proto-oncogenes such as *fms* is also relevant [98]. Many effects may be anticipated from the administration of GM-CSF besides neutrophil recovery, including synchronisation of malignant cells prior to cycle-specific CT and perhaps also direct maturation induction of leukaemic cells [99]. However, the utilisation of HGFs, and more specifically GM-CSF, in the setting of BMT (Allo, Auto) for AML is still in its infancy. Many myeloid/monocytic leukaemia cells have receptors for the late-acting HGFs, and promyelocytic leukaemia cells have them in the highest degree for G-CSF [100]. The administration of GM-CSF was found useful to expedite neutrophil recovery after aggressive CT in aged patients, in whom the danger of leukaemia activation was thought less important than the persistence of pancytopenia [101].

Granulocyte colony stimulating factor (G-CSF) was administered to 15 patients with non-myeloid malignancies who were treated with HDCT and AutoBMT. Neutrophil recovery exceeded 0.5×10^9/l at a mean of 11 days after marrow infusion compared to 20 days for historical controls [102].

A third important application is in the area of the graft failure/rejection complex after AlloBMT. Despite conventional therapy, the majority of patients who experience graft failure die, and only 15% of them will be alive 1 year later. The first clinical studies seem promising [88].

It is becoming clear that the HGFs will be used in combination to obtain maximal effect [91,92,103,104]. Since the "late" HGFs act only on committed progenitors, thus potentially depleting the earlier ones, the combined utilisation of "early" HGFs such as IL-1 and IL-3 and "late" ones appears to be promising. In an illuminating animal study, the administration, first of IL-3 and subsequently of GM-CSF, was followed by prompt and marked elevation of all peripheral nucleated cells, including eosinophils [105].

Finally, recent trials are focussing on the ability of IL-2 to contribute to the elimination of minimal residual disease (MRD), both by its direct activity [106] and by its known boosting effect on NK and LAK cytotoxic effectors [107].

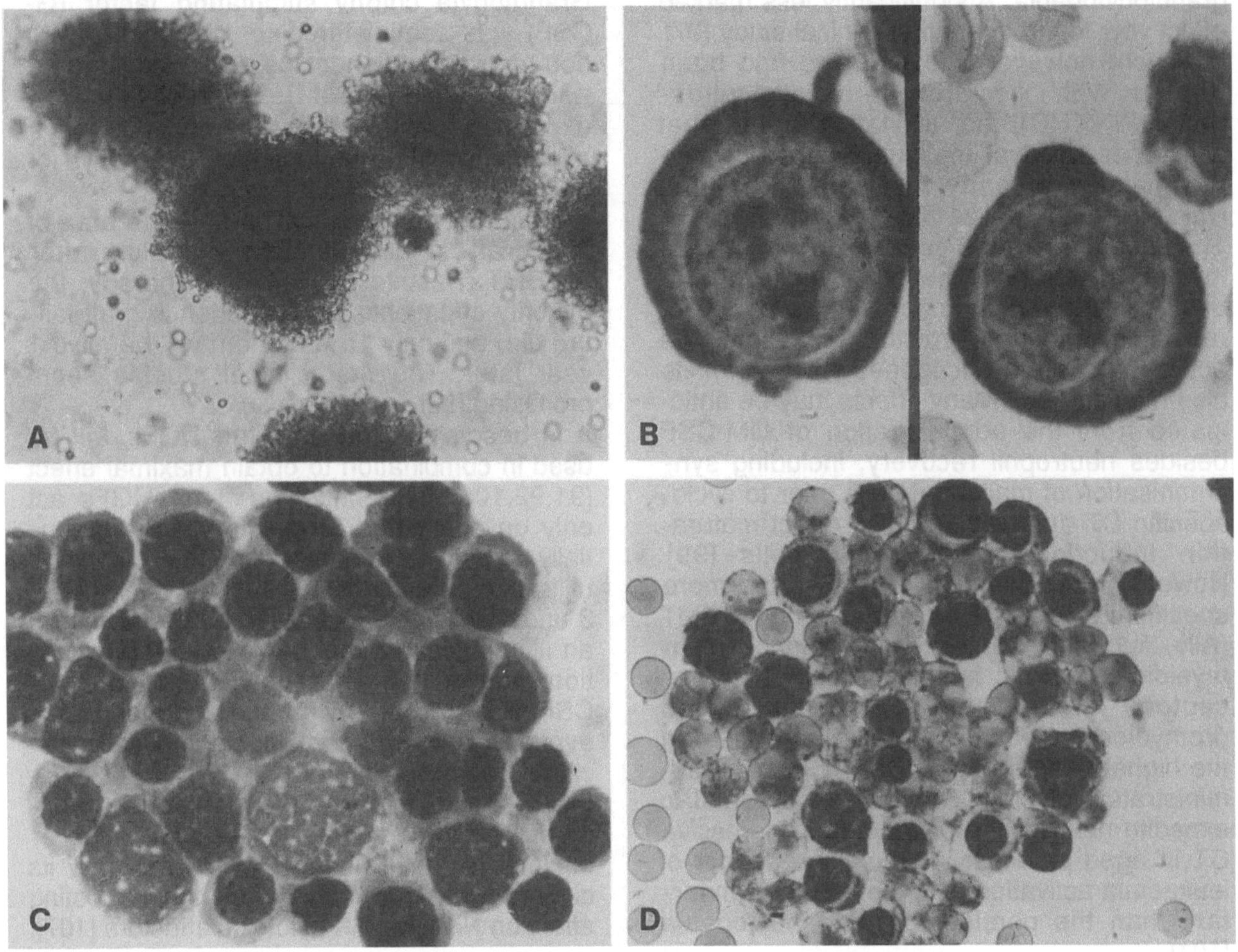

Fig. A. Burst-forming units, erythroid (BFU-E) in a bone marrow culture obtained 1 month after AlloBMT.

Fig. B. Primitive erythroid precursors ("proerythroblasts") in a myeloaspirate 1 week after transplant. Supravital preparation stained with an admixture of kresyl violet and new methylene blue. Note the size and morphology of the deeply basophilic nucleoli.

Fig. C. A typical erythroblastic island with a central macrophage. These formations may be considered as the equivalent of colony-forming units, erythroid (CFU-E) *in vivo*.

Fig. D. Erythroblastic island with gradual depletion of erythroblasts and marked early reticulocytosis. Supravital preparation stained with brilliant kresyl blue.

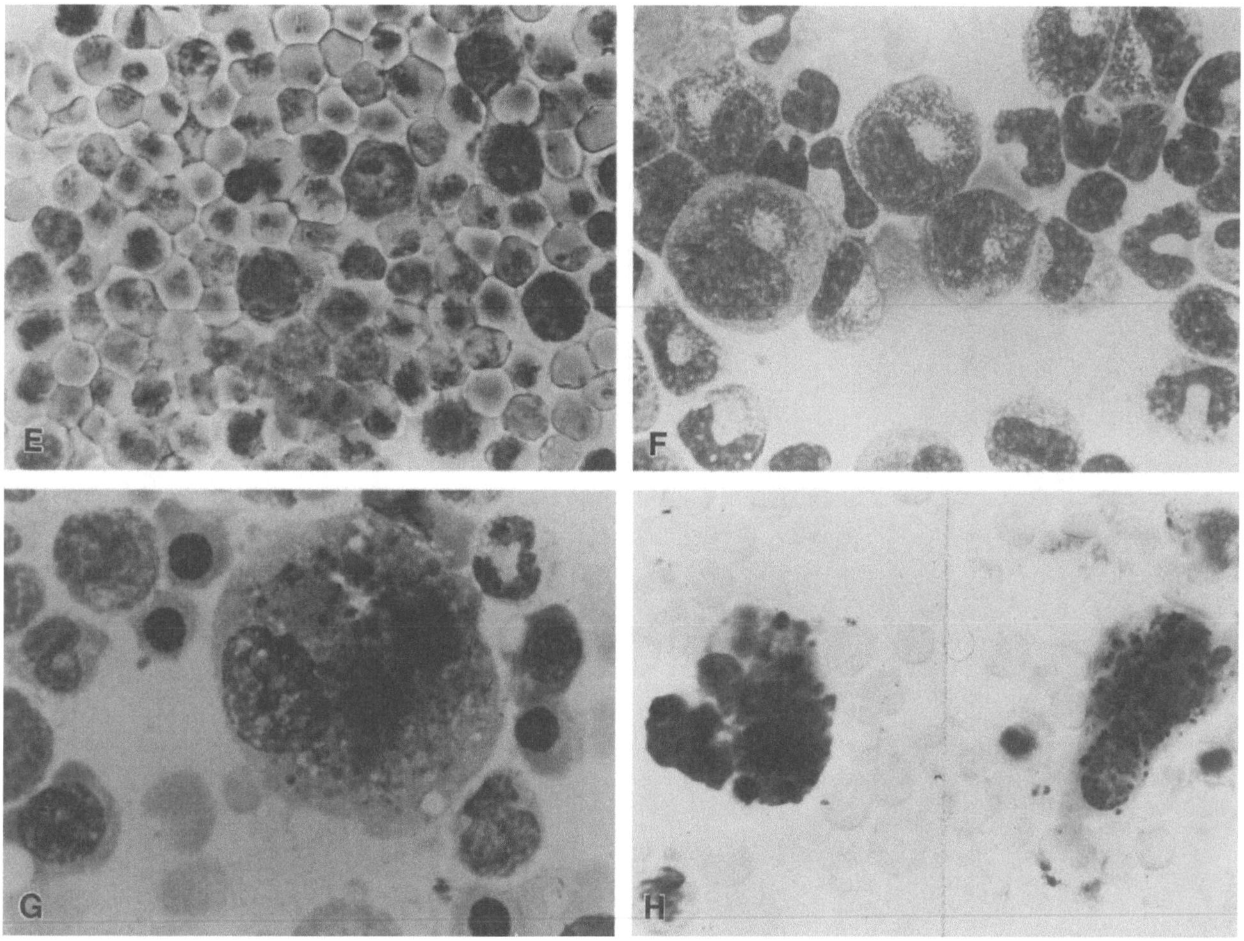

Fig. E. Supravital preparation of a myeloaspirate showing extreme reticulocytosis with some scattered erythroblasts. This preparation comes from a case of major ABO incompatibility between donor and recipient. Initial erythroid hypoplasia was superseded by explosive erythropoiesis after repeated plasma exchange.
Staining with an admixture of kresyl violet and new methylene blue.

Fig. F. Intensive granulocytopoiesis in a myeloaspirate performed 2 weeks after transplant. Note the conspicuous Golgi areas in the paranuclear cytoplasm of the granulocytic precursors.
Cytocentrifuge preparation.

Fig. G. Macrophage engulfing all sorts of cellular debris. These aspects indicate the massive cell destruction which takes place after conditioning regimens.

Fig. H. Macrophages engulfing haemoglobin degradation products. This type of macrophagic reaction is most frequent after major ABO incompatible transplants.

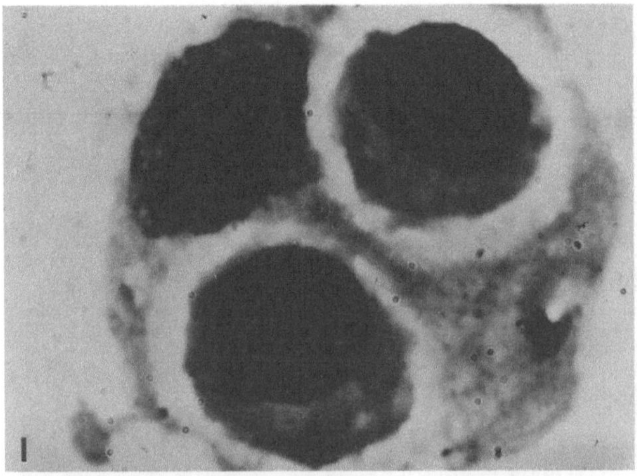

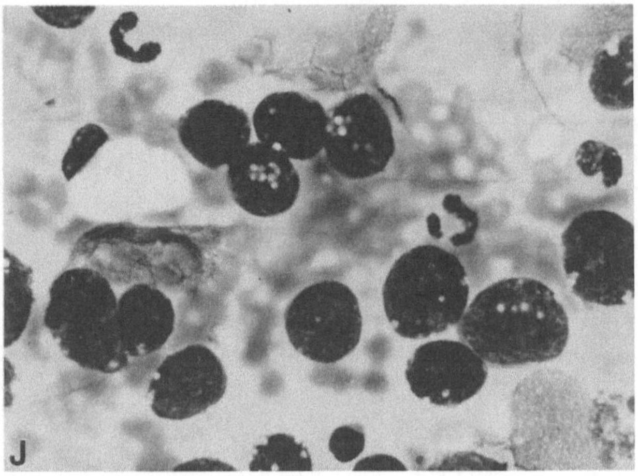

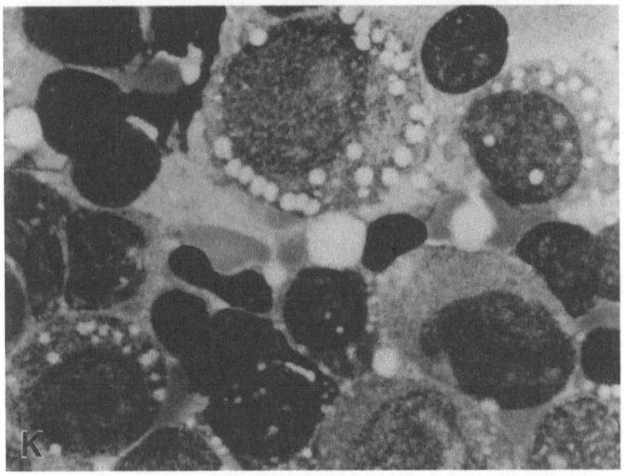

Fig. I. Macrophage phagocytosing 2 apparently discrete erythroblasts. All these "early" macrophages were found to be of recipient origin when Y body studies could be performed.

Fig. J. Myeloaspirate showing relapse after AlloBMT for acute lymphoblastic leukaemia (ALL). The multiple small vacuoles throughout the cytoplasm, sometimes overlying the nucleus, are reminiscent of the B or Burkitt type ALL. However, this was a typical case of T-ALL, complete with mediastinal enlargement at presentation.

Fig. K. Myeloaspirate showing relapse after AlloBMT for acute myeloblastic leukaemia (FAB M2). Multiple cytoplasmic vacuoles are prominent, but cytoplasmic "myeloid' granules are also discernible. Vacuolisation, which reflects the dissolution of lipoprotein granules by the ethanol-containing May-Grünwald reagent, indicates a deeply disturbed cellular metabolism.

Allogeneic Bone Marrow Transplantation

Introduction

The archetypal blood malignancy, leukaemia [13], continues to be the main indication for AlloBMT worldwide [14,16,33,108,109]. Other haematological malignant diseases include chronic lymphocytic leukaemia, multiple myeloma, acute myelofibrosis, malignant histiocytosis and, perhaps more importantly, the myelodysplastic syndromes. While the acute leukaemias (AL) were the principal indication until a few years ago, the constant improvement of CT and also of AutoBMT have rendered this whole area somewhat controversial [110-112]. On the other hand, CML has become the principal indication for AlloBMT, followed by the spectrum of MDS and secondary AML. It is clear that eradication of the malignant clonogenic cells is not strictly related to the pre-transplant conditioning, but may also be achieved with non-chimaerising procedures, while the lack of genuinely normal HSCs makes the administration of donor HSCs mandatory. This is also the reason for which mismatched (generally 1 locus) family members and matched unrelated donors are utilised.

Statistical studies of the EBMT clinical material have confirmed that remission status (first complete remission-CR1 for the AL patients and first chronic phase-CP1 for CML patients) is the main factor influencing leukaemia-free survival (LFS), which was 50% if AlloBMT was performed at this stage for all 3 leukaemias, independently of the diagnostic category (AML, ALL or CML), compared with 30% if the transplant was performed at a later stage of the disease [108,109]. Age was also an important factor adversely influencing LFS and transplant-related mortality (TRM), and similarly so the donor-recipient sex combination of female to male [113]. There was no significant improvement in the outcome for patients with the 3 types of leukaemia transplanted in Europe over the past 7 years [14,109]. A small improvement in the overall leukaemia-free survival was found in an IBMTR 10-year progress report analysing data from 4034 patients transplanted between 1978 and 1987 [114].

AlloBMT for leukaemia should not be regarded as a "special" treatment, and insulated from, or even worse, opposed to other therapies. It is highly probable that it will be superseded eventually by other methods of treatment [115]; however, paraphrasing the controversy that has been taking place for ALL in children, it may well be a passing phase in the management of all types of leukaemia [116], but its time is far from gone [117]. There is still place for much improvement [118]. Before discussing results in single diseases, a summary of problems specifically associated with AlloBMT will be given.

Immunology

Histocompatibility

A patient can be considered for allogeneic BMT only in the presence of a suitable donor. Whether a donor is suitable is decided on the basis of testing for human leukocyte antigens (HLA) of class I (HLA A and B) and of class II (HLA DR, DP, DQ), and on the degree of donor/recipient matching. The inheritance of HLA antigens in the family is studied by analysing the parental "haplotypes". This term refers to the HLA antigens carried on each of the parental chromosomes: a/b and c/d will thus identify the 4 parental haplotypes. Short but informative reviews for the use of haematologists have been published [119-122].

HLA A, B and DR typing is usually performed by serology; problems may arise in very severe aplastic anaemia because of the scarcity of B-lymphocytes, and in CML. In the latter form, lowering of the leucocyte count is generally adequate; however, in some cases difficulties may persist. The introduction of new, specific probes for DR, DP and DQ has done much to obviate these problems. After HLA typing has been completed, donor and recipient cells are tested in mixed lymphocyte cultures (MLR); however, the relevance of MLR has been debated. In the setting of genotypically HLA A, B, DR matched siblings, the MLR is almost always negative, though the relative response index (RRI) may vary from 0% to 10% and there does not seem to be a difference within this range of reactivity [124,125]. However, in the setting of partially mismatched donors, the RRI may vary from 0% to 100%. A recent report of the European Bone Marrow Transplant (EBMT) Immunology Working Party [126] suggests that in partially mismatched BMT a negative MLR is a favourable prognostic factor for survival.

Donor Selection

Any healthy individual between the age of 18 and 60 is a potential marrow donor. Children down to the age of one have been successfully used as donors. Donors may be syngeneic twins, HLA-identical siblings, family donors other than the former and matched unrelated donors (MUDs). In the first instance there are no immunological complications, but the lack of a GvL effect may be detrimental (see later). Most transplants are carried out between siblings who have inherited the same 2 haplotypes from the parents, and are therefore genotypically HLA identical, and non-reactive in MLR. The chance that a sibling will be identical with the patient is 1/4.
When parents share one HLA haplotype, they can be phenotypically identical with a son and non-responsive in MLR. When such phenotypically identical grafts are performed, transplant-related mortality (TRM) is comparable to that seen in the HLA-identical sibling situation. When one of the parents is homozygous for all HLA antigens (a very rare situation), then either one of the paternal chromosomes will confer the same haplotype to the children, and 2 children may thus be phenotypically identical. Also in this rare situation TRM is acceptable. When the donor and the recipient share one haplotype but differ for one or more antigens on the other haplotype, then TRM is significantly increased, both because of a higher incidence of rejection and of acute graft-versus-host disease (GvHD). The assessment of TRM in 1-antigen mismatched grafts may differ greatly according to the underlying disease: in leukaemia it has been reported to be similar to HLA-identical grafts [123], but in severe aplastic anaemia (SAA) it is clearly higher [124].

Non HLA Identical Siblings

Leaving aside identical twins, 2 different sources of HSCs have been utilised, that is, mismatched related donors and MUDs. The first results from Seattle in this respect were moderately encouraging, inasmuch as patients receiving transplants from family member donors mismatched at a single antigen had more GvHD than matched patients but survived equally well [123]. However, survival becomes poorer with increasing mismatch [125]. Two important recent studies have addressed the question, the first from the EBMT [126] and the second from the IBMTR [127]. In the European experience, the overall survival out of 242 non-identical transplants was 29%. Out of 117 remission patients, there was a 41% survival after AlloBMT with unmanipulated marrow, as compared to 27% survival after TCD. The IBMTR study included 438 patients with leukaemia who were transplanted from related, non-HLA identical donors. The risks of graft failure and grade II-IV aGvHD increased progressively in a reciprocal way. For patients with early leukaemia the age-adjusted 2-year probability of survival was 56%, 35%, 33% and 21% for patients with genotypically identical, phenotypically identical, 1-locus, 2-loci and 3-loci disparate donors, respectively. In conclusion, the risk of TRM correlated strongly with the degree of HLA disparity between donor and recipient.
Finally, MUDs chosen from large panels have been increasingly used over the past few years [128,129]. Most panels contain only HLA A and B typing data, with DR typing being performed once an HLA A and B match has been found. Most centres require in addition a negative MLC before transplanting. Usually, the degree of matching required includes full class I and class II matching in order to obtain a successful outcome. The frequency of cytotoxic T-cells with recipient specificity may vary greatly within the MUD situation, and correlates with TRM. It is now possible to match UDs by class I HLA serology, class II HLA-specific probes, MLR, and cytotoxic T-cell frequencies. However, it has been pointed out that the HLA typing techniques may be inadequate to define the high

level of phenotypic identity that may be necessary, and that MLCs, which are useful in the identical sib setting, are much less so in the MUD situation [130]. Progress has been made both with 2-dimensional electrophoresis for class I antigens and in characterising class II genes by RFLP analysis and more recently with allele-specific oligonucleotide probes in conjunction with the polymerase chain reaction (PCR) [130]. Leaving aside such degrees of sophistication, the highly polymorphic nature of the HLA antigen severely reduces the probability that any 2 unrelated individuals will be matched at any given HLA locus. In a recent study it was calculated that, with registries containing 1000, 10,000 or 100,000 donors, the average probabilities of finding an HLA-A, B, Dr, Dw match were 3.8%, 14% and 32.2%, respectively [131]. An increase in donor pool size to 1 million would still leave 50% of patients without a fully matched donor [131]. Thus far, about 200 transplants using well or less well MUDs have been performed worldwide [133]. Notwithstanding former encouraging results, the more recent ones appear to be somewhat inferior to a matched patient population receiving HLA-identical sibling donor transplants. It is therefore of great interest that, following the former endeavours of the EBMT [134,135], a merger of 12 different bone marrow donor registries, called "Bone Marrow Donors Worldwide" (BMDW), has been compiled by J.J. van Rood. There are 224,000 HLA-A,B typed donors in the 1990 collection, comprising 30,710 phenotypes; in addition, there are 96,000 HLA-A,B,DR donors (54,500 phenotypes), making up a total of 320,000. The participating registries are listed in Table 1. More panels are planned to join this International Project, and it is hoped that, through cooperation, files of close to 1,000,000 individuals will soon be established.

It must be remarked that the search for MUDs should be primarily restricted for those patients in whom no autologous residual stem cells can be expected, such as inborn errors, the myelodysplastic syndromes (MDS) and CML, in which the situation has not changed appreciably notwithstanding recent, exciting results [136]. AutoBMT and aggressive CT are to be considered in the first place before programming a UD AlloBMT for the ALS.

Table 1. Marrow donor registries participating in the BMDW

Anthony Nolan Research Centre, London, U.K.
UKBTS, Bristol, U.K.
Europdonor Foundation, Leiden, The Netherlands
GMFT, Paris, France
Bone Marrow Donors Ulm, Ulm, F.R.G.
IBMDR, Genoa, Italy
Moscow, U.S.S.R.
NMDP, St. Paul, Minnesota, U.S.A.
Austrian Bone Marrow Donors, Vienna, Austria
National Marrow Donor Program, Brussels, Belgium
Swiss UBMR, Bern, Switzerland
UBMDR, Vancouver, Canada

Conditioning and Conditioning Regimens

The term *conditioning* has superseded the perhaps more correct terminology of pretransplant preparative regimen(s). The consensus is that the ideal preparative regimen for AlloBMT in leukaemia should have the following properties: 1) adequate "space-making" and immunosuppressive properties to allow full and sustained engraftment of the allogeneic marrow; 2) adequate antileukaemic properties to prevent leukaemia relapse (for the sake of clarity, the antileukaemic properties of the allograft are not considered here); 3) minimum of short-term extra marrow toxicities; 4) minimum of late toxicities [137,138]. The combination of all these factors is extremely complex, and it has been demonstrated that even a slight degree of additional toxicity may produce an unacceptable increase in overall toxicity that might negate improved antileukaemic effects.

Conditioning regimens for AlloBMT in leukaemia can be divided into 3 categories: 1) combined modalities (CT-RT); 2) combination CT; 3) new and still experimental methods.

The combination of high-dose cyclophosphamide (CY: 60 mg/kg for 2 consecutive days) followed by total body irradiation (TBI: 10 Gy in a single dose) is the original Seattle regimen [139], which is the standard of comparison for all other conditioning regimens. Modifications of the CY 120 - TBI 10 Gy regi-

Table 2. CY-TBI conditioning regimens

Agents	Dosage	Timing	Centre	Ref.
CY STBI	120 mg/kg 10 Gy	2 days 1 day	Seattle	140
CY FTBI	120 mg/kg 12 Gy	2 days 6 days	Seattle	141
HFTBI CY	13.20 Gy 120 mg/kg	4 days 2 days	MSKCC New York	144-146
CY FTBI	120 mg/kg 9.90 Gy	2 days 3 days	Genoa (AML)	142
CY HFTBI	120 mg/kg 12 Gy	2 days 6 days	Genoa (ALL)	147

men have been introduced concerning both the RT and the CR arm.

There have been 2 different trends, the first of which was favourable to fractionated irradiation (fTBI) with a clearly protective effect on the incidence of interstitial pneumonitis (IPn), cataracts and veno-occlusive disease of the liver (VOD), without loss of antileukaemic effect [140-142]. Hyperfractionated TBI followed by CY was utilised at Memorial Sloan Kettering Cancer Center (MSKCC) in children with ALL in CR2 with a 5-year 64% LFS [143-145]. Similar results were obtained in Genoa without altering the classical CT-RT sequence [146], so that the better results of HfTBI versus fTBI should not be interpreted as an effect of schedule reversal, but of the hyperfractionation procedure itself. However, fast-dose single-fraction TBI is essential to control the increased graft failure and relapse rate observed after TCD [147], as will be discussed later. Another way of increasing the total radiation dose is incorporated in the split TBI VVRAPID-X regimen, leaving aside the CT component (vincristine, daunorubicin, cytarabine, teniposide), which was effective in reducing the graft-failure rate following TCD BMT [148]. Some of the most commonly used CY-TBI regimens are shown in Table 2.

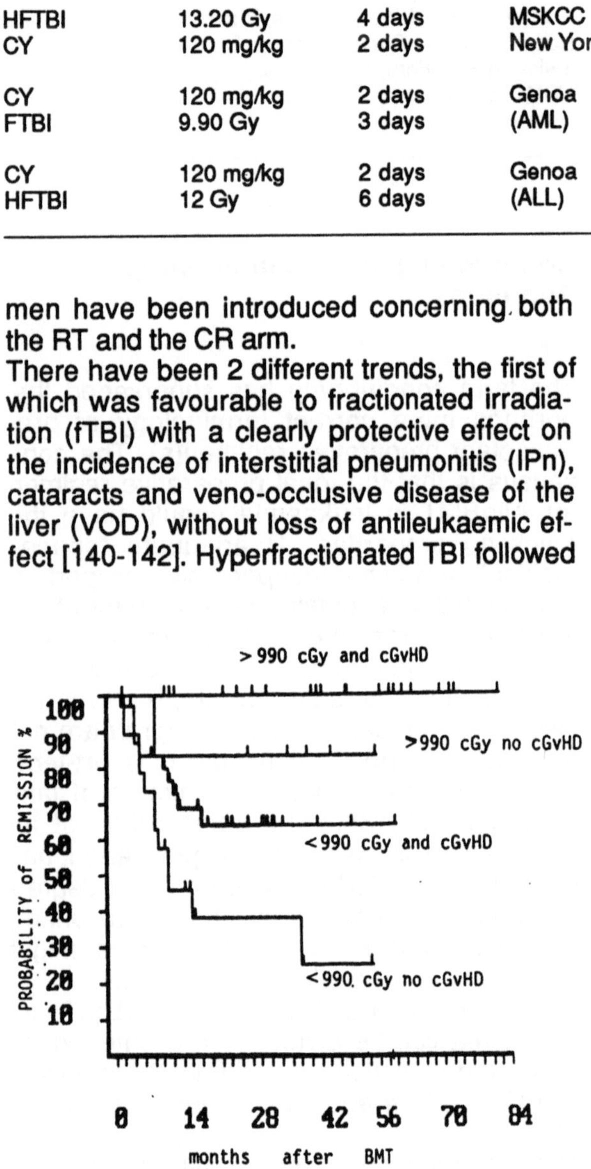

Fig. 2. The effect of efficient (>990 cGy received) versus inefficient (<990 cGy received) and chronic GvHD on relapse. High radiation dosage and chronic GvHD offered the best protection. From [150], with permission

The advantages and disadvantages of STBI versus the fractionated schedules will ideally depend upon the radiobiological properties and the radiosensitivity (Do) of a given leukaemic population [149]. For example, 1 log cell kill corresponds to between 2 and 3 Do on the exponential part of the radiation survival curve of lymphocytes. It is well known that survival and LFS in allotransplanted patients depends on a combination of not intolerable procedure toxicity, conditioning intensity and still poorly characterised immunological reactions constituting the GvHD/GvL complex (see further). In a recent study of 175 transplanted patients in Genoa, it could be

Table 3. Conditioning regimens combining other chemotherapeutic agents with TBI

Agents	Dosage	Timing	Centre	Ref.
FTBI Etoposide	13.20 Gy 60 mg/kg	4 days 2 days	Duarte	151
Piperazinedione FTBI	50 mg/m^2 8 Gy	2 days 2 days	Houston	152
Cytarabine FTBI	3 g/m^2 12 Gy	6 days 6 days		153
Melphalan FTBI	110 mg/m^2	1 day	Royal Marsden London	154

shown that, after stratifying for chronic GvHD and TBI dose, the dose effect of TBI on relapse was evident in patients with and without GvHD [150]. This means that both effects, the radiobiological and the immunological, are active and combined in eradicating leukaemia (Fig. 2).

Another type of variation of the CT-TBI regimen consists in the substitution or integration of CY with other chemotherapeutic agents such as cytarabine, etoposide, melphalan, piperazinedione (PIP) [151-154] and others. Although combination CT with TBI theoretically appears more attractive than single-agent CT, this must be balanced, as usual, against the increase in toxicity [155,156], and also, as with anthracyclines, against a slower haematopoietic recovery [157]. The better known alternative CT-TBI regimens are shown in Table 3.

Long before the debate whether TBI is really indispensable for cytoreductive regimens prior to BMT [158], the alternative CT-only approaches were centered upon the combination of busulfan (BU) and CY: in the original parent regimen BU 4 mg/kg of ideal body weight was followed by CY 50 mg/kg IV daily x 4 (= 200 mg/kg). The Baltimore experience with this regimen was reviewed recently [159,160]. A similar experience in Pesaro was also published very recently [162], while a slight reduction in the BU arm (3.5 mg/kg) was employed in the same centre for homozygous thalassaemia [162]. A reduction in the CY arm was used in Columbus (120 mg/kg in 2 days), with very good results in AML [163] but also in the accelerated phase of CML [164] and in multiple myeloma [165]. The BU-CY regimen has also been employed preferentially for second transplants, especially if the patients had received TBI for the first. Also, a combination of etoposide and BU was utilised in this situation [166].

Finally, the need for preparatory regimens with greater antitumour effect, greater immunosuppression and less toxicity has led to 2 types of selective radiotherapy employing radionuclides. In the first, high doses of ^{131}I linked to antimyeloid antibodies were used in the canine model, and it was estimated that 15 mCi/kg delivered at least 15 Gy to the marrow. In the second, a rare earth radionuclide, 166-Holmium, was linked to an aminophosphoric acid that binds avidly to bone and therefore exposes the marrow to its low penetrating, ß-emission. Both approaches are still experimental [138,167].

Complications

The complications of AlloBMT are multiple, and it is often difficult to distinguish between the toxic effects caused by the conditioning regimen, and those more specifically related to the transplant *per se*. The first group is generally considered under the heading of toxicity, which is both haematological (pancytopenia and, more significantly, neutropenia and thrombocytopenia) and non-haematological. This early toxicity, together with aGvHD, graft failure, interstitial pneumonitis (IPn), acute respiratory distress syndrome (ARDS), veno-occlusive disease of the liver (VOD) and others all contribute to what is generally known as TRM. TRM is the cause of the first and precipitous drop of survival curves following AlloBMT. Reducing early deaths is a clear objective that might be achievable over the next 10 years [118].

Leukaemia Relapse

Although leukaemia relapse cannot be considered as a complication of AlloBMT, but rather as its failure, it may be appropriately discussed under this heading, since all treatment failures are interconnected in a complex relationship and, as will be discussed later, prophylactic regimens against GvHD may unfavourably affect the risk of leukaemia relapse [168-172]. Conversely, the severity of GvHD correlates directly both with the risk of infection [173] and with the risk of IPn [174] and inversely with the probability of relapse [175-178]. The implications of this phenomenon will be discussed later.

The first year following the transplant is the period of greatest risk of treatment failure, including TRM and relapse [179]. Patients who survive this critical interval have an excellent chance of long-term LFS [180]. In a recent IBMTR study it was found that, in early leukaemia, the median interval from transplant to relapse was 7.8 months, in intermediate leukaemia 6.4 months and in advanced leukaemia 3.3 months [179]. In another multicentre retrospective study of the EBMT on 117 patients relapsing after AlloBMT for acute leukaemia (41 AML and 76 ALL), it was found that relapse occurred between 3 and 30 months after transplant [181]; when investigated, the leukaemia was found to have relapsed in recipient cells. Of 74 patients who received additional treatment for leukaemia, 32 achieved a complete remission, and donor marrow was shown to be responsible for haemopoietic recovery. Mixed chimaerism is often a feature of these situations [182,183], although much more frequent after TCD (see later). There is evidence for a competition between donor and recipient haemopoiesis [184,185].

Seventeen late relapses were reported in 232 transplanted leukaemic patients, occurring between 2 and 6.3 years after grafting [186]. Although the suspicion of *de novo* leukaemias occurring in the donor's haemopoiesis was entertained, relapse in the original host cells has been documented 5 [187] and almost 7 [188] years after transplantation.

Relapse in donor lineage cells has been reported in at least 8 cases of AL and in 2 cases of CML [189-193]; it has been estimated that cases of donor-derived leukaemia may account for up to 5% of all relapses occurring after AlloBMT [194]. Different mechanisms have been proposed to explain this phenomenon, among which the transfection of a dominant oncogene from the DNA of a degenerating host leukaemic cell to a developing donor cell. However, the whole question of donor relapse is now a subject of revision, since there have been recent reports showing a discrepancy between cytogenetic (indicating donor cells) and molecular (by restriction fragment length polymorfism: RFLP: indicating host cells) studies [195]. Those data strongly suggest that careful and critical DNA probes should be made before assigning the leukaemic cell lineage in such cases [195].

Secondary Neoplasms

Malignancies arising after AlloBMT may conceptually be divided into 4 categories [189]: 1) relapses of the original leukaemia, which are by far the most frequent; 2) the rare relapses in donor cells; 3) non-Hodgkin's lymphomas, generally of B type and associated with Epstein-Barr virus; 4) solid tumours. In a recent survey from Seattle comprising all patients receiving Allo- or AutoBMT for leukaemia and aplastic anaemia, the age-adjusted incidence of secondary neoplasms, including non-Hodgkin lymphomas, leukaemias and solid tumours was 6.9 times higher than that of primary cancers in the general population [196]. The predictors of any type of secondary cancer were aGvHD treated with either antithymocyte globulin (ATG) or anti-CD3 MoAb, TCD and HLA mismatch. The risk was found to be significant but low, and similar to malignant tumour inci-

Table 4. Acute complications of AlloBMT

Pancytopenia
Mucositis and other oral complications
Gastroenteritis and diarrhoea
Urotoxicity
Hepatic damage
Cutaneous toxicity
Neurotoxicity
Cardiotoxicity
Interstitial pneumonia, ARDS
Fluid and electrolyte imbalance

dence after combined modality treatments. Secondary leukaemias are to be expected more in TCD transplants [196]. It is remarkable that no secondary cancer, with the one exception of a cytogenetically donor-type relapsed leukaemia [197], was found in Genoa in about 600 patients having undergone either Allo- or AutoBMT.

Acute Complications

The acute complications of AlloBMT are given in Table 4, which is taken from a recent monograph by Deeg et al. [20] where all acute complications are dealt with. Only some major complications will be discussed here.

The Graft-Failure/Rejection Complex

Since most transplants for malignancies have been made using HLA/D-DR matched sibling donors, preparative regimens employing TBI and unmanipulated marrows, graft rejection, differently from severe aplastic anaemia, was very rare, occurring in less than 1% of cases. The situation has changed for the worse while striving for improvement: enlargement of the donor pool by inclusion of familiar mismatched donors has increased rejection to 5% for 1-antigen mismatch, and to 15-20% for 2-antigen mismatch. In addition, TCD was also found to be associated with the graft-failure/rejection complex, as will be discussed later.

Graft failure in the setting of GvHD has been described; aGvHD grade II or more was shown to be the single most significant factor associated with failure to maintain sustained haemopoiesis following normal engraftment [85]. The association of thrombocytopenia with chronic GvHD has also been described, and was shown to be of poor prognostic value [198].

Graft-versus-Host Disease

Notwithstanding some diversity in the evaluation of both acute [199] and chronic [200] GvHD, the general consensus is that aGvHD occurs in 45% of transplant recipients, and is fatal in about 25% [23,201]. Apart from being the most important expression of the immune conflict between donor and host cells after AlloBMT, GvHD is an extremely important clinical complication and has been studied extensively, both in its acute [202-204] and chronic [206,207] forms. The latter is remarkable because of its predominantly autoimmune physiopathology [206-209].

Although the pathogenesis of GvHD is multifactorial [210], requiring an array of complex interactions that include antigenic differences, host factors and environmental conditions [202], it is commonly accepted that the pivotal cells are T-lymphocytes [211], which are of host origin and survive after conditioning [212]. There is now evidence for an interactive, 2-phase pathogenesis [213], with CD4+ cells initiating GvHD in man against non-major HLA antigens [214], and activated LGL/NK cells, with phenotypic and functional characteristics similar to CD3+ gamma/beta cells, which normally mediate immunological surveillance of epithelial cells [215], exerting cytolytic effects [216]. These effects seem to be mediated by their lysosome-like granules, which are exocytosed over the target cells and produce pore-forming proteins (perforins) capable of inducing lethal membrane lesions [217,218]. The activation of the effector cells appears to be a cytokine-mediated phenomenon [219,220]. The cellular and humoral processes involved in GvHD represent a complicated network of interactions [221]. Candidate cells with GvHD activity are listed in Table 5 [221].

The threshold dose of T-lymphocytes for causing GvHD in humans in HLA-matched recipients was found to be $2x10^5$ clonable T-cells/kg of recipient body weight [222], but it

Table 5. Candidate cells involved in the GvHD network

Cell type	Initiator	Effector
Suppressor lymphocytes (T8)	+	+
Helper lymphocytes (T4)	+	+
Natural killer cells	-	+
Natural suppressor cells	-	+ (?)
Langerhans' cells of the skin	+ (?)	+ (?)

was pointed out that each donor-recipient pair may have a different threshold [223]. This is, indeed, clearest in recipients of unmanipulated marrows from HLA-identical transplants, 55% of whom never develop GvHD. On the basis of an extensive database, an informative evaluation of risks was prepared by the IBMTR [201]. Age of the patient was a significant risk factor, but the age gradient was modest, and if parous or transfused female-male transplants were excluded, it was not a significant factor (Fig. 3). The donor's age

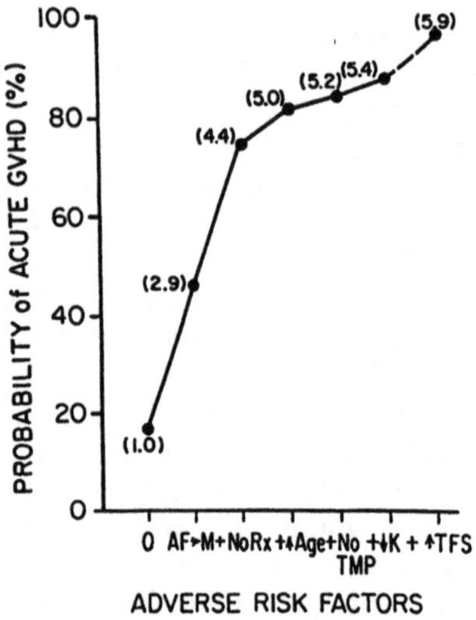

Fig. 3. Multivariate cumulative relative risk (numbers in parentheses) and cumulative percent probability of moderate to severe acute graft-versus-host disease. When one of the significant adverse risk factors identified in this study was present, a risk of 1.0 was used. First adverse risk factor = alloimmune female/male transplants; second = no prophylaxis against graft-versus-host disease; third = older patients; fourth = trimethoprim-sulphamethoxazole not given; fifth = lower pretransplant performance ratings; sixth = larger number of post-transplant transfusions. Reproduced from [201], with permission

came out as the most significant risk factor in a recent analysis in Genoa.

Leaving aside former conflicting reports, the female to male sex match was an important predictive factor in the IBMTR analysis [201], and it was markedly increased if female donors for male recipients were previously pregnant or transfused (RR 2.9, $p < 0.0001$).

In a recent EBMT study [224] on 1915 patients, it was found that females have better LFS and less TRM than males. The effect of sex-mismatching was disease dependent, with no effect in AML (except in bad risk AML), marginal in CLL and very significant in CML. Confirming the former findings, recipient male - donor female was the worst combination, resulting in more cGvHD ($p=0.0001$) and IPn ($p=0.01$).

Patients with post-transplant cytomegalovirus (CMV) infection and with CMV-positive donors not only had an increased risk of developing cGvHD [225], but showed some evidence of a GvL effect independent of GvL [226]. This is another, somewhat unexpected, confirmation both of the association of GvH and GvL effects in man, and of the possible dissociation between the two [227-229], which will be discussed later. The role of ABO matching has also been explored [230]. In the Seattle experience, aplastic anaemia patients had less GvHD when transplanted from B 8+ donors, and more of it with B18+ donors [231]. An interesting predictive mixed lymphocyte skin test has been developed [232]. In addition, in skin explant cultures the percentage of CD4+ population influenced the degree of GvHD [233].

Chronic GvHD, which may follow aGvHD or develop independently, has an even more complex physiopathology, with a distinct switch to autoimmunity [205-209]. It may mimic various connective tissue disorders, but most markedly progressive systemic sclerosis (PSS) and Sjögren's disease, which may progress to corneal perforation and blindness.

Both acute and chronic GvHD have been described extensively [202,221,234], and they are still scored according to the original Seattle criteria [234], although some modifications appear to be indicated [20]. Continuing educational interchange among centres has been advocated for a more uniform evaluation both of acute [199] and chronic [200] GvHD.

Prevention and Treatment

GvHD prevention has been and is still being attempted by means of a great variety of procedures, which include physical, chemical and immunological treatment of the explanted marrow in order to reduce the T-lymphocyte subpopulations which recognise and react against the recipient's tissue antigens. It is quite obvious that all these procedures compromise both engraftment and GvL; since both effects have been observed most markedly in CML, immunological T depletion will be discussed in that section.

Recently, an interesting approach was made by means of exposure of the marrow to ultraviolet B light, which is capable of inactivating marrow T-lymphocytes while sparing HSCs [235]; however, no clinical studies have been performed yet.

Soybean lectin agglutination and rosetting with sheep blood cells are being used effectively at MSKCC to eliminate T-cells from the inoculum [236]; however, an enhancement of both rejections and relapses was observed, which was partially obviated through the use of T-cell specific immunosuppressive measures administered in the early post-transplant period. Counterflow centrifugation to deplete marrow lymphocytes has also been employed, either alone [237] or in combination with the subsequent administration of irradiated donor buffy coat [238]. It appears that T-cell depletion by means of physical means has a less favourable influence on leukaemia relapse [170]. Full discussions of these problems have been published [173,239].

The treatment of established GvHD consists of additional immune suppression, most generally with high doses of corticosteroids. New approaches include ATG, monoclonal antibodies, immunotoxins [240] and, for the chronic form, thalidomide [241].

Pulmonary Complications

Pulmonary complications of AlloBMT have been divided in "early" and "late" [242]; the early ones include severe mucositis, the pulmonary oedema syndromes including the capillary leak syndrome and the adult respiratory distress syndrome (ARDS) [243], and IPn. The risk factors for IPn have been assessed carefully [244,245], and it has been established that the use of MTX for the prevention of GvHD, the dose rate of TBI given in a single dose and the severity of GvHD were all associated with increased risk for IPn. However, the experience with T-cell depletion indicates that severe IPn may appear even in the absence of GvHD [170]. IPn has been divided into idiopathic and secondary to viral infections, the most important of which is cytomegalovirus (CMV). The outlook for patients with this complication has improved considerably in relation both to earlier diagnosis with new techniques and to the combination of high-dose immune globulins and gangiclovir (DHPG) [246,247], although late progressive pulmonary deterioration has been reported [248].

Chronic obstructive lung disease (COLD) [249] is an infrequent late complication that has been recognised lately [250,251]; it affects approximately 10% of patients with cGvHD, but may uncommonly occur in the absence of clinical GvHD [252]. Lung function tests indicate worsening obstructive airway disease; the airflow obstruction tends to be progressive, and most patients die within 3 years [252]. However, immunosuppressive treatment may be beneficial.

Liver Complications

Liver dysfunction following AlloBMT may occur in over 80% of patients [253], ranging from mild and transient enzyme elevation to fulminant hepatic failure. The major causes of liver damage include conditioning toxicity, GvHD, infections (especially viral and fungal), drug-induced liver injuries (parenteral nutrition, CyA, antibiotics) and the effects of bacteraemia and hypotension [254]. Liver abnormalities in acute and chronic GvHD include cholestasis and hepatocellular necrosis of variable degrees. A diagnosis of liver aGvHD is likely to be correct when a typical multisystem GvHD develops and no signs of VOD (sepsis, shock, viral disease and drug injury) can be detected. Viral hepatitis may be caused by different agents (B, Δ, non-A, non-

B), and its incidence in these patients may be over 40%, owing to the extreme immune suppression and to blood transfusions [255]. The histological differentiation between hepatic GvHD and non-A non-B hepatitis is often difficult [256,257]. In a recent study on 186 patients, actuarial survival was not significantly better in patients with normal as opposed to abnormal transaminases pre-transplant. Evidence of compensated hepatitis was not a relative contraindication for AlloBMT [258].

The prognosis of VOD is generally severe, and in some centres it was found to be a major cause of liver-related morbidity and mortality [259,260]. Recent data indicate that CyA plus MTX and increasing doses of fTBI are associated with a higher incidence of VOD [261]. These data, together with the findings in Genoa [258], suggest that a lower and slower TBI is more important than pre-transplant normal transaminase values in preventing VOD.

Chronic Myelogenous Leukaemia

Chronic myelogenous leukaemia (CML) has become the major indication for AlloBMT [13,14,33,108,114,262] for 3 main reasons: 1) despite recent, exciting advances in the knowledge on the molecular biology of the disease [263-267] and the provocative perspectives of treatment with alpha-IFN [269], there is not (yet?) any evidence of a medical cure of CML; 2) there is, instead, hard evidence that AlloBMT is capable of curing the disease [262,263,269-272]; 3) there is no real competition (yet?) between Allo- and AutoBMT, despite new, highly sophisticated techniques [136,272].

An estimated collection of 1500 patients with CML have been treated with AlloBMT; 1202 are registered at the IBMTR and over 200 in Seattle [271]. Six hundred and sixteen patients are in the EBMT registry [14]; they overlap with the IBMTR data, but were analysed separately. The Genoa experience has been published and discussed elsewhere [262,273]

The great majority of these patients were transplanted from HLA-D/DR identical sibling donors, and conditioned by the Seattle-model CY-TBI regimen (120 mg/kg CY followed by 10-15.75 Gy, fractionated). However, there is no clear evidence that RT forms an essential component of the preparative regimen, and equally good results are obtained with the BU-CY protocol, and with its CY 120 reductive modification [164]. Indeed, it would be quite unexpected if busulfan, which is the most typical stem cell suppressive drug, would not be active in suppressing the Ph-positive clone; on the other hand, one must also consider the potential pulmonary (and systemic) toxicity which might supervene in patients already treated for years with the same drug.

Splenectomy, performed in a small group of patients, was followed by quicker engraftment, most probably due to the lack of HSCs being trapped in the spleen, but aGvHD appeared to be more severe [274]. In a retrospective study of 210 patients with CML transplanted between 1980 and 1985, 105 splenectomised and 105 not, neither splenectomy nor irradiation were found to alter survival and relapse significantly [275]. It was concluded that debulking was of no value, and that routine splenectomy should be abandoned; however, this does not mean that the occasional large spleen resistant to all treatments should not be removed before performing transplantation. In addition, adjunct radiotherapy to the spleen has been found beneficial in some centres, e.g., in Genoa [273]. There is a prospective, randomised EBMT study that is specifically aimed at answering this question. No difference has been found.

Quite a number of problems have arisen from the worldwide experience [262,265,266,269-271], some of which were resolved, while others are still controversial.

Timing of AlloBMT

It is firmly established that the best results can be expected when AlloBMT is performed in CP, while survival and LFS are significantly worse in the accelerated (AP) and blastic (BP) phases. This is clearly shown in the IBMTR material (Fig. 4). After metamorphosis [276], not more than 15-20% of patients are capable of becoming long-term survivors

[265], although an encouragingly good estimated 55% LFS was obtained recently in 21 patients conditioned with the BU-CY2 regimen [164]. However, other data emphasise once again the increased risk and relatively poor results that occur when transplantation is deferred until signs of acceleration appear [277] (Figs. 4 and 5).

Two new aspects may be added to the decision making for AlloBMT in advanced CML. Firstly, while a cohort of patients with no additional cytogenetic abnormalities had a 3-year risk of relapse of 31%, this rose to 73% in patients with trisomy 8, double Ph or variant Ph [278]. Secondly, since in patients with lymphoid BC a CR may be induced with comparative ease and without excessive toxicity, deferral of transplantation is warranted until remission is achieved.

An unresolved controversial issue remains timing within the chronic phase (CP); since TRM is still excessively high (about 30%), it would appear reasonable to defer transplantation for 2 or 3 years, especially in those cases which appear to have a slower pace of disease, as deduced from staging [279], duration of first remission [230] and sensitivity to busulfan [265,269]. A computerised, decision-assisting programme has been proposed by Segel et al. [281], but is not widely utilised. It has been consistently reported from Seattle that there was a better LFS associated with a shorter interval from diagnosis to transplant [271,282]; however, this aspect has not been confirmed in the most recent IBMTR study [283]. A comparison of these data is shown in Table 6.

In a subset of 29 patients conditioned with CY 120 and fTBI 12 Gy, given MTX and CyA and transplanted within a year of diagnosis, the probability of survival at 5 years was over 95% [271].

If the duration of CP could really be assessed by means of molecular abnormalities of *bcr* and c-*abl*, as has been suggested [284-286], then clinicians would have an important intrinsic factor indicating the evolution of the disease. However, conflicting studies have been published [267,287,288].

In spite of extensive research, the precise role of oncogenes in the pathogenesis of human leukaemia is fairly unknown [289]. However, the recent demonstration that a myeloproliferative syndrome mimicking human CML resulted from reconstituting irradiated mice with marrow infected with a retrovirus encoding P 210 *bcr/abl* has shown that this hybrid protein may indeed cause irreversible clonal myeloid cell proliferation [290]. Notwithstanding this exciting breakthrough, the timing of transplantation is still, in the end, both a medical and a philosophical decision [16].

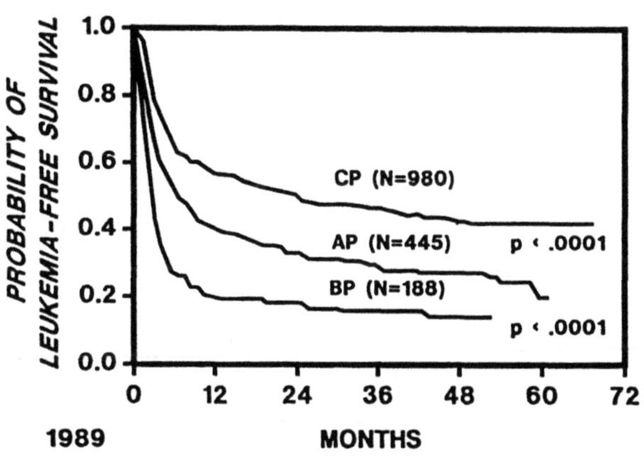

Fig. 4. Probability of leukaemia-free survival for 1613 patients with CML transplanted from HLA-identical siblings worldwide. CP = chronic phase, AP = accelerated phase, BP = blastic phase. The influence of the phase of disease on outcome is highly significant. Data from the IBMTR

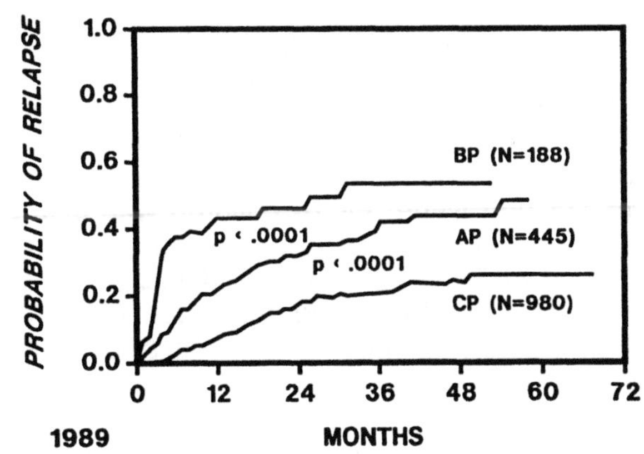

Fig. 5. The effect of disease status at transplant on relapse. Data from the IBMTR

Table 6. Comparison of actuarial data from the Seattle and the IBMTR series of patients transplanted for CML in chronic phase

	IBMTR	SEATTLE
No. of patients	405	190
Probability of survival	0.55	0.65
Probability of relapse	0.19	0.24
Probability of survival		
Diagnosis to transplant < 17 months*	0.57	0.73
Diagnosis to transplant > 17 months*	0.54	0.54

* IBMTR: 202 patients in each group; Seattle: 115 patients < 17 months and 75 patients > 17 months

Age

There is no doubt that the younger the patient, the better the outcome [261,264,270]. This relates primarily to the higher incidence of complications (TRM, GvHD, IPn) in the older patients. However, when survival was analysed by decade, no significant difference was seen in the IBMTR analysis between results of AlloBMT in the third, fourth and fifth decades of life [282] (Fig. 6). The upper age limit is, at present, undefined. Juvenile CML, although superficially resembling "genuine" CML, is an entirely different myeloproliferative disease, and is mentioned here only because of the age issue. Of 14 children with JCML between the ages of 2 and 5 years who received AlloBMT (6 from HLA-identical siblings and 8 from HLA-non-identical family members), 6 survive in continuous remission [288].

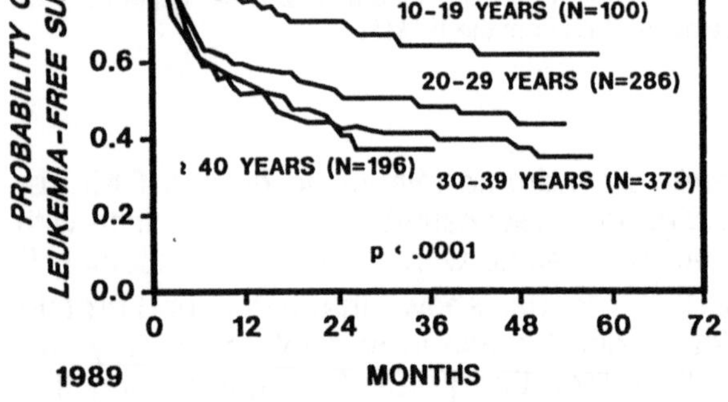

Fig. 6. The influence of age on leukaemia-free survival after AlloBMT for CML in chronic phase. Note that the difference between the 4th decade and beyond is almost negligible. Data from the IBMTR

Relapses

While the probability of relapse is high after transplantation for patients in AC/BP, it is significantly lower in CP for patients given unmanipulated marrow. In these patients, if pure cytogenetic relapses are excluded (see later), the probability of relapse may be estimated at 20%, but it may attain higher rates with the passing of time. While relapses in patients having been transplanted in advanced CML are typically of the blastic phase, 3 different patterns have been identified for those relapsing after AlloBMT in CP [265,269]. *Cytogenetic* relapse indicates those cases in which a varying proportion of marrow of recipient origin again displays Ph positivity. This pattern may progress to full-blown *haematological* relapse, which is the second pattern, but may also recede [292,293]. Reversal from cytogenetic relapse (recipient) to normal (donor) marrow may occur after discontinuation of CyA [294], thus confirming the down-regulating effect of this immunosuppressive drug on the post-transplant adoptive immunosurveillance (Fig. 7). Encouraging results have been obtained utilising alpha-IFN in full dosage [295,296]. In a cohort of 18 patients relapsed after TCD AlloBMT and treated with alpha-2b IFN, although no patient with haematological relapse became Ph-negative, 8 out of 14 patients with cytogenetic relapse did not progress to haematological relapse, and 2 achieved complete cytogenetic remission with disappearance of the *bcr* rearranged band [297].

Finally, there may be a straightforward *blastic* relapse, which occurred, in a Genoa case, 5 years after AlloBMT, indicating that the rare

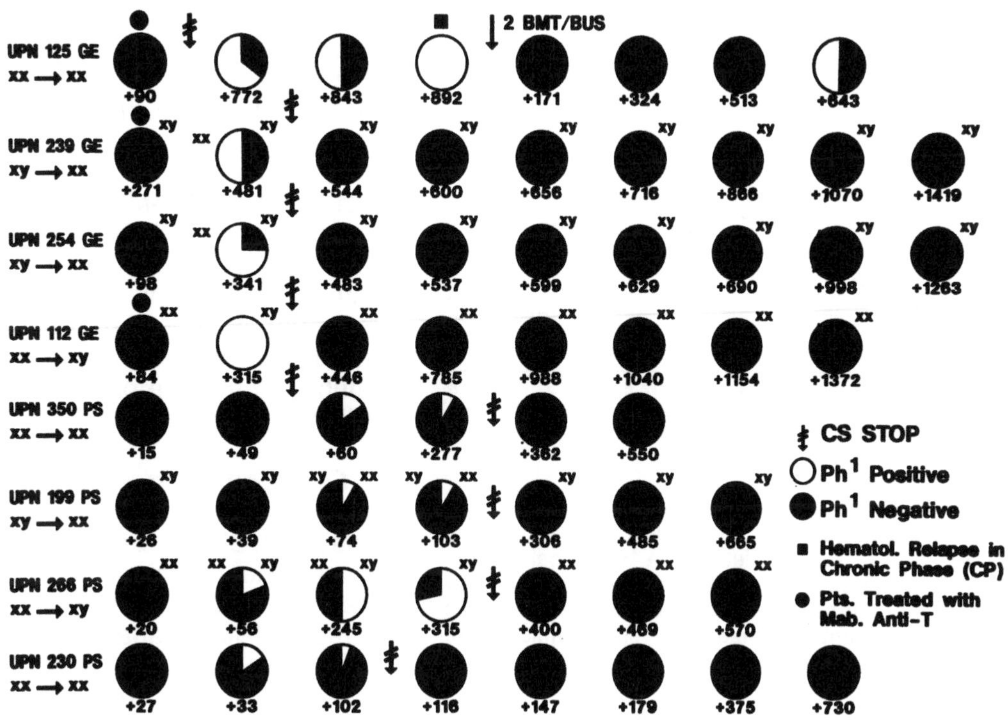

Fig. 7. Cytogenetic patterns after AlloBMT for CML in CP observed in Genoa (GE) and in Pesaro (PS). In some cases, discontinuation of cyclosporin (CS) was attended by reversal from Ph-positivity to negativity. This behaviour was more frequent in T-cell depleted transplants

surviving host Ph-positive cells had undergone a silent transformation, just as they were programmed to do according to the natural history of the disease.

A fourth type of relapse was identified recently, which could be defined as *molecular* relapse. Since the demonstration that *bcr-abl* translocation could be detected by the polymerase chain reaction (PCR) modified to use mRNA as the starting material, thus detecting the specific RNA transcript with a sensitivity (in clinical material) evaluated as 100 or 1000 times greater than that of cytogenetic techniques [298], many studies have been published, often with conflicting results [299-306]. In a number of patients no *bcr-abl* message could be found after transplantation, thus suggesting, but not proving, that long-term survivors are truly cured [298]. However, in 11 out of 12 patients in clinical and cytogenetic remission, the *bcr-abl* transcript was detected 3 months to 6 years after transplantation [303]. The hypothesis that a Ph-positive "lanthanic" microclone may persist, held in check by the GvL effect, is strongly reinforced by the observation that the same group that had obtained negative findings after unmanipulated AlloBMT found positive PCR reactions in patients who had received TCD marrows [303]. However, even in these cases a slow evolution of the relapsed leukaemia has been observed in some cases, suggesting a "low grade" disease because of an alteration of the biological tempo, conceivably induced by other donor-derived lymphoid cells [304].

Cytogenetic and molecular genetic methods, including Southern blot analysis of DNA, complement rather than replace each other for the detection of residual Ph-positive cells after AlloBMT. However, the sensitivity of the PCR reactions has been further enhanced by the introduction of the 2-step technique [301]. Since it appears that in a significant number of patients the leukaemic clone may survive for several years after AlloBMT before it is actually eradicated, the finding of residual leukaemia by PCR in the first years after transplantation could have less ominous prognostic significance than believed previously [305] (Fig. 8).

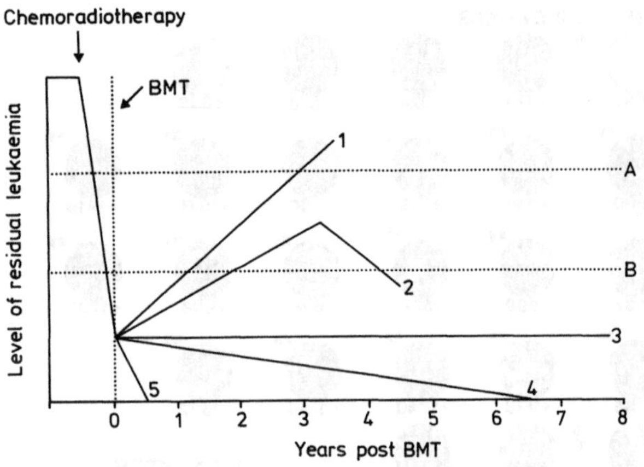

Fig. 8. The various alternative fates of the leukaemic clone after BMT for CML. Line A denotes the threshold for detection of residual leukaemia by clinical criteria. Line B denotes the threshold for detection by cytogenetic criteria. 1, steady increase in leukaemic clone and eventual relapse; 2, leukaemic clone increases above threshold of detection by cytogenetics but does not progress to clinical relapse; 3, leukaemic clone persists and is never eradicated; 4, leukaemic clone gradually eliminated over years; 5, leukaemic clone rapidly eliminated. Patterns 1 and 2 are known to occur, while patterns 3-5 are hypothetical. From [305], with permission

Unrelated Marrow Donors

Since the majority of CML patients lack HLA-identical siblings, suitably matched, unrelated donors (MUDs) have been utilised. In the most recent experience of 4 centres [132], 82 patients, 44 of whom in CP and 38 in AP, received AlloBMT from unrelated donors. The Kaplan-Meier estimates of survival at 2 years for the entire group (All) and for the matched and mismatched groups are shown in Table 7. This report has been updated very recently to comprise 102 patients [307].

In a former contribution, the results appeared to be comparable for CP patients whether the donor was fully matched or 1-locus mismatched [132]. In the London Hammersmith experience, the actuarial survival at 2 years of 22 patients (20 in CP and 2 in AP) is 35% [130]. In a large IBMTR study of 470 unrelated transplants (for all diseases), it was confirmed that increased HLA disparity was associated with decreased disease-free survival [308]. However, if there will be no major breakthrough in alternative directions, there is no doubt that the use of MUDs for CML patients will steadily increase.

T-Cell Depletion and the GvL Effect

These problems are common to all 3 main types of leukaemia [168-170,211]; however, they are most prominent in CML [309,310]. In a recent IBMTR analysis, the highest probability of remaining in remission (>90%) was found for patients with mild to severe cGvHD having received a T-replete marrow, while the lowest was found in patients having received TCD marrows and not having developed any type of GvHD [283]. The influence of higher doses of TBI in this context for prevention of relapse was ascertained in a retrospective study in Genoa [150].
In addition, although not exclusively in CML, 3 other, different but intimately related phenomena were shown to be associated with TCD, i.e., delayed haemopoiesis of donor origin, thus allowing a growth advantage to the residual leukaemic cells [311,312], the presence of radiation-induced chromosomal abnormalities in recipient cells [313] and haemopoietic mixed chimaerism [182,183]. It has been postulated that the host biology and the disease burden are different in CML [314], in which the disease is not minimal at the time

Table 7. Unrelated AlloBMT for CML: experience of 4 centres

Group	No.	Median age	Percentage surviving	95% Confidence interval	P
All	82	29	32%	17-47%	
Matched	44	31	40%	20-60%	0.20
Mismatched	38	27	22%	2-42%	

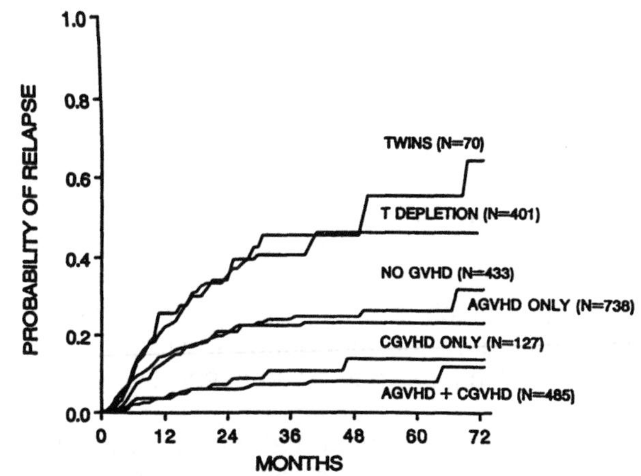

Fig. 9. The different effects of GvHD, T-cell depletion and identical twin transplantation on the probability of leukaemia relapse. From [320], with permission

of transplantation. Treatment with alpha-IFN *before* AlloBMT in order to obtain real MRD would not seem unreasonable [315]. However, preliminary observations seem to indicate a slower haemopoietic reconstitution in patients so treated, perhaps in association with the marrow fibrosis induced by IFN.

There is no doubt that the immune-related mechanisms connected with the graft are active in eradicating MRD surviving cytotoxic marrow ablation, and contribute substantially to the ultimate therapeutic effect [175,227, 229,317,318]. However, although in rodent models GvL and GvH reactivity are manifested by separate as well as overlapping cell subpopulations [228,317,318], the situation is more complex in man, where this type of dissection was attempted more indirectly (Fig. 9). Three separate components were postulated to exert this additional antileukaemia effect: 1) antileukaemia activity associated with clinically evident GvHD; 2) antileukaemia activity mediated by allogeneic (but not syngeneic) donor cells that can operate in the absence of GvHD; and 3) antileukaemia activity independent of GvHD mediated by both allogeneic and syngeneic donor cells, that is, weakened or abrogated by TCD [320]. The GvL effect was evaluated differently, and it was proposed that it may represent 50-150% of the magnitude of the conditioning procedure [318]. However, in a recent study it was calculated that it contributes the equivalent of 1 log cell kill to the eradication of MRD surviving after conditioning [321]. In considering the relapse rates of 4 types of transplants (HLA-identical, TCD grafts; twin transplants; HLA-identical, T-replete transplants with or without GvHD), the following evaluation of the 3 components mentioned above was presented recently [322] (Table 8).

Although it is still impossible to exploit "controlled" GvHD in man [333], the intentional induction of an autoimmune syndrome mimicking cGvHD by means of CyA was attempted in AutoBMT for malignant lymphomas [324]. Whether this will turn out to be significantly beneficial remains to be ascertained. Reverting to AlloBMT, and more specifically in the related, non HLA-identical setting, it was found that, although TCD did not improve DFS, there was no significant increase in relapse rates. This was related to the fact that, unlike aGvHD, cGvHD was not significantly different for the T-replete and TCD cohorts (Fig. 10 and 11).

Table 8. Effect of 3 different, immune-related components of AlloBMT on leukaemia relapse [from 322]

	T-cells	GvL	GvHD
ALL	++	++	++++
AML	+	++++	++++
CML	++++	+	++++

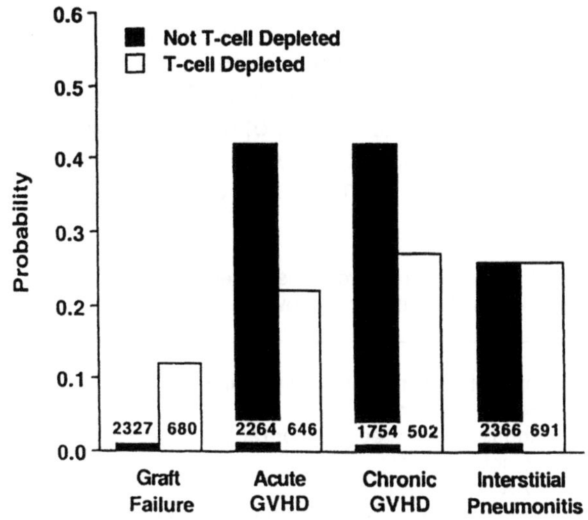

Fig. 10. The effect of T-cell depletion on graft failure, acute and chronic GvHD, and interstitial pneumonitis. From [170], with permission

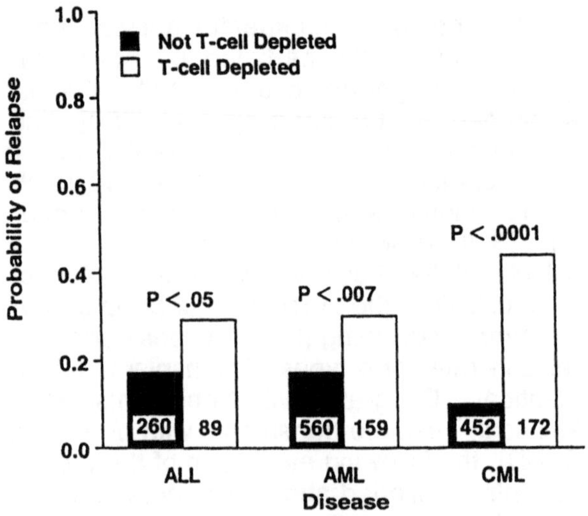

Fig. 11. The effect of T-cell depletion on relapse in early leukaemia. This effect is particularly outstanding in CML. From [170], with permission

Be this as it may, it is certain that the most unfavourable impact of TCD on leukaemia relapse after AlloBMT is found in CML, and that the procedure should be attempted only in special circumstances with high risk factors for GvHD, and even so with appropriate compensating procedures. These are shown in Table 9, taken from Goldman [265], with some modifications.

In a computerised model developed in an already mentioned IBMTR study [170], the optimisation of the controllable variables that influence the outcome of TCD AlloBMT, such as the technique of TCD and of post-transplant IS, was attempted; in the best situation, with all 6 variables optimised, LFS was predicted to be 62%. This is, of course, a theoretical calculation, but it may turn out to be useful in selecting both patients and procedures.

Table 9. Possible approaches to reduce relapse for recipients of TCD donor marrows

1. Intensified conditioning, including TBI
2. Partial or selective TCD
3. Addition of titrated fresh or radiated T-cells, or of selected subpopulations
4. LAK cells post BMT
5. Alpha-IFN post BMT (timing and dosage to be determined)
6. GM-CSF or IL-3 post BMT
7. Other lymphokines
8. Programmed optimisation of variables (see below)

The Acute Leukaemias

Acute Myeloid Leukaemia

The number of patients who have undergone AlloBMT for AML is now quite high: as of 1989 there are over 2000 cases in the IBMTR files, which also contain data from the EBMT Registry, which in turn includes 754 patients [14]. Including the independent Seattle data, over 3000 cases may be conservatively estimated.

This cumulative clinical material is, of course, quite heterogeneous, since it comprises patients of all ages, in different stages of their disease (early, intermediate and advanced), with different subtypes of AML, different tumour burden and pace of disease, and with different types of conditioning and prophylaxis for GvHD. Although the great majority of these patients have received the CY-TBI basic protocol, with the modified regimens that have been discussed previously, the solely chemotherapeutic BU-CY regimen has produced superimposable, if not occasionally superior, results, both in its original [156,160] and modified [163] versions. The importance of an effective adequate irradiation dose in the CY-TBI regimen has been demonstrated [150].

Factors Influencing the Outcome of Transplantation

Foremost among the intrinsic factors, remission status is the main factor influencing LFS, independently from leukaemia category (AML, ALL, CLL) and subtype.

Transplantation performed in advanced leukaemia is penalised both by excessive TRM and relapse incidence (RI), so that it is quite impressive that, of the original 54 patients with end-stage, refractory AML who were transplanted between 1970 and 1975 in Seattle, 6 are alive and well 11-15 years after grafting [325]. However, the same group transplanted AML patients in CR1 as early as 1979, 58% of whom are alive between 9 and 10 years after transplantation [16,326]. In another update of 20 patients with AML, the actual 4-year and actuarial 10-year survival was 60%, with a 4- and 10-year RI of 14% [327],

thus confirming the rarity of the late and very late relapses that were discussed previously [181,186]. The key role of CR1 status in ensuring a favourable outcome has been confirmed and stressed in all recent surveys [11,14-16,23,33,108-110,328], and is shown most clearly in Fig. 12, reporting the most recent IBMTR data. The RI between 10% and 20% of these CR1, adequately induced and subsequently transplanted patients suggests that there is a hard core of very malignant leukaemia which is not curable at this time. When it comes to patients relapsed after CR1, it has been shown that there is no advantage to reinduce them into CR2 rather than giving them a straightforward transplant [16,329].
Age is certainly the second most important factor influencing outcome. There is an increase of TRM decade by decade, with a marked increase above the age of 20-25 [16,33,108-110,328-330]. Although this is a general rule, some experiences differ. In a recent Minnesota study, the overall LFS was almost identical (52%) in children and adults with AML; it must be pointed out, however, that the age cutoff was 18 [331]. In other clinical studies specifically dealing with children and adolescents, the outcome has been even better [332], attaining a 59% LFS at 2 years and beyond [333-334].
Coming to other risk factors, a high number of WBC (>75x10^9/l) was an important risk factor in a recent IBMTR analysis [112]; the relative risk of relapse (RR) for patients with initial WBC above 75x10^9/l was 2.28 (p<0.04) compared with those with counts below that level (RR=1). Counts were correlated with FAB subtype, being significantly higher in the M4-M5 subtypes than in the M1-M3 ones. Organ impairment at the time of transplant was also a significant adverse factor.
Among the extrinsic factors, which are partially or totally dependent on the physicians, the adverse effect of the female-to-male combination was found to be minimal in AML, except in "bad risk" cases [113]. The effects of CMV infection are somewhat contradictory [225-226].
Differently from ALL, as will be discussed later, GvHD prophylaxis with CyA rather than MTX is a significant favourable factor [14,33,109]. The adverse effect of TCD on RI has already been discussed previously, and it

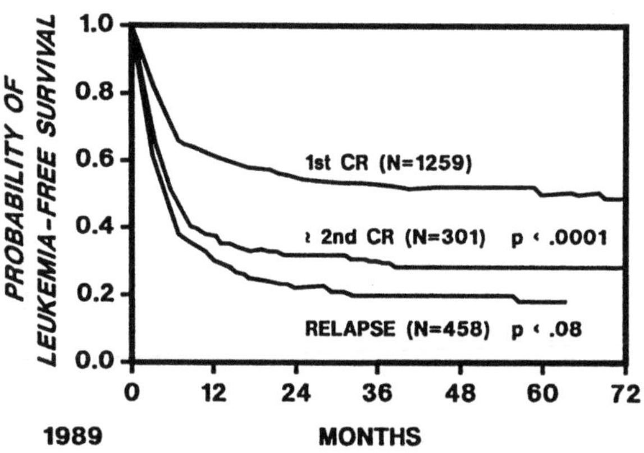

Fig. 12. The effect of disease status at transplantation in 2018 patients with AML. The difference between patients in CR2 and in first relapse is not significant. Data from the IBMTR

has been pointed out that it is significantly less than in CML.
A study on regional differences in outcome has been recently performed in Europe [335]. There were clear differences in diagnostic categories and leukaemia subtypes, as well as in the time intervals between diagnosis and transplant for AML and CML-CP patients. No centre effect could be detected, and TRM was identical in all regions if the major risk factors were taken into consideration. Relapse incidence was, however, greater in the southern region, yet the number of patients originating from the same region was small when compared with the data collected subsequently, so that another study specifically addressed to this issue is in progress.

Transplant or Chemotherapy. Timing and Incorporation in an Integrated Study

A three-pronged attack against the ALs, and most particularly against AML, is currently being performed by means of aggressive multidrug CT, AlloBMT and AutoBMT. There is much debate in favour or against each of these 3 procedures [16,27,110-112,336,337]. It has been pointed out that there is considerable overlap, and factors such as patient selection and loss of bad-risk patients before transplant may have overshadowed evaluation [111,112]. In addition, each of the 3 procedures is gradually improving, so that the results of prospective studies may reflect more the past than the present. As recently stated by Santos, "Further trials of chemotherapy versus allogeneic marrow transplantation for ANLL will add little to satisfy those critics who are on one side or the other of the issue" [328].

Out of a number of single-centre studies [338,339], the most significant comes, again, from Seattle, with a subsequent 5-year follow up. The patients were compared in 3 ways, and significantly more patients are alive in CCR at ≥5 years in the transplant group [340,341]. However, improved recent results with high-dose cytarabine and daunorubicin as consolidation have again emphasised the areas of overlap [342,343]. An illuminating, albeit only retrospective, analysis of the EBMT-EORTC has compared LFS from CR1 in 236 patients treated with CT (EORTC AML-5 and AML-6), 453 patients having undergone AlloBMT and 182 AutoBMT [344]. The age at diagnosis was restricted to between 15 and 45. The results of the proportional hazards of CT as compared to AlloBMT and AutoBMT in terms of LFS are shown in Table 10.

In considering an overall strategy for AML, since the majority of results worldwide indicate about 30% LFS in patients transplanted in first relapse and/or in CR2 [111,112], a strategy has been proposed to delay transplantation to the situation mentioned above, in order to avoid transplanting potentially cured patients. However, since organ impairment is an important risk factor [344], and cumulative toxicity from consolidation CT plus intensive conditioning may be hazardous, no conclusive guidelines may be given. Two concomitant EORTC prospective trials are attempting to answer these questions.

Second Transplants

Second AlloBMTs in patients with any type of leukaemia having relapsed after a first transplant are justified by the practically inexistent curative potential of repeat CT. A first group of attempts met with variable results [345-349]. Subsequently, 26 patients received second transplants in Seattle [350], and other 90 have been assembled in an EBMT report [351], so that one may now estimate that there are over 150 worldwide. The subject is discussed in this section because the greatest number of patients were affected by AML, followed by CML and ALL.

Most of the patients received a BU-CY regimen for conditioning, although in a few cases a repeat CY-TBI regimen was applied. Perhaps the most important finding of the Seattle study [350] was that the interval between the first and the second transplant is an important factor in determining outcome. TRM, including VOD, was very high in those patients who underwent AlloBMT <1 year after the first transplant, while those who sur-

Table 10. Proportional hazard analysis of CT as compared to Allo- and AutoBMT. Leukaemia-free survival from CR is analysed

	Regression coefficient	p	Relative risk* RR	95% confidence intervals RR
Allogeneic BMT vs. chemotherapy within 6 months of transplant	-0.083	0.52	0.92	0.71-1.19
Allogeneic BMT vs. chemotherapy after 6 months of transplant	-0.727	<0.01	0.48	0.34-0.68
Autologous BMT vs. chemotherapy within 6 months of transplant	-0.262	0.13	0.77	0.54-1.09
Autologous BMT vs. chemotherapy after 6 months of transplant	-0.242	0.27	0.79	0.51-1.21

* Risk of relapse or death relative to chemotherapy at equivalent times after first complete remission

vived 1 or more years after the initial transplant had less TRM and improved survival after the second one.

In the EMBT survey [351], factors significantly favouring survival and probability of LFS were: an interval greater than 1 year between first AlloBMT and relapse, and second transplant carried out in remission of AL or in CP of CML. While overall survival was meagre (11.5%), and nil for patients transplanted within 1 year from first transplant, it grew to 35% for patients transplanted >1 year, and attained 55% for patients transplanted >1 year and in CR/CP. Both studies pointed out that the procedure is similar to a syngeneic transplant, but, nevertheless, there was significant GvHD [350]. Low-toxicity conditioning regimens were recommended.

In a 22-year old female patient with CML in CP1 transplanted from an HLA-identical sister after TCD in Genoa [345], a first cytogenetic and subsequently haematological relapse took place starting on day +772. She was given a second, unmanipulated transplant 1074 days after the first, after a complete BU-CY regimen, but has relapsed again starting on day +843. A third transplant is currently being evaluated.

Myelodysplastic Syndromes (MDS) and Secondary (Therapy-Related) Syndromes

There are many reasons for discussing these conditions under a single heading: secondary or therapy-related AML (sAML) is generally preceded by a prolonged myelodysplastic and/or oligoblastic stage [352-354], and both conditions are characterised by the paucity or near absence of normal HSCs, so that aggressive CT is more likely to produce irreversible aplasia rather than a remission. The toxicity of aggressive CT is substantial, and no study has demonstrated an overall survival advantage [355]. This is especially true for the therapy-related MDS-AML syndrome, with its well-known defects of chromosomes 7 and 5, the latter implying deletion of genes critical to haemopoiesis [356-358]. In all these situations, the administration of allogeneic HCSs is indicated, and there is much less competition both from CT and AutoBMT.

In spite of all this, there are still reasons for making a separation between the idiopathic and the therapy-related conditions. Apart from the strategic chromosomal abnormalities, which have been pointed out previously, these patients have already been heavily treated with CT and RT, and are more susceptible to being saddled with multiple, even if not prominent, organ impairment. There is more affinity between therapy-related MDS and ANLL than between the former and idiopathic MDS. For these reasons, the 2 conditions will be discussed separately.

The Myelodysplastic Syndromes

Although there is considerable heterogeneity in the FAB classification, which lumps together such widely differing entities as the refractory and sideroblastic anaemias (RA and RARS) and RAEB-T, with its marked overlap with oligoblastic AML, it will be adhered to for clarity [357].

Since there are important prognostic differences between the genuine *anaemias* and the *oligoblastic states* [360,361], most patients have been transplanted for the latter conditions. Little more than 20 patients with RA/RARS have been transplanted worldwide [362,363]; relapses are significantly rarer than in the oligoblastic states [364], but have occurred [362]. Relapses have also occurred in oligoblastic MDS when conditioning had been limited to CT with CY only [364]. It is accordingly essential to distinguish hypoplastic MDS from aplastic anaemia, since the preparative regimen for MDS should be as for leukaemia patients [365].

A series of single-centre studies have reported long-term LFS in approximately half of the patients [367-369]. Two important surveys have been performed [363,369], one of which is still being perfected [363]. In the EMBT study, including 78 patients transplanted in Europe between 1982 and 1988, 2-year LFS was 58% for untreated RA, 64% for untreated RAEB and 50% for untreated RAEB-T [369]. In the therapy-related states (MDS/ANLL), the best results were obtained when the patients were transplanted in CR obtained with CT, but it was recognised that patients with hypocellular or myelofibrotic marrow are not likely to respond favourably to CT. The IBMTR study includes 123 patients; preliminary data

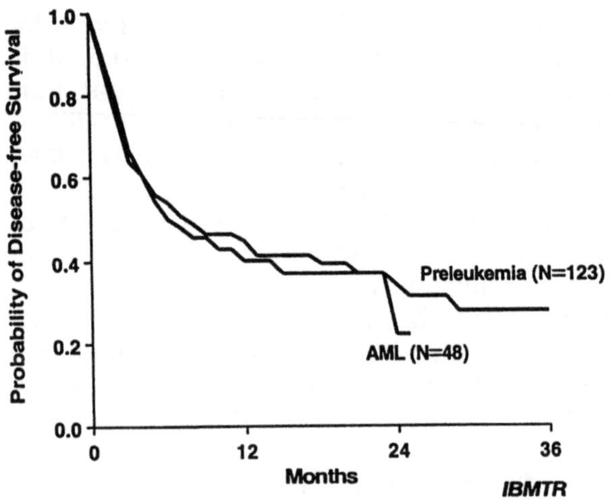

Fig. 13. Probability of leukaemia-free survival for patients transplanted (HLA-identical sibling donors) for myelodysplastic syndromes without or with overt leukaemia. Data from the IBMTR

indicated that the best results of BMT are likely to occur when patients are transplanted in the preleukaemic stage rather than after evolution into AML [363] (Fig. 13).

Secondary Leukaemias

The main question for sAML, and more generally the sMDS/AML syndrome, is whether the transplant should be performed after having achieved CR by means of CT, or directly. The EBMT data are in favour of the first type of strategy [369]; however, there are single case reports in which straightforward AlloBMT was followed by success [370,371]. In a preliminary analysis performed on 17 published patients, data indicated that AlloBMT was successful in half of the cases with overt disease; in addition, TRM, rather than relapse, was the main cause of death. No strict policy should be adhered to in sAML. When the cytologic, cytokinetic and cytogenetic features mimic *de novo* AML, and the tumour burden is high, there is little doubt that the induction of remission should be attempted before transplant. When the disease follows an indolent, smouldering course, an upfront transplant may be performed without running into the risks of a complicated remission induction with CT [371].

Acute Lymphoblastic Leukaemia

ALL is the most frequent childhood cancer, perhaps also in relation to the cellular development of immunity [373], and accounts for approximately 20% of adult AL [373]. The disease is markedly heterogeneous, and the most striking clinical feature is the therapeutic dichotomy between childhood and adult ALL. Recent trials indicate 80-90% 3- to 5-year LFS in children with standard risk disease, and also in high-risk patients intensive CT has improved results to approximately 70% [374,376]. In adults, however, it is a common notion that LFS is approximately 35% [377]. The reasons for this discrepancy are still unclear, but intrinsic characteristics of the leukaemic cells (higher proportions of B-Cell and CALLA-positive ALL in childhood versus more T-cell and null-cell, and more frequent Ph-positivity in adults) and perhaps also a greater tolerance to drugs in children may account for the difference [378]. In addition, hybrid ALL is significantly more frequent in adults [379].

Acute Lymphoblastic Leukaemia in Children

Over 2,000 AlloBMTs have been performed for patients with ALL, but only selected children with very poor prognosis have been transplanted in CR1. These typically include very high WBC and infants of less than 1 year of age; however, a recent evaluation of the BFM groups considers only the categories which are shown in Table 11 [380].
The presence of myeloid markers, indicating hybrid leukaemia [379], should perhaps also be considered [381]. Single-centre studies have given reasonably good results for this high-risk group of patients, with LFS ranging

Table 11. High-risk groups of ALL in children for which AlloBMT should be considered in CR1

- Late responders
- Steroid nonresponders to initial corticotherapy
- Ph-positive ALL
- Certain translocations (e.g., t(4;11))

from 40% to 76% [382,383]. This has been confirmed in multicentre studies [384], and most particularly in a recent IBMTR analysis in which, despite very poor prognostic factors, there was a 5-year 56% LFS in 56 children who had been transplanted in CR1 [385].

It is not surprising, then, that the great majority of transplants for children with ALL has been performed in CR2, where initial studies had shown a clear advantage of AlloBMT over CT [386-388]. However, improved salvage protocols have changed the situation once again, and it is widely accepted that the date of relapse, whether within or after 18 months post-remission, dictates further policy, that is, towards transplantation (<18 months) or CT (>18 months) [375,388,389]. This is clearly related to what Barrett has called "pace of disease" [390], i.e., intrinsic faster tumour cytokinetics. However, to rely entirely on CT for relapsed ALL children is perhaps unjustified and, as already stated, AlloBMT may be a passing phase in the management of AL in childhood, particularly in ALL, but its time has not yet gone [116,117].

As already indicated, ALL in adults carries a much poorer prognosis, so that transplantation in CR1 is certainly more justified [146,391] (Fig. 14). In the first IBMTR study, in which most of the patients were adults and many had additional risk factors, LFS after AlloBMT was approximately 45% in CR1 and 20% in CR2 [384]. In the second study, 5-year LFS was 39% in adults transplanted in CR1, while for both children and adults in CR2 5-year LFS was 26% [385]. The utilisation of a hyperfractionated TBI regimen has already been discussed in the section on conditioning, and has been found useful both at MSKCC [143-145] and in Genoa [146].

Somewhat surprisingly, the IBMTR study has shown a significantly higher risk of relapse associated with the use of CyA and TCD to prevent GvHD as compared with methotrexate (MTX) in both CR1 and CR2 transplants [385,392]. The question of TCD favouring relapse has already been discussed in the section on CML, where this effect is most apparent; in any case, it is much less evident in ALL [147,168-170] than in the ALs in general [393]. MTX was associated with a 5-fold decrease in RI in CR1 transplants and a 3-fold decrease in CR2. However, no improvement in LFS was observed in the MTX-treated patients due to increased mortality from IPn. Corticosteroids combined with MTX or CyA were associated with a 2.8-fold increase in LFS in CR1 adult transplants. The reduced RI in patients treated with MTX was interpreted as being due to the drug's direct antileukaemia effect, since it persisted after correcting the data for incidence and severity of GvHD [385,392]. Closely similar results have been reported by a Swedish group [394]. However, that this may perhaps not be the whole story is suggested by a recent, randomised study from Genoa, where the actuarial risk of relapsing for 38 patients grafted in CR1, 19 with 1mg/kg and 19 with 5mg/kg, was 7% and 42%, respectively, with no clear correlation with the incidence of GvHD [395].

Transplant versus Chemotherapy

The situation is in even greater flux that in AML, mainly because direct comparison of the results of CT and AlloBMT trials is hampered by the differences in patient selection and exclusion of patients from transplant series whose remission is too brief to allow a transplant to be performed [337,396]. An important clinical study combining the IBMTR results for 252 ALL patients transplanted in CR1 and the German Multicentre ALL Therapy Trials (GMATT) results for approximately 400 patients treated with the 1988 Hoelzer protocol [397] is being completed [398]. The probabilities for LFS have been

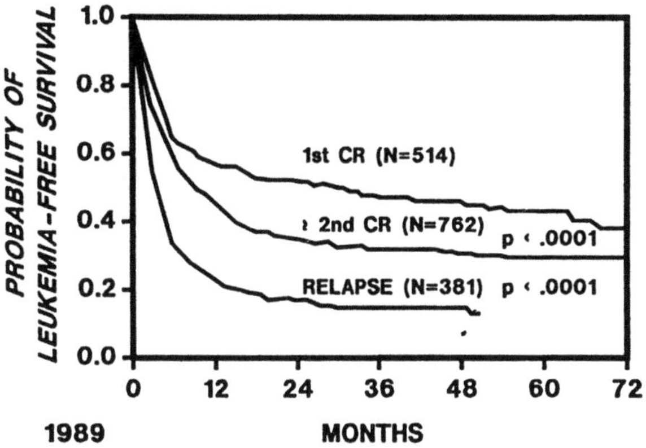

Fig. 14. The effect of disease status for 1657 patients with acute lymphoblastic leukaemia. Data from the IBMTR

Table 12. Transplantation versus chemotherapy in ALL[1]

COHORT	Transplant 1st			Chemotherapy 1st		
	Trans-plant	Rescue[2]	Total	Chemo-therapy	Rescue	Total
Children[3]	55%	5%	60%	60-70%	10%[4]	70-80%
Adults	45%	5%	50%	35%	15%[5]	50%

1 Data are summarised from the literature cited and the IBMTR
2 Assumes a 30% relapse rate with a 10% outcome of chemotherapy rescue
3 High-risk only
4 Assumes a 30-40% relapse rate with a 35% outcome of transplant in second remission
5 Assumes a 65% relapse rate with a 20% outcome of transplant in second remission

calculated after adjustment for number of patients, disease characteristics, and censoring of early relapses for the transplant group, and the results suggest that CT and AlloBMT are comparable for adults with ALL in CR1. In contrast, transplants in adults in CR2, which result in a minimum of 20% 3-year LFS, are clearly superior to CT.

Notwithstanding considerable controversy [375,377,399,400], the present situation is adequately synthesised by Butturini and Gale [396] in Table 12.

Similarly to what has already been discussed in the section on AML, it appears that 2 alternative strategies may be developed for ALL. In the first, AlloBMT is performed in CR1, and CT is used to rescue relapsed patients; second transplants may also be considered, and MUDs can and must be searched for when it is perceived that transplantation offers more chances than CT. The alternative strategy advocates initial aggressive CT, with AlloBMT, when feasible, as a rescue measure for patients who relapse. Results of these alternative approaches are indicated in Table 13, taken from the same authors [396].

Other Haematological Malignancies

Lymphoproliferative Diseases

Chronic lymphocytic leukaemia (CLL) is most generally treated by medical means [401-403], and there are few indications for AlloBMT. However, 9 patients have been reported recently by Michallet et al. [404]: 8 were in advanced, refractory stages while 1 patient was transplanted as primary treatment. In all cases, there was evidence of CR with successful engraftment. Five patients are in LFS with a median follow up of 20 months, 1 relapsed and 2 died of transplant-related toxicity. CLL is a disease of the elderly, and it is quite unlikely that a patient should undergo transplantation; however, it appears that it is feasible for very special cases.

There has been little progress in the treatment of patients with multiple myeloma, and the average survival time is still only about 3 years [405]. AlloBMT is up to now the only therapeutic measure capable of achieving

Table 13. Alternative strategies of transplantation versus chemotherapy in ALL in first remission

	3-5 year leukaemia-free survival	
	Chemotherapy	Transplants
1st Remission		
Children (high risk)	60-70%	55%
Adults	35%	45%
2nd Remission		
Children (< 18m)[1]	<5%	20%
Children (> 18m)	20-40%	30-40%
Adults	<5%	20%
> 3rd Remission	0	15%

1 1st remission < or > 18 months

long-term disease-free survival. There have been many single-centre studies, and both the modified BU-CY regimen [165] and high-dose multi-agent chemo-radiotherapy [406-410] have been employed. The most important clinical material has been assembled by the EBMT [409,410]. Out of 50 patients, 36 of whom in stage III, about 40% achieved CR and about 34% remained disease free [410].
AlloBMT has also been resorted to in very few cases of hairy-cell leukaemia [411,412]; however, the excellent results obtained with the new medical treatments (IFN-alpha, pentostatine) have made this practice obsolete.

Myeloproliferative and Histiocytic Diseases

Agnogenic myeloid metaplasia is the most typical myeloproliferative disorder, and patients of suitable age and with histocompatible sibling donors could be considered as suitable candidates for AlloBMT [413]. Indeed, successful transplantations were performed in a few, selected, cases of acute "malignant" myelosclerosis [414,415].
Marrow fibrosis in general is considered to be a risk factor for marrow colonisation by the circulating stem cells; however, both in this condition and in severe fibrosis associated with long-standing CML, AlloBMT has been capable of reversing fibrosis [416]. The hypothesis that the spleen might represent an essential intermediate station for marrow seeding in the presence of marrow fibrosis is rendered improbable by reports of equally successful transplants in previously splenectomised patients [371,417].
Malignant histiocytosis is a rare haematological malignancy affecting the monocyte-macrophage lineage. Few children have been transplanted, and there have been both long-term remissions [418-420] and relapses [421]. A case from our own clinical material is particularly enlightening. A 17-year old male (UPN 253) had been diagnosed as affected by malignant histiocytosis in 1981. At that time, he had superficial and mediastinal enlarged lymph nodes. He was brought into CR by CT, but relapsed with skin and marrow involvement in February, 1985. He obtained a third remission in March of the same year, and was transplanted in CR3 from a male HLA-identical sibling on 22 March, 1985, after conditioning with CY (120 mg) and TBI (330 Gy x 3). He is in unmaintained CCR since that date (5 years).
Although, as already indicated, malignant histiocytosis is an infrequent haematological malignancy, there is no doubt, considering also the young age of patients, that AlloBMT should be resorted to whenever possible. The search for MUDs is also warranted.

Autologous Bone Marrow Transplantation

Introduction

Bone marrow autotransplantation consists of the administration of extremely high doses of CT and/or RT (generally TBI), followed by "rescue" with autologous cryopreserved [43], but also fresh HSCs. Since the patient acts as his own donor, immunological interactions are absent, and rejection, GvHD and GvL do not occur. Indeed, some effort to elicit this last, beneficial type of reaction is being made both in man [324] and in animals [422], via the generation of a GvHD-like, cyclosporin-mediated immune reaction.

Autologous HSCs are generally harvested with the bone marrow multiple aspirate, but peripheral HSCs are increasingly utilised [1-5,423-425]. Special procedures, such as eliciting a wave of circulating HSCs after high doses of CY in cancer patients together with the administration of GM-CSF, are being performed [426], although these procedures are more indicated for solid tumours and lymphomas than for leukaemia. The identification of the CD34+ surface membrane antigen on such cells is a reliable indicator of their stem cell nature [427], although it may also be expressed by highly undifferentiated leukaemia cells [428]. Marrow and/or blood collections are cryopreserved with special procedures [429]. The clinical toxicity of cryopreserved marrow infusions has been investigated recently [430], but is seldom prohibitive.

The reinfusion of autologous HSCs is determining for the utilisation of very high doses of CT, which are critical for its efficacy, without concern for myelotoxicity. As opposed to conventional CT, the procedure allows a much greater utilisation of dose intensity, i.e., by a factor of 2-3 times. However, major limitations may derive from non-haematological, single and/or multiorgan toxicity. The outcome of phase I dose escalation studies with AutoBMT [431] is reported in Table 14.

The criticism has been made that patients already cured by CT may be among those who undergo "successful" AutoBMT, thus inflating the percentage of positive outcomes [432]. The impact of including these cases, which are included in CT trials, would be to discount the reported efficacy of AutoBMT by sizeable figures [433]. However, notwithstanding the time-censoring issue, more recent multicentre studies suggest that AutoBMT, with or without purging, may increase the probability of LFS in leukaemia over and above treatment with CT alone.

As has been pointed out recently [36,38,115], whether leukaemia is indeed curable by AutoBMT will depend upon (a) the risk of reinfusing residual leukaemia clonogenic cells and (b) the incomplete eradication of leukaemia by the conditioning regimen. The absence of alloreactivity is tantamount to the loss of the spectrum of GvL reactions [320,322], although it has been proposed that some benefit could be preserved by endogenous activated killer cells [115]. Incomplete

Table 14. Outcome of phase I escalation studies with AutoBMT

Agent	Maximum dose with marrow support	Non-haemopoietic dose-limiting toxicity
Cyclophosphamide	210 mg/kg	Cardiac
Etoposide	2100 mg/m^2	Mucositis
Mitomycin C	40 mg/m^2	Gastrointestinal, hepatic, cardiopulmonary
Melphalan	180 mg/m^2	Gastrointestinal
Carmustine (BCNU)	1200 mg/m^2	Hepatic, pulmonary

haemopoietic reconstitution, that is, autologous graft failure, is an uncommon complication, although there generally are prolonged platelet reconstitution times. Although the marrow inoculum is exposed to the combined injuries of previous myelotoxic therapy, cryopreservation and, most importantly of all, purging procedures, infusion of as few as 5 x 10^7 nucleated cells/kg, equivalent to 4 x 10^4 CFU-GM/kg, is sufficient to restore complete haemopoiesis [434]. This issue is at the moment considerably influenced not only by the powerful beneficial impact of haemopoietic growth factors, as already discussed [87-104, 435,436], but also by a more careful stem cell sparing procedure based on the determination of the maximum tolerated dose of mafosfamide by very early HSCs in culture [437,438].

However, the most important point consists in the risk of infusing residual leukaemia cells. Whether these cells are responsible for relapse, compared to other residual leukaemia cells not residing in the marrow inoculum, is a matter of debate, but, as has been aptly remarked, "there is a natural reluctance to inject any malignant cell into a patient who has received therapy designed to eradicate disease *in vivo* [115]. This issue will be discussed further on.

The utilisation of AutoBMT has increased rapidly [439,440], and it seems that over 1500 such transplants per year are performed worldwide. The most frequently treated diseases included non-Hodgkin's lymphoma (22%), AML (19%), ALL (15%), Hodgkin's disease (15%) and neuroblastoma (5%). There were striking differences in the utilisation of AutoBMT between North America and Europe [440], in the sense that lymphomas and solid tumours were the main indication in North America, while leukaemia was the main indication in Europe. A number of reviews [23,38,39,115,441,442] and two outstanding volumes [35,36] have been published.

Comprehensive reports on AutoBMT for malignant lymphomas [443-445], with special emphasis on the Hodgkin [446-448] and non-Hodgkin [449,450] categories, neuroblastoma [451] and other chemosensitive solid tumours [452,453] have also appeared recently. However, these last issues will not be pursued any further.

Minimal Residual Disease and Its Detection

Remission-inducing CT will cause an average 4 log leukaemia cell kill, which can be further increased by the consolidation-intensification procedures. Different calculations have been made to determine this minimal leukaemia residue in the explanted bone marrow, but the figure of 1.5 x 10^6 leukaemia cells in a graft containing a total of 1.5 x 10^{10} cells has been postulated [115]. However, studies on Brown Norway myelocytic leukaemia (BNML) of the rat have shown that not more than 1% of *in-vivo* clonogenic residual leukaemia cells survive cryopreservation [454,455]. Accordingly, only 15-150 clonogenic leukaemic cells out of 1.5 x 10^3 would be reinfused with the graft. Assuming an ED 50 value for human leukaemia of 1 x 10^3 - 1 x 10^4 clonogenic cells, which seems to be realistic based on previous BNML studies [454,455], it can be calculated that the chance of reinfused leukaemic cells causing leukaemia is 1-10% or 1-1%, respectively. For these reasons, more emphasis is placed on the so-called *in-vivo* purging, that is, a reduction of the patient's leukaemia cells to a truly minimal residue [456]. This concept has been extended to other chemosensitive, relapsed lymphomatous diseases [457].

The ability to detect minimal residual leukaemia (MRD) in the marrow of patients in conventional complete remission has been hampered, up to now, by the lack of sensitive assays and the identification of reliable, specific, tumour cell markers. In Burkitt's lymphoma, visual microscopic examination permits detection of up to 10^{-4} MRD cells in an apparently normal marrow [458]. In an artificial model, the detection of as few as 10^{-6} residual malignant cells stained with the vital dye Hoechst 342 was made possible by computerised analysis [459]. Most recent procedures include the PCR reaction, which has already been discussed when dealing with CML, in this case, however, detecting the RNA transcription of proto-oncogenes *sis*, *raf*, and especially *myc* [460]. Another technique involving immune selection followed by immunoglobulin or T-cell receptor gene rearrangement analysis has allowed the detection of 1 tumour cell out of 1000 normal marrow cells in B and/or T ALL patients [461]. However, perhaps the most sensitive and reasonably feasible technique for detecting MRD of lymphoblastic cells is a double immunofluorescence staining procedure for TDT and B or T-lineage antigens [462]. A general comment regarding these studies is that they need not be performed by all clinical teams performing AutoBMT for leukaemia and/or other malignant neoplasms, but that they are a yardstick for evaluating the biological efficacy of various purging procedures.

Purging Techniques

When considering bone marrow purging, the consensus is that one should distinguish between physical, chemical and immunological methods [115,463]; however, biophysical purging, which is based on differences in cell density or size [464] on percoll or bovine serum albumin (BSA) gradients is complex and rarely used. Counterflow centrifugation is specifically utilised for TCD in AlloBMT [237]. UV irradiation of the graft is also proposed for the same setting [235]. Procedures based on photosensitisation utilising a vital dye such as merocyanine 540 [465], represent a physicochemical technique. The two fundamental methods are pharmacological and immunological.

Pharmacological Purging

Ex vivo marrow purging with the activated oxazolphosphorine derivatives 4-hydroxyperoxycyclophosphamide (4HC) and INN mafosfamide (Asta-Z 7557) has been used most extensively after the pioneering Baltimore studies [466]. Mafosfamide is generally considered to be the best agent, and has been analysed in depth [467], also with reference to its differential effects upon normal and leukaemic stem cells [468]. The *in-vitro* chemosensitivity of leukaemic progenitor cells (AML-CFU) to a combination of mafosfamide lysine (Asta-Z 7654) and etoposide was studied, and it was found that the chemosensitivity of AML-CFU closely mimicked that of normal CFU-GM [469]. Although a fixed dose was used more commonly, another, more laborious, adjusted dose procedure has been utilised subsequently [438,470]. The use of still other drugs has been analysed [471], but none of them competes favourably with mafosfamide in the general practice, although etoposide was found to be a suitable agent [472].

Immunological Purging

According to this procedure, unwanted cells are specifically targeted by monoclonal antibodies (MoAbs), and then destroyed by means of different effector mechanisms [473]. While chemical purging is generally used for AML, immunological methods are utilised more specifically for ALL because of the better individualised antigenic properties of the leukaemic cells. A brief description of the principal immunological methods is given in the following.

Complement-Mediated Lysis

MoAbs (IgM and/or IgG2a isotypes) lyse targeted cells in the presence of rabbit complement [474]. Some of these MoAbs, such as the rat antibodies Campath-1 and many other mouse MoAbs, are lytic also with human complement [311]. In a recent, already mentioned study [462], MoAbs CD10, CD19 and their mixture were able to eliminate > 3 logs of B ALL cells in 84%, 75.5% and 90% of cases, respectively. When human complement was substituted for the rabbit's, the same reagents eliminated 26.8%, 0% and 45%, respectively. MoAb CD7 eliminated > logs of T ALL blasts with both sources of complement in 73% of cases.

Immunomagnetic Depletion

The use of paramagnetic microbeads, which may be linked to target cells by an antibody bridge, is utilised for the purging of tumour cells and/or lymphocytes from the marrow [475,476]. The efficacy of immunomagnetic bone marrow was found to be dependent upon matching of the targeting MoAb and the secondary antibodies that link to the surface of the microbeads [477].

Immunotoxins

MoAbs may be conjugated to various plant toxins [478]. Ricin is the one most commonly utilised in clinical studies [479-481], and acts by a double mechanism, the toxic A chain penetrating into the cell and inhibiting protein synthesis by the ribosomes, and the B chain permitting cell entry. Such an immunotoxin has been employed recently for the prophylaxis of GvHD in AlloBMT [482], and has yielded the usual advantages and disadvantages. The dramatic therapeutic effect of this type of immunotoxin on steroid-resistant GvHD has already been reported [240]. Other phytotoxins have also been utilised [482].

Is Purging Necessary?

In order to establish whether purging is capable of producing significant benefits in AutoBMT, two questions must be asked [115]. Does it effectually remove malignant cells from the bone marrow? and, Does it increase the probability of patient cure? It appears that we are somewhat closer to the answers than when the questions were formulated (1988).
Starting with the first question, reduction of leukaemic cell contamination marrows collected in CR or in artificial marrow-tumour cell mixtures has been demonstrated not only in animal experiments [462,465,477], but also in human leukaemia [461]. An illuminating recent study from Baltimore has shown, in a syngeneic transplant model for rats affected by Brown-Norway AML (BNML), a 58% cure rate after BU-CY conditioning and subsequent administration of an IgM MoAb binding both with human and rat AML cells and activating complement. All controls, that is, leukaemic rats conditioned and transplanted in the same way, died of leukaemia relapse [483].
To establish, despite the lack of prospective randomised studies, whether patient survival is improved, some retrospective clinical studies, among which an important EBMT survey, indicate that purging is valuable [484]. They will be discussed in the following sections.

Acute Myeloblastic Leukaemia

A considerable number of single-centre studies on AutoBMT for AML have been published. As for AlloBMT, the first trials were performed in relapsed patients. Out of 63 patients who were in first or second relapse and were reconstituted with CR1 marrow at 5 different centres, 70% went into CR, but the median duration of remission was only 6 months, and only 5% of the patients experienced a long-term benefit [485]. Another study on patients in first relapse was performed soon after [486].
All subsequent studies, however, were performed in remission, most often in CR1 but also in CR2 [487-490]. An excellent overview appeared in 1986 [491]. A 2-year LFS of nearly 50% for patients in CR1 was generally obtained. In the large retrospective EORTC/EBMT study which has already been discussed [344], AutoBMT was found to have a relative relapse risk versus AlloBMT of 0.77 within 6 months of transplant, and of 0.79 after 6 months of transplant.
Up till now, two basic questions have stood in the way of AutoBMT for acute leukaemia, but these are gradually finding their answers. The first concerns the problem of purging. All the Baltimore studies on AutoBMT for AML have been performed with marrow purged with 4-hydroxyperoxycyclophosphamide (4-HC).
Their results are encouraging, showing that the relapse rate is similar to that estimated for syngeneic BMT, and that LFS is comparable to that reported for AlloBMT [308,492]. An indirect demonstration of the importance of dose effect in the *ex-vivo* purging with 4-HC has been furnished by the same group recently [493]. However, the most compelling evidence comes, after a series of dubious reports [487,494], from the most recent EMBT survey [484].
In this report, 335 patients with AML (M1-M5 FAB subtype) were autografted in CR1 or CR2 between January 1st, 1981 and December 31st, 1987. In CR1, 235 patients were classified as standard risk (SR) and 32 as high risk (HR). In CR2, 65 patients were SR and only 3 HR. A variety of conditioning regimens were utilised, thus somewhat impairing the study's significance. The majority of patients, i.e., 237 (70.7%), received un-

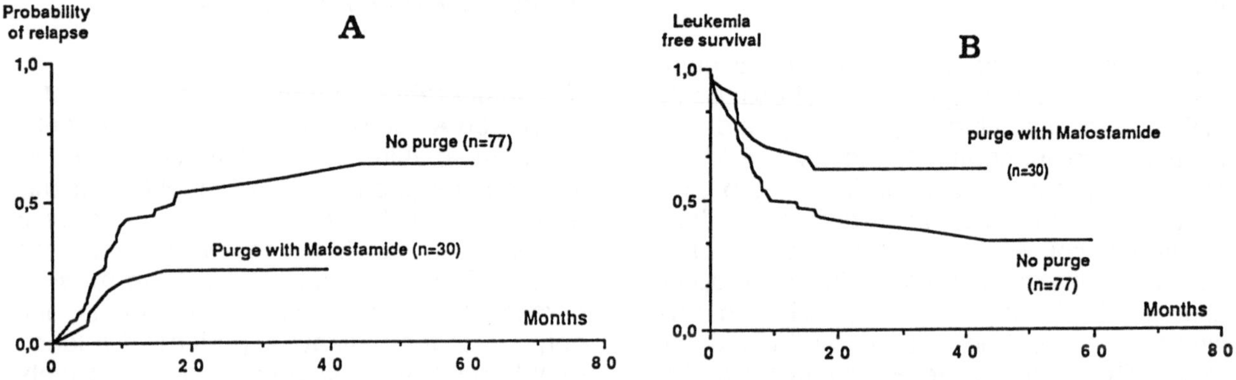

Fig. 15. Cumulative probability of relapse (A) and of leukaemia-free survival (B) in patients with standard risk AML autografted in CR1 following chemo-radiotherapy, according to whether or not the marrow was treated *in vitro* with mafosfamide ($p<0.05$ and $p<0.005$, respectively, in multivariate analyses). From [484], with permission

purged marrow, while 98 patients (29.3%, 69 in CR1 and 29 in CR2) had their marrow purged with mafosfamide, either at standard or individually adjusted levels [438,470].

Leukaemia-free survival was better in certain FAB subclasses, in patients transplanted more than 9 months post-CR (a well-known knotty point in AutoBMT) and, obviously, in the SR patients. Considering marrow purging SR, patients with AML in CR1 having been conditioned with a TBI incorporating regimen and receiving marrow treated with mafosfamide, had a significantly better LFS than those receiving unpurged marrow (LFS at 4 years: 63% + 8 vs. 34% + 7; p=0.05) (Fig. 15).

As for AlloBMT, there are multiple conditioning regimens, although the two major models of purely chemical and CT-TBI type predominate. Among the CT regimens, the BAVC (BCNU, Amsacrine, VP-16, ARA-C) Rome protocol is probably the most effective. In a very recent study including 39 AML patients in CR1, 25 were conditioned with BAVC and 14 with the standard CY-TBI regimen. The probability of remaining in CCR was significantly higher in the CY-TBI cohort, indicating the greater eradicating power of this regimen; however, there was a larger number of toxic deaths. The overall LFS of the 39 patients after a median follow-up of 47 months was 51% [495]. The modified BU-CY regimen has been utilised recently: acute toxicity was notable, but a 55% LFS was obtained in 20 AML patients [496].

A novel approach to obtain a greater ablation of the pathological marrow consists in double autografts [497,498]. Although the number of cases is small, and the patients are a selected group, the incidence of relapse appears to be reduced [497]. Even after purging with mafosfamide, the cryopreserved marrow was capable of reconstituting haemopoiesis twice in children who were double-autografted for solid tumours [499].

Autotransplantation versus Allotransplantation

This is one of the fundamental contemporary problems in the treatment of AL. It has been discussed previously, and only a single, important clinical study [500] will be analysed here. The comparative values of Allo- and AutoBMT were assessed in 117 15- to 60-year old consecutive patients with AML following remission-induction therapy. AlloBMT was performed in 23 eligible patients, AutoBMT in 32, and the remaining patients were treated with CT. Three-year overall survival was 66% after AlloBMT and 37% after AutoBMT, whereas the LFS at 3 years was 51% and 35%, respectively. Patients treated with CT alone had a 3-year LFS of 9%.

Although this well-constructed study has shown an advantage of Allo- vs. AutoBMT, more extensive prospective trials are clearly needed. A comparison between allotransplanted and autotransplanted patients treated with the same induction and consolidation protocols in Genoa has up to now failed to show any significant difference.

Acute Lymphoblastic Leukaemia

The heterogeneity, age-dependent therapeutic responsiveness and all other factors that make the choice between CT and transplantation controversial, have been discussed in the chapter on AlloBMT. Therapeutic options have been examined [373,377,501], and the arguments as to which form of transplantation, let alone CT, is superior for patients with ALL, parallel those already raised and discussed for AML [16]. A series of single-centre studies have recently been reviewed by Carella [502], and there is also the large EBMT study [503]. Only some of them will be considered here.

In the most recent Minnesota study including 91 high-risk ALL patients in CR1, long-term LFS survival was obtained in 27% of patients who had been allotransplanted and in 20% of those who had been autotransplanted [504]. Interestingly but not unexpectedly, a 79% probability of relapse was found both for patients autotransplanted and for those not having developed GvHD after AlloBMT.

In a joint study of the Royal Free Hospital, London, the University Hospital, Uppsala and the Royal Hospital for Sick Children, Glasgow, 54 patients with high-risk ALL were treated with AutoBMT using marrow purged with selected MoAbs. Leukaemia-free survival at 4 years was 64% for 21 patients transplanted in CR1 [505]. Twelve patients achieved inversion (that is, a CR longer than the previous one), seven other patients having the potential to achieve it. Inversion is a powerful indicator of a more effective treatment.

In a very recent study from Boston, 44 children with ALL who had relapsed were intensively treated with CT, had remission marrow purged with MoAbs (J5 CALLA and J12/gP26), were conditioned with a CT-TBI protocol and were then infused with their own purged marrow [506]. Event-free survival (EFS) at 5 years was 29%, and, for the 20 patients whose CR1 had been longer than 2 years, 51%.

In the latest EBMT study, 560 patients underwent AutoBMT for ALL [503]. The median age was 15 years (range 1-55); 43% were children (<15) and 47% adults, of whom 3% over 45. Thirteen patients had a Ph chromosome. The marrow was purged in 55% of SR patients in CR1, 79% of HR patients in CR1 and SR patients in CR2, and 85% of HR patients in CR2. Leukaemia-free survival at 5 years was 42% for patients autografted in CR1 (SR + HR) and 25% for patients in CR2 (SR + HR). Survival for patients in CR2 was significantly ($p < 0.05$) superior in children (42% at 52 months) compared to adults (20% at 24 months). Once again, better LFSs were found in patients with a longer interval from CR1 to transplant, reflecting, as already discussed, the lower pace of disease. A trend was seen in favour of HR patients in CR1 who were autografted with their marrow purged with mafosfamide at adjusted levels.

In the end, it appears that studies in second and subsequent remissions may be more useful for resolving some of the most burning issues [507,508].

Chronic Myelogenous Leukaemia

As remarked previously, AlloBMT is, up to now, the only cure for CML. There are, however, some new and interesting developments, which have been reviewed recently [509].

Many approaches have been devised for eliminating the Ph-positive stem cells in the autograft, including long-term marrow cultures [136,510,511), *ex-vivo* exposure of the marrow to cyclophosphamide derivatives [272], long-term treatment of patients with IFN-alpha and still other methods, but none of them has produced consistently reproducible results [509]. Also *ex vivo* marrow incubated with IFN-gamma has been utilised [512]. That the infusion of cryopreserved autologous marrow harvested in CP is capable of producing a second CP when infused in patients with BC after eradicative conditioning is well known [513-516]. Much work and much enthusiasm were put into these endeavours, but the second CP which could thus be obtained was distressingly short, with few exceptions

[509,516,517]. About 150 patients received such AutoBMTs but, while 40% to 50% of them showed some recovery of Ph-negative haemopoiesis, usually these HSCs were completely replaced by Ph-positive cells within 1 year after transplant [509]. Whether relapse is caused by residual blast cells, or by a shorter chronic life-span of the reinfused, Ph-positive stem cells, is a matter for conjecture. For those rare cases that had Ph-negative haemopoiesis up to 3 years after autografting, it has been postulated that the cytoreductive treatment might have "irreversibly" damaged the leukaemic clone, but other explanations are possible.

About 50 patients in CP received AutoBMTs. Most returned to chronic phase post-transplant. Few subjects progressed to transformation, but the follow-up is short. About 60% became partly or totally Ph negative, some for more than 4 years. Two to 3-year LFS, that is, freedom from Ph-positivity, is <10%, and overall survival is about 70%. About 10% of patients died of TRM [509].

A possibly more promising approach is based on the ability to harvest the patients' Ph-negative, peripheral blood HSCs emerging after intensive CT, and to utilise them for autografting. Some encouraging reports have appeared [518,519]. In a pilot study performed in Genoa, peripheral blood Ph-negative HCSs, harvested immediately after intensive CT in CML patients in BC, were able to restore Ph-negative haemopoiesis after subsequent ablative CT in 3 out of 4 patients [520]. Follow-up is too short to evaluate long-term results, but it must be emphasised that these were patients in BC with a severely adverse prognosis. Whether this approach may be extended to patients in CP lacking histocompatible donors is a matter for discussion.

The review of recent data on treatment with IFN-alpha, allogeneic transplants and autografting shows how difficult treatment discussions for CML have become [517]. There is no doubt, however, that allogeneic HSCs, whatever their origin (siblings, twins, MUDs), still offer the greatest chance of cure for these patients.

REFERENCES

1 McCarthy DM, Goldman JM: Transfusion of circulating stem cells. CRC Crit Rev Clin Lab Sci 1984 (20):1-24
2 Bell AJ, Hamblin TJ, Oscier DG: Peripheral blood stem cell autografting. Hematol Oncol 1987 (5):45-55
3 Reiffers J, Marti G, Boiron JM et al: The role of peripheral blood stem cells as rescue after myeloablative therapy. Bone Marrow Transpl 1989 (4 Suppl 1):212-214
4 Körbling M, Dorken B, Ho DA et al: Autologous transplantation of blood-derived hemopoietic stem cells after myeloablative therapy in a patient with Burkitt's lymphoma. Blood 1986 (67):529-532
5 To LB, Haylock DN, Thorp D et al: The optimization of collection of peripheral blood stem cells for autotransplantation in acute myeloid leukemia. Bone Marrow Transpl 1989 (4):41-47
6 To LB, Russel J, Moore S, Juttner CA: Residual leukemia cannot be detected in very early remission peripheral blood stem cell collections in acute nonlymphoblastic leukemia. Leuk Res 1987 (11):327-330
7 Chang J, Morgenstern GR, Coutinho LH et al: The use of bone marrow cells grown in long-term culture for autologous bone marrow transplantation in acute myeloid leukaemia: an update. Bone Marrow Transpl 1989 (4):5-9
8 Dausset J: Préfation. In: Gorin NC, Duhamel G (eds) L'Autogreffe de Moelle. Masson, Paris 1987
9 Silverstein MN: Foreword. In: Blume KG, Petz LD (eds) Clinical Bone Marrow Transplantation. Churchill-Livingstone, New York-Melbourne, 1983
10 Santos G: History of bone marrow transplantation. Clin Haematol 1983 (12):611
11 Marmont AM: Il Trapianto di Midollo Ematopoietico. Pozzi, Rome 1984
12 Bortin MM, Rimm AA: Increasing utilization of bone marrow transplantation. Transplantation 1986 (42):229-234
13 Advisory Committee of the International Bone Marrow Transplantation Registry: Report from the International Bone Marrow Transplant Registry. Bone Marrow Transpl 1989 (4):221-228
14 Gratwohl A, Hermans J, Lyklema A, Zwaan F: Bone marrow transplantation for leukaemia in Europe. Bone Marrow Transpl 1989 (4 Suppl 2):1-2
15 Appelbaum F, Thomas ED: The role of marrow transplantation in the treatment of leukemia. In: Bloomfield CD (ed) Chronic and Acute Leukemias in Adults. Nijhoff, Boston 1985 pp 229-262
16 Appelbaum F: Allogeneic marrow transplantation for malignancy - Current problems and prospects for improvement. In: Magrath I (ed) New Directions in Cancer Treatment. UICC. Springer Verlag, Berlin-Tokyo, 1989 pp 143-165
17 Marmont AM: Il trapianto di midollo allogenico in Italia. It J Med 1989 (80):537-542
18 Blume KG, Petz LD: Clinical Bone Marrow Transplantation. Churchill-Livingstone, New York 1983
19 Van Bekkum DW, Löwenberg B: Bone Marrow Transplantation. Biological Mechanisms and Clinical Practice. Dekker, New York-Basle 1985
20 Deeg HJ, Klingemann HG, Phillips GL: A Guide to Bone Marrow Transplantation. Springer Verlag, Berlin-Tokyo 1988
21 Nathan DG (ed): Bone marrow transplantation. Clin Haematol 1983 (12):9-11
22 Jaffé ER (ed): Bone marrow transplantation. Sem Hematol 1984 (21):1
23 Petersen FB, Buckner CD: Allogeneic and autologous bone marrow transplantation for acute leukemia and malignant lymphoma. Hematol Oncol 1987 (5):233-243
24 Gale RP, Fox CF (eds): Biology of Bone Marrow Transplantation. Academic Press, New York 1980
25 Gale RP (ed): Recent Advances in Bone Marrow Transplantation. Alan R Liss Inc, New York 1983
26 Gale RP, Champlin R (eds): Progress in Bone Marrow Transplantation. Alan R Liss Inc, New York 1987
27 Gale RP, Champlin RD (eds): Bone Marrow Transplantation: Current Controversies. Alan R Liss Inc, New York 1989
28 Bone Marrow Transpl 1,Suppl 1, 1986; ibid 2,Suppl 1, 1987; ibid 3,Suppl 1, 1988; ibid 4,Suppl 2, 1989
29 Baum SJ, Santos GW, Takaku F (eds): Recent advances and future directions in bone marrow transplantation. Exp Hematol Today 1987 Springer Verlag, New York
30 Thomas ED: The role of marrow transplantation for the eradication of malignant disease. Cancer 1982 (49):1963
31 Möller G: Allogeneic bone marrow transplantation. Immunol Rev 1983 (71)
32 O'Reilly RJ: Allogeneic bone marrow transplantation: Current status and future directions. Blood 1983 (62):941-946
33 Gratwohl A, Gahrton G: Allogeneic bone marrow transplantation in leukemia. Acta Oncol 1988 (27):557-565
34 Marmont AM: Il trapianto di midollo in oncoematologia. Le Scienze. Milano 1989 pp 971-981
35 Gorin NC, Duhamel G: L'Autogreffe de Moelle. Masson, Paris 1987
36 Goldstone AH (ed): Autologous bone marrow transplantation. Clin Haematol 1986 (15):1-269
37 Dicke KA, Spitzer G, Zander AR: Autologous Bone Marrow Transplantation. Proceedings of the First (1985), Second (1987) and Third (1988) International Symposia. Univ of Texas, MD Anderson Hospital and Tumor Institute of Houston
38 Marmont AM, Carella AM: Autologous bone marrow transplantation in haematologic malignancies. Haematol 1986 (71):1-12
39 Cheson BD, Lacerna L, Leyland-Jones B et al: Autologous bone marrow transplantation. Current status and future directions. Ann Intern Med 1989 (110):51-65
40 Rizzoli V, Mangoni L, Carella AM et al: Drug-mediated marrow purging: mafosfamide in adult acute leukemia in remission. The experience of the Italian study group. Bone Marrow Transpl 1989 (4 Suppl 1):190-194

41 Marmont AM: Bone marrow transplantation and stem cell reseeding. Haematol 1980 (65):141-150
42 Gordon MY: Annotation. Adhesive properties of haemopoietic stem cells. Br J Haematol 1988 (68):149-151
43 Gordon MY, Greaves MF: Physiological mechanisms of stem cell circulation in bone marrow transplantation and haemopoiesis. Bone Marrow Transpl 1989 (4):335-338
44 Aizawa S, Tavassoli M: Molecular basis of the recognition of intravenously transplanted hemopoietic cells in bone marrow. Proc Natl Acad Sci USA 1988 (85):3180-3183
45 Aizawa S, Tavassoli M: In vitro homing of hemopoietic stem cells is mediated by recognition system with galactosyl and mannosyl specificities. Proc Natl Acad Sci USA 1987 (84):4485-4489
46 Aizawa S, Tavassoli M: Marrow uptake of galactosyl-containing neoglycoproteins: implications in stem cell homing. Exp Hematol 1988 (16):811-813
47 Gordon MY, Riley GP, Clarke D: Heparan sulfate is necessary for adhesive interactions between early hemopoietic progenitor cells and the extracellular matrix of the marrow microenvironment. Leukemia 1988 (2):804-809
48 Chamberlain JK, Lichtman MA: Marrow cell egress: specificity of the site of penetration into the sinus. Blood 1978 (52):959-968
49 Zipori D: Stromal cells from the bone marrow: evidence for a restrictive role in regulation of hemopoiesis. Eur J Haematol 1989 (42):225-232
50 Mintz B, Anthony K, Litwin S: Monoclonal derivation of mouse myeloid and lymphoid lineages from totipotent hematopoietic stem cells of the mouse. Nature 1982 (310):476
51 Abkowitz JL, Oh RM, Holly RD, Adamson JW: Clonal evolution following chemotherapy-induced stem cell depletion in cats heterozygous for glucose-G-phosphate dehydrogenase. Blood 1988 (71):1687-1692
52 Fialkow P, Singer JW, Raskind WH et al: Clonal development, stem-cell differentiation and clinical remissions in acute nonlymphocytic leukemia. N Engl J Med 1987 (317):468-473
53 Nash R, Storb R, Neiman P: Polyclonal reconstitution of human marrow after allogeneic bone marrow transplantation. Blood 1988 (72):2031-2037
54 Turhan AG, Humphries RK, Phillips GL et al: Clonal hematopoiesis demonstrated by X-linked DNA polymorphisms after allogeneic bone marrow transplantation. New Engl J Med 1989 (320):1655-1661
55 Török-Storb B: Cellular interactions. Blood 1988 (72):373-385
56 Johnson A, Dorshkind K: Stromal cells in myeloid and lymphoid long-term marrow culture can support multiple hemopoietic lineages and modulate their production of hemopoietic growth factors. Blood 1986 (68):1348-1354
57 Singer JW, Keating A, Wight TN: The human hematopoietic microenvironment. In: Hoffbrand AV (ed): Recent Advances in Haematology. Churchill-Livingstone, Edinburgh 1985 pp 1-24
58 Gulati GL, Ashton JK, Hyun BH: Structure and function of the bone marrow and hematopoiesis. Hematol Oncol Clin North Am 1988 (2):495-511
59 Metcalf D: Haemopoietic growth factors I. Lancet 1989 (i):825-827
60 Dexter TM: Regulation of hemopoietic cell growth and development: experimental and clinical studies. Leukemia 1989 (3):469-474
61 Ogawa M: Effects of hemopoietic growth factors on stem cells in vitro. Hematol Oncol Clin North Am 1989 (3):453-464
62 Gordon MY: The origin of stromal cells in patients treated by bone marrow transplantation. Bone Marrow Transpl 1988 (3):247-251
63 Keating A, Singer JW, Killen PD et al: Donor origin of the in vitro haematopoietic microenvironment after marrow transplantation. Nature 1982 (298):280-283
64 Marmont AM: Transplantation haemopoiesis. Nouv Rev Fr Hématol 1979 (21):133-146
65 Thomas ED, Marmont AM, Sale GE: Aplastic anemia and hematopoiesis after marrow transplantation. In: Zucker-Franklin D, Greaves MF, Grossi CE, Marmont AM (eds) Atlas of Blood Cells. Functions and Pathology. Edi-Ermes, Lea A Febiger, Milano-Philadelphia 1988 pp 733-760
66 Loutit JF, Marshall MJ, Nisbet NW, Vaugan JM: Versatile stem cells in bone marrow. Lancet 1982 (ii):1090-1092
67 Thomas ED, Ramberg RE, Sale GE et al: Direct evidence for a bone marrow origin of the alveolar macrophage in man. Science 1976 (192):1016-1017
68 Gale RP, Sparkes RS, Golde DW: Bone marrow origin of hepatic macrophages (Kuppfer's cells) in humans. Science 1978 (201):937-938
69 Volc-Platzer B, Stingl G, Wolff K et al: Cytogenetic identification of allogeneic epidermal Langerhans cells in a bone marrow graft recipient. N Engl J Med 1983 (310):1123
70 Loutit JF, Nishet NW: The origin of osteoclasts. Immunobiol 1982 (161):193-198
71 Barrett AJ: BMT for metabolic disorders: a review. In: Gale RP, Champlin R (eds) Progress in Bone Marrow Transplantation. Alan R Liss Inc, New York 1987 pp 937-949
72 Marmont AM, Frassoni F, Van Lint MT et al: Isohemagglutinin induced pure red cell aplasia following major ABO incompatible marrow transplant for severe aplastic anemia. Resolution after plasma exchange. Exp Hematol 1983 (11 Suppl 13):51-53
73 Harrison DE, Astle CM: Loss of stem cell repopulating ability upon transplantation procedure. Effects of donor age, cell number, and transplantation procedure. J Exp Med 1982 (156):1767-1772
74 Mauch P, Hellman S: Loss of hematopoietic stem cell renewal after bone marrow transplantation. Blood 1989 (74):872-875
75 Atkinson K: Reconstruction of the haemopoietic and immune systems after marrow transplantation. Bone Marrow Transpl 1990 (5):209-226
76 Thomas ED, Storb R: Technique for human marrow grafting. Blood 1970 (36):507-515

77 Freedman MH, Weizman S, Chang LJ: Surgical procurement of bone marrow for transplantation. J Cell Biochem 1983 (Suppl 7A) abstr
78 Lucas PJ, Quinones RP, Moses RD et al: Alternative donor sources in HLA-mismatched transplantation: T cell depletion of surgically resected cadaveric marrow. Bone Marrow Transpl 1988 (3):211-220
79 Bortin MM, Buckner CD: Major complications of marrow harvesting for transplantation. Exp Hematol 1983 (11):916-921
80 Buckner CD, Clift RA, Sanders JE et al: Marrow harvesting from normal donors. Blood 1984 (64):630-634
81 Hill HF, Chapman CR, Jackson TL, Sullivan KM: Assessment and management of donor pain following marrow harvest for allogeneic bone marrow transplantation. Bone Marrow Transpl 1989 (4):157-161
82 Gale RP, Feig S, Ho W: ABO blood group system and bone marrow transplantation. Blood 1978 (50):165-173
83 Bacigalupo A, Avanzi G, Strada P et al: Major ABO incompatible bone marrow transplantations. Haematol 1980 (62):2
84 Gilmore MJM, Prentice HG, Blacklock HA: A technique for rapid isolation of bone marrow mononuclear cells using Ficoll-metrizoate and the IBM 2991 blood cell processor. Br J Haematol 1982 (50):619-626
85 Peralvo J, Bacigalupo A, Pittaluga PA et al: Poor graft function associated with graft-versus-host disease after allogeneic marrow transplantation. Bone Marrow Transpl 1987 (2):279-285
86 Bensinger W, Petersen FB, Banaji M et al: Engraftment and transfusion requirements after allogeneic marrow transplantation for patients with acute non-lymphocytic leukemia in first complete remission. Bone Marrow Transpl 1989 (4):409-414
87 Metcalf D: Haemopoietic growth factors 2: clinical applications. Lancet 1989 (i):885-886
88 Appelbaum FR: The clinical use of hematopoietic growth factors. Sem Hematol 1989 (26 Suppl 3):7-14
89 Dexter TM: Haemopoietic growth factors. Br Med Bull 1989 (45):337-369
90 Golde DW (ed): Hematopoietic growth factors. Hematol Oncol Clin North Am 1989 (3):369-553
91 Sieff CA: Haemopoietic growth factors: in vitro and in vivo studies. In: Hoffbrand AB (ed) Recent Advances in Haematology 5. Churchill-Livingstone, Edinburgh-New York 1989 pp 1-18
92 Groopman JE, Molina JM, Scadden DT: Haemopoietic growth factors. Biology and clinical applications. N Engl J Med 1989 (321):1449-1459
93 Graber SE, Krantz SB: Erythropoietin: biology and clinical use. Hematol Oncol Clin North Am 1989 (45):369-400
94 Goodnough LT, Rudnick S, Price TH et al: Increased preoperative collection of autologous blood with recombinant human erythropoietin therapy. N Engl J Med 1989 (321):1163-1168
95 Nemunaitis J, Singer JW, Buckner CD et al: Use of recombinant human granulocyte-macrophage colony-stimulating factor in autologous marrow transplantation for lymphoid malignancies. Blood 1988 (72):834-836
96 Gianni AM, Siena S, Bregni M et al: Granulocyte macrophage colony stimulating factor to harvest circulating haemopoietic stem cells for autotransplantation. Lancet 1989 (2):580-584
97 Blazar BR, Kersey JH, McGlave PB et al: In vivo administration of recombinant human granulocyte/macrophage colony-stimulating factor in acute lymphoblastic leukemia patients receiving purged autografts. Blood 1989 (73):849-857
98 Demetri GD, Griffin JD: Hemopoietins and leukemia. Hematol Oncol Clin North Am 1989 (3):535-553
99 Mitsuyasu RT, Golde DW: Clinical role of granulocyte-macrophage colony-stimulating factor. Hematol Oncol Clin North Am 1989 (3):411-425
100 Metcalf D: The molecular control of blood cells. Harvard Univ Press, Boston 1988
101 Büchner Th, Hiddemann W, Koenigsmann M et al: Human recombinant granulocyte macrophage colony stimulating factor (GM-CSF) for acute leukemia in aplasia and at high risk of early death. Haematol 1988 (73 Suppl 1):41
102 Sheridan WP, Morstyn G, Wolf M et al: Granulocyte colony-stimulating factor and neutrophil recovery after high-dose chemotherapy and autologous bone marrow transplantation. Lancet 1989 (ii):891-895
103 Gabrilove J: Biology and clinical applications of human recombinant granulocyte colony stimulating factor. Proc Am Assoc Cancer Res 1989 (30):638-640
104 Garnick MB, O'Reilly RJ: Clinical promise of new hematopoietic growth factors: M-CSF, IL-3, IL-G. Hematol Oncol Clin North Am 1989 (3):495-509
105 Donahue RE, Seehra J, Metzger M et al: Human IL-3 and GM-CSF act synergistically in stimulating hematopoiesis in primates. Science 1988 (241):1820-1823
106 Heslop HE, Gottlieb DJ, Bianchi ACM et al: In vivo induction of gamma interferon and tumor necrosis factor by interleukin-2 infusion following intensive chemotherapy or autologous bone marrow transplantation. Blood (in press)
107 Gottlieb DJ, Brenner MK, Heslop HE et al: A phase I clinical trial of recombinant interleukin-2 following high dose chemo-radiotherapy for haematological malignancy: applicability to the elimination of minimal residual disease. Br J Cancer 1989 (60):610-615
108 Gale RP: Analysis of bone marrow transplantation data in man. Bone Marrow Transpl 1986 (1):3-9
109 European Group for Bone Marrow Transplantation: Allogeneic bone marrow transplantation for leukaemia in Europe. Lancet 1988 (1):1379-1382
110 Champlin R and Gale RP: Bone marrow transplantation for acute leukemia: recent advances and comparison with alternative therapies. Sem Hematol 1987 (24):55-67
111 Butturini A and Gale RP: Annotation. Chemotherapy versus transplantation in acute leukaemia. Br J Haematol 1989 (72):1-8

112 International Bone Marrow Transplant Registry: Transplant or chemotherapy in acute myelogenous leukaemia? Lancet 1989 (i):1119-1121
113 Zwaan FE, Hermans J, Gratwohl A: The influence of donor-recipient sex mismatching on the outcome of allogeneic BMT in leukaemia. Bone Marrow Transpl 1989 (4 Suppl 2):8
114 Horowitz M, Bach FH, Barrett AJ et al: Ten-year progress report of allogeneic bone marrow transplantation for leukemia. Submitted for publication
115 Prentice HG, Brenner MK: Recent advances in bone marrow transplantation in the treatment of leukaemia. In: Hoffbrand AV (ed) Recent Advances in Haematology 5. Churchill-Livingstone, Edinburgh-New York 1988 pp 153-177
116 Pinkel D: Allogeneic bone marrow transplantation in children with acute leukemia: a practice whose time has gone. Leukemia 1989 (3):242-244
117 Chessels JM: A reply to D. Pinkel. Allogeneic bone marrow transplantation in childhood leukemia: another form of intensive treatment. Leukemia 1989 (3):543-544
118 Editorial: How can results of bone marrow transplantation be improved? Bone Marrow Transpl 1988 (3):1-4
119 Miller MV: The human histocompatibility complex: a review for the hematologist. In: Brown EB (ed) Progress in Hematology. Grune & Stratton, New York-San Francisco-London 1977 pp 173-191
120 Hansen J, Thomas ED: HLA and marrow transplantation. In: Ferrone S, Solheim B (eds) HLA Typing: Methodological and Clinical Apects. CRC Press, Cleveland 1982 p157
121 Yunis EJ, Awdeh Z, Raum D, Alper CA: The MHC in human bone marrow allotransplantation. Clin Haematol 1983 (12):641-680
122 Hansen JH: Donor selection for marrow transplantation: HLA polymorphism and matching. In: Gale RP, Champlin R (eds) Bone Marrow Transplantation: Current Controversies. Aland R Liss Inc, New York 1989 pp 607-618
123 Beatty PG, Clift RA, Mickelson EM et al: Marrow transplantation from related donors other that HLA identical siblings. N Engl J Med 1985 (313):765-771
124 Hows JM, Kaminski E, Brookes P et al: Unrelated and mismatched transplants for aplastic anaemia. In: Gale RP, Champlin R (eds) Bone Marrow Transplantation: Current Controversies. Alan R Liss Inc, New York 1989 pp 9-18
125 Marrow transplantation from relatives other than HLA identical siblings. In: Gale RP, Champlin R (eds) Bone Marrow Transplantation: Current Controversies. Alan R Liss Inc, New York 1989 pp 619-624
126 Irlé C, Damaro J, van Rood JJ: Mismatched related BMT for remission leukemia. Bone Marrow Transpl 1989 (4 Suppl 2):39
127 Horowitz MM, Ash RC, Bach FH et al: Bone marrow transplantation using related donors other than HLA identical siblings. Bone Marrow Transpl 1989 (4 Suppl 2):38
128 van Rood JJ, Zwaan FE, Willemze R: The unrelated bone marrow donor. Bone Marrow Transpl 1988 (3):371-377
129 Ash RC, Casper J, Manitove J et al: Evolving role of the closely HLA-matched unrelated marrow donor: HLA matching considerations for alternative donor transplantation. In: Gale RP, Champlin R (eds) Bone Marrow Transplantation: Current Controversies. Alan R Liss Inc, New York 1989 pp 629-640
130 Goldman JM, Mackinnon S: Bone marrow transplantation for chronic myeloid leukaemia using matched unrelated donors. Bone Marrow Transpl 1989 (4 Suppl 3):
131 Beatty PG, Dahlberg S, Mickelson EM et al: Probability of finding HLA-matched unrelated marrow donors. Transplantation 1988 (45):714-718
132 Beatty PG, Ash R, Hows JM and McGlave PB: The use of unrelated bone marrow donors in the treatment of patients with chronic myelogenous leukemia: experience of four marrow transplant centers. Bone Marrow Transpl 1989 (4):287-290
133 Goldman JM: Allogeneic bone marrow transplantation (BMT) with HLA-identical unrelated donors (UD). Exper Hematol 1989 (17):476 (abstr)
134 van Rood JJ, de Planque M, van Leeuwen A et al: Unrelated bone marrow donor files. Bone Marrow Transpl 1989 (4 Suppl 2):6 (abstr)
135 McCullough J, Hansen J, Perkins H et al: Establishment of the National Bone Marrow Donor Registry. In: Gale RP, Champlin R (eds) Bone Marrow Transplantation: Current Controversies. Alan R Liss Inc, New York 1989 pp 641-658
136 Barnett MJ, Eaves CJ, Phillips GL et al: Successful autografting in chronic myeloid leukaemia after maintenance of marrow in culture. Bone Marrow Transpl 1989 (4):345-351
137 Santos GW: Workshop summary: Regimens for allogeneic bone marrow transplantation in leukemia. In: Gale RP, Champlin R (eds) Progress in Bone Marrow Transplantation. Alan R Liss Inc, New York 1987 pp 113-119
138 Appelbaum FR, Petersen FB, Buckner CD et al: New preparative regimens prior to marrow transplantation for acute nonlymphoblastic leukemia. In: Gale RP, Champlin R (eds) Bone Marrow Transplantation: Current Controversies. Alan R Liss Inc, New York 1989 pp 107-116
139 Thomas ED, Storb R, Clift RA et al: Bone marrow transplantation. N Engl J Med 1975 (292):832-838
140 Thomas ED, Clift RA, Hersman J et al: Marrow transplantation for acute nonlymphoblastic leukemia in first remission using fractionated or single dose irradiation. Int J Radiat Oncol Biol Phys 1981 (7):1695-1701
141 Vitale V, Bacigalupo A, van Lint MT et al: Fractionated total body irradiation in marrow transplantation for leukemia. Br J Haematol 1983 (55):547-554
142 Vitale V, Scarpati D, Frassoni F, Corv R: Total body irradiation: single dose, fractions, dose rate. Bone Marrow Transpl 1989 (4 Suppl 1):233-235
143 Shank B, Hoplan S, Kim JH et al: Hyperfractionated total body irradiation for bone marrow transplantation. I. Early results in leukemia

patients. Int J Rad Oncol Biol Phys 1981 (7):1109-1115
144 Dinsmore R, Kirkpatrick D, Flomberg N: Allogeneic bone marrow transplantation for patients with acute lymphoblastic leukemia. Blood 1983 (62):381-387
145 Brochstein JA, Kernan NA, Groshen S et al: Allogeneic bone marrow transplantation after hyperfractionated total-body irradiation and cyclophosphamide in children with acute leukemia. N Engl J Med 1987 (317):1618-1624
146 van Lint MT, Bacigalupo A, Frassoni F et al: Bone marrow transplantation (BMT) for acute lymphoblastic leukemia (ALL) in remission. Haematol 1986 (71):135-138
147 Prentice HG, Brenner MK, Gottlieb D: T cell depleted bone marrow transplantation in acute myeloblastic leukaemia: the way ahead. Bone Marrow Transpl 1989 (4 Suppl 1):225-232
148 Davis HP, Revell P, Giangrande P et al: Safe application of a 13-Gy split dose total body irradiation schedule prior to bone marrow transplantation. Bone Marrow Transpl 1988 (3):349-356
149 Van Bekkum DW: From radiation chimaeras to 1988. Bone Marrow Transpl 1989 (4 Suppl 1):216-221
150 Frassoni F, Bacigalupo A, Vitale V et al: The effect of total body irradiation dose and chronic graft-versus-host disease on leukaemic relapse after allogeneic bone marrow transplantation. Br J Haematol 1989 (73):211-216
151 Blume KG, Forman SJ, O'Donnell MR et al: Total body irradiation and high-dose etoposide: a new preparative regimen for bone marrow transplantation in patients with advanced hematologic malignancies. Blood 1987 (69):1015-1020
152 Horwitz LJ, Kantarjan HM, Jagannath S et al: Piperazinedione plus total body irradiation: an alternative preparative regimen for allogeneic bone marrow transplantation in advanced phases of chronic myelogenous leukemia. Bone Marrow Transpl 1989 (4):101-105
153 Coccia PF, Strandjord SE, Warkentin PI et al: High-dose cytosine arabinoside and fractionated total-body irradiation: an improved preparative regimen for bone marrow transplantation in children with acute lymphoblastic leukemia in remission. Blood 1988 (71):888-893
154 Helenglass G, Powles RL, McElwain TJ et al: Melphalan and total body irradiation (TBI) versus cyclophosphamide and TBI as conditioning for allogeneic matched sibling bone marrow transplants for acute lymphoblastic leukaemia in first remission. Bone Marrow Transpl 1988 (3):21-29
155 Petersen FB, Appelbaum FR, Buckner CD et al: Simultaneous infusion of high-dose cytosine arabinoside with cyclophosphamide followed by total body irradiation and marrow infusion for the treatment of patients with advanced hematologic malignancy. Bone Marrow Transpl 1988 (3):619-624
156 UCLA Bone Marrow Transplant Group: Bone marrow transplantation with intensive combination chemotherapy/radiation therapy (SCARI) in acute leukemia. Ann Intern Med 1977 (86):155-161
157 Van der Lely N, De Witte T, Raemaekers J et al: Anthracyclines added to the conditioning regimen for allogeneic bone marrow transplantation are associated with a slower haematopoietic recovery. Bone Marrow Transpl 1989 (4):163-166
158 Kanfer EJ, McCarthy DM: Annotation. Cytoreductive preparation for bone marrow transplantation in leukemia: to irradiate or not? Br J Haematol 1989 (71):447-450
159 Santos GW, Tutschka PJ, Brookmeyer R et al: Marrow transplantation for acute nonlymphocytic leukemia after treatment with busulfan and cyclophosphamide. N Engl J Med 1983 (309):1347-1353
160 Geller RB, Saral R, Piantadosi S et al: Allogeneic bone marrow transplantation after high-dose busulfan and cyclophosphamide in patients with acute nonlymphocytic leukemia. Blood 1989 (73):2209-2218
161 Angelucci E, Polchi P, Lucarelli G et al: Allogeneic bone marrow transplantation for hematological malignancies following therapy with high doses of busulphan and cyclophosphamide. Haematol 1989 (74):455-461
162 Lucarelli G, Polchi P, Delfini C et al: Marrow transplantation for thalassaemia following busulphan and cyclophosphamide. Lancet 1985 (1):1335-1337
163 Tutschka PJ, Copelan EA, Klein PJ: Bone marrow transplantation for leukemia following a new busulphan and cyclophosphamide regimen. Blood 1987 (70):1382-1388
164 Copelan EA, Tutschka PJ: Marrow transplantation following busulfan and cyclophosphamide for chronic myelogenous leukaemia in accelerated or blastic phase. Br J Haematol 1989 (71):487-491
165 Copelan EA, Tutschka PJ: Marrow transplantation following busulfan and cyclophsophamide in multiple myeloma. Bone Marrow Transpl 1988 (3):363-365
166 Blume KG, Forman SJ: High dose busulfan/etoposide as a preparatory regimen for second bone marrow transplants in hematologic malignancies. Blut 1987 (55):49-53
167 Storb R, Appelbaum FR, Badger C et al: New conditioning regimens. Bone Marrow Transpl 1989 (4 Suppl 2):15
168 Butturini A, Gale RP: T cell depletion in bone marrow transplantation for leukemia: current results and future directions. Bone Marrow Transpl 1988 (3):185-192
169 Marmont AM, Gale RP, Butturini A et al: T-cell depletion in allogeneic bone marrow transplantation: progress and problems. Haematol 1989 (74):235-248
170 Marmont AM, Horowitz MM, Gale RP et al: T-cell depletion of HLA-identical transplants in leukemia. Submitted for publication
171 Backman L, Ringdèn O, Tollemar J, Lonqvist B: An increased risk of relapse in cyclosporin-treated compared with methotrexate-treated patients:

long-term follow up of a randomized trial. Bone Marrow Transpl 1988 (3):463-471
172 Storb R, Deeg HJ, Pepe M et al: Methotrexate and cyclosporine versus cyclosporine alone for prophylaxis of graft-versus-host disease in patients given HLA-identical marrow grafts for leukemia: long-term follow-up of a controlled trial. Blood 1989 (73):1729-1734
173 Bowden RA, Myers JD: Infectious complications following marrow transplantation. Plasma Ther Transfusion Tech 1985 (6):283-302
174 Weiner RS, Bortin MM, Gale RP: Interstitial pneumonitis after bone marrow transplantation: assessment of risk factors. Ann Intern Med 1986 (104):168-175
175 Butturini A, Bortin MM, Gale RP: Graft-vs-leukemia following bone marrow transplantation. Bone Marrow Transpl 1987 (2):233-242
176 Weiden PL, Flournoy N, Thomas ED et al: Antileukemic effect of graft-versus-host disease in human recipients of allogeneic marrow grafts. N Engl J Med 1979 (300):1068-1073
177 Bacigalupo A, van Lint MT, Frassoni F, Marmont AM: Graft-versus-leukaemia effect following allogeneic bone marrow transplantation. Br J Haematol :749-751
178 Sullivan KM, Weiden PL, Storb R et al: Influence of acute and chronic graft-versus-host disease on relapse and survival after bone marrow transplantation from HLA-identical siblings as treatment for acute and chronic leukemia. Blood 1989 (73):1720-1728
179 Bortin MM, Ringden O, Horowitz M et al: Temporal relationships between the major complications of bone marrow transplantation for leukemia. Bone Marrow Transpl 1989 (4):339-344
180 Thomas ED: Long-term results of marrow transplantation for leukemia. Bone Marrow Transpl 1986 (Suppl 1):175-176
181 Frassoni F, Barrett AJ, Granena A et al: Relapse after allogeneic bone marrow transplantation for acute leukaemia: a survey by the EBMT of 117 cases. Br J Haematol 1988 (70):317-320
182 De Witte T, Schattenberg A, Salden M et al: Mixed chimaerism and the relation with leukaemic relapse after allogeneic bone marrow transplantation. Bone Marrow Transpl 1987 (Suppl 1):11-12
183 Petz LD, Yam P, Wallace B et al: Mixed hematopoietic chimerism following bone marrow transplantation for hematologic malignancies: incidence, characterization, and implications for GVHD and relapse. In: Gale RP, Champlin R (eds) Progress in Bone Marrow Transplantation. Alan R Liss Inc, New York 1987 pp 121-134
184 Frassoni F, Repetto M, Podestà M et al: Competitive survival/proliferation of normal and Ph1 positive haemopoietic cells. Br J Haematol 1986 (63):135-141
185 Waldmann H, Hale G, Cobbold SP: The immunobiology of bone marrow transplantation. In: McMichael (ed) Leucocyte Typing III. OUP, Oxford 1987 p 932
186 Witherspoon R, Flournoy N, Thomas ED et al: Recurrence of acute leukemia more than two years after allogeneic marrow grafting. Exp Hematol 1986 (14):178-181
187 van 't Veer-Korthof ETh, van Weel-Sipman MH, Hahlen K et al: Leukemia relapse in host cells after bone marrow transplantation for acute non-lymphocytic leukemia in first complete remission. Bone Marrow Transpl 1988 (3):647-651
188 Kamani N, Lange B, August CS, Nowell P: Leukemic relapse in host cells almost 7 years after bone marrow transplantation for acute promyelocytic leukemia in first complete remission. Bone Marrow Transpl 1989 (4):455-456
189 Marmont AM: La réapparition de leucémie dans les cellules hématopoietiques du donneur après transplantation de la moelle osseuse. Med Hyg 1985 (43):1592-1594
190 Witherspoon RP, Schubach W, Neiman P et al: Donor cell leukemia developing six years after marrow grafting for acute leukemia. Blood 1985 (65):1172-1174
191 Schmitz N, Johannson W, Schmidt G et al: Recurrence of acute lymphoblastic leukemia in donor cells after allogeneic bone marrow transplantation associated with a depletion of the long arm of chromosome 5. Blood 1987 (70):1099-1104
192 Fieg SA, Dreazen O, Simon M et al: B cell acute lymphoblastic leukemia (ALL) in donor cells following bone marrow transplantation for T cell ALL. Bone Marrow Transpl 1988 (3):331-337
193 Smith JL, Heerema NA, Provisor AJ: Leukemic transformation of engrafted bone marrow cells. Br J Haematol 1985 (60):415-422
194 Boyd CN, Ramberg RC, Thomas ED: The incidence of recurrence of leukemia in donor cells after allogeneic bone marrow transplantation. Leuk Res 1982 (6):833-836
195 Stein J, Zimmerman PA, Kochera M et al: Origin of leukemic relapse after bone marrow transplantation: comparison of cytogenetic and molecular analyses. Blood 1989 (73):2033-2040
196 Witherspoon RP, Fisher LD, Schoch G et al: Secondary cancers after bone marrow transplantation for leukemia or aplastic anemia. N Engl J Med 1989 (321):784-789
197 Marmont AM, Frassoni F, Bacigalupo A et al: Recurrence of Ph1-positive leukemia in donor cells after marrow transplantation for chronic granulocytic leukemia. N Engl J Med 1984 (310):903-905
198 Anasetti C, Rybka W, Sullivan KM et al: Graft-vs-host disease is associated with autoimmune-like thrombocytopenia. Blood 1989 (73):1054-1058
199 Atkinson K, Horowitz MM, Biggs JC et al: The clinical diagnosis of acute graft-versus-host disease: a diversity of views amongst marrow transplant centers. Bone Marrow Transpl 1988 (3):5-10
200 Atkinson K, Horowitz MM, Gale RP et al: Consensus among bone marrow transplanters for diagnosis, grading and treatment of chronic graft-versus-host disease. Bone Marrow Transpl 1989 (4):247-254

201 Gale RP, Bortin MM, van Bekkum DW et al: Risk factors for acute graft-versus-host disease. Br J Haematol 1987 (67):397-406
202 van Bekkum D: Graft-versus-host disease. In: van Bekkum DW, Lowenberg B (eds) Bone Marrow Transplantation: Biological Mechanisms and Clinical Practice. Marcel Dekker, New York 1985 pp 147-212
203 Gale RP: Graft-versus-host disease. Immunol Rev 1985 (88):193-213
204 Sullivan KM: Acute and chronic graft-versus-host disease in man. Int J Cell Cloning 1986 (Suppl 1):42-93
205 Shulman HM, Sullivan KM: Graft-versus-host disease: allo- and autoimmunity after bone marrow transplantation. In: Cruse JM, Lewis RE Jr (eds) Cellular Aspects of Autoimmunity. Concepts in Immunopathology 1988 (6):141-165
206 Tutschka PJ: Mechanisms of chronic GvHD. In: Gale RP, Champlin R (eds) Progress in Bone Marrow Transplantation. Alan R Liss Inc, New York 1987 pp 457-472
207 Atkinson K: Chronic graft-versus-host diesase. Bone Marrow Transpl 1990 (5):69-82
208 Parkman R, Declerck Y, Champagne Y, Walker S: Chronic graft versus host disease is an autoimmune disease. In: Gale RP, Champlin R (eds) Progress in Bone Marrow Transplantation. Alan R Liss Inc, New York 1987 pp 497-504
209 Rouquette-Gally AM, Boyeldein D, Prost AC and Gluckman E: Autoimmunity after allogeneic bone marrow transplantation. Transplantation 1988 (40):238-240
210 De Gast G, Gratama JW, Ringden O and Gluckman E: The multifactorial etiology of graft-versus-host disease. Immunol Today 1987 (8):209-212
211 Poynton CH: T cell depletion in bone marrow transplantation. Bone Marrow Transpl 1988 (3):265-279
212 Butturini A, Seeger RC and Gale RP: Recipient immunecompetent T lymphocytes can survive intensive conditioning for bone marrow transplantation. Blood 1986 (68):954-956
213 Ferrara J, Marion A, Murphy G and Burakoff SJ: Acute graft-versus host disease: pathogenesis and prevention with a monoclonal antibody in vivo. Transpl Proc 1987 (19):2662-2663
214 Atkinson K, Cooley M, Farrelly H et al: CDA+ T cells appear capable of initiating graft-versus-host disease across non-major histocompatibility complex (MHC) barriers in man. Bone Marrow Transpl 1987 (2):79-84
215 Janeway CA, Jones B and Hayday A: Specificity and function of T cells bearing receptors. Immunol Today 1988 (8):73
216 Ferrara JL, Guillen FJ,van Dijken P et al: Evidence that large granular lymphocytes of donor origin mediate acute graft-versus-host disease. Transplantation 1989 (47):50-54
217 Podack ER: The molecular mechanism of lymphocyte-mediated tumor cell lysis. Immunol Today 1985 (6):21-27
218 Sale GE, Callucci BB, Schubert MM et al: Direct ultra-structural evidence of target-directed polarization by cytotoxic lymphocytes in lesions of human graft-versus-host disease. Arch Pathol Lab Med 1987 (111):333-336
219 Cohen J: Cytokines as mediators of graft-versus-host disease. Bone Marrow Transpl 1988 (3):193-197
220 Piguet PF, Gram GE and Vassalli P: The role of cytokines in the pathogenesis of GvHD. Bone Marrow Transpl 1989 (4 Suppl 2):83
221 Barrett AJ: Graft-versus-host disease: Clinical features and biology. Bone Marrow Transpl 1990 (4 Suppl 4):18-21
222 Kernan NA, Collins NH, Juliana L et al: Clonable T lymphocytes in T-cell depleted bone marrow transplants correlated with development of graft-versus-host disease. Blood 1986 (68):770-773
223 Gale RP, Butturini A: Comments on T-cell depletion in allogeneic bone marrow transplantation. In: Marmont A (moderator) T-cell Depletion in Allogeneic Bone Marrow Transplantation. Haematologica 1989 (74):235-248
224 Zwaan FE, Hermans J, Gratwohl A: The influence of donor-recipient sex mismatching on the outcome of allogeneic BMT in leukaemia. Bone Marrow Transpl 1989 (Suppl 2):8
225 Jacobsen N, Andersen HK, Skinhoj P et al: Correlation between donor cytomegalovirus immunity and chronic graft-versus-host disease after allogeneic bone marrow transplantation. Scand J Haematol 1986 (36):499-508
226 Jacobsen N, Lonquist B, Ringden O et al: Graft-versus-leukaemia activity associated with cytomegalovirus seropositive bone marrow donors but separated from graft-versus-host disease in allograft recipients with AML. Eur J Haematol 1987 (38):350-355
227 Okunewick JP, Meredith RF (eds) Graft-versus-Leukemia in Man and Animal Models. CRC Press, Boca Raton 1981
228 Slavin S, Naparstek E, Or E, Weiss L: Prevention of GvHD and induction of graft-versus-leukemia effects: will it ever be possible? Bone Marrow Transpl 1988 (3 Suppl 1):208
229 Boranovic M: Graft versus leukemia in bone marrow transplantation. Blut 1988 (57):57-63
230 Bacigalupo A, van Lint MT, Occhini D et al: ABO compatibility and acute graft-versus-host disease following allogeneic bone marrow transplantation. Transplantation 1988 (45):1091-1094
231 Storb R, Anasetti C, Appelbaum FR et al: Predictive facts and prevention of acute graft-versus-host disease: the Seattle experience. Bone Marrow Transpl 1988 (3 Suppl 1):7-10
232 Vogelsang G, Hess AD, Beckman AW et al: An in vitro predictive test for graft-versus-host disease in patients with genotype HLA-identical bone marrow transplants. N Engl J Med 1985 (313):643-646
233 Dickinson AM, Sviland L, Carey P et al: Skin explant culture as a model for cutaneous graft-versus-host disease in humans. Bone Marrow Transpl 1988 (3):323-329
234 Deeg HJ, Storb R: Graft-versus-host disease: pathophysiological and clinical aspects. Ann Rev Med 1984 (35):11-24

235 Deeg HJ, Bazar L, Sigaroudinia M, Cottler-Fox M: Ultraviolet light inactivates bone marrow T lymphocytes but spares hematopoietic precursor cells. Blood 1989 (73):369-371
236 O'Reilly RJ, Kernan N, Cunningham I et al: Allogeneic transplants depleted of T cells by soybean lectin agglutination and E rosette depletion. Bone Marrow Transpl 1988 (3 Suppl 1):3-6
237 De Witte T, Hoogenhout J, De Pauw B et al: Depletion of donor lymphocytes by counterflow centrifugation successfully prevents acute graft-versus-host disease in matched allogeneic marrow transplantation. Blood 1986 (67):1302-1308
238 Gratwohl A, Tichelli A, Wursch A et al: Irradiated donor buffy coat following T-cell depleted bone marrow transplants. Bone Marrow Transpl 1988 (3):577-582
239 Martelli MF, Grignani F, Reisner Y (eds): T-cell Depletion in Allogeneic Bone Marrow Transplantation. Serono Symp Rev 1988 (13)
240 Kernan N, Byers V, Scannon PJ et al: Treatment of steroid-resistant acute graft-vs-host disease by in vivo administration of an anti-T cell Ricin A chain immunotoxin. JAMA 1989 (259):3154-3156
241 Vogelsang GB, Hess AD, Santos GW: Thalidomide for treatment of chronic graft-versus-host disease. Bone Marrow Transpl 1988 (3):393-398
242 Buckner CD, Meyers JD, Springmeyer SC et al: Pulmonary complications of marrow transplantation. Review of the Seattle experience. Exp Hematol 1984 (12 Suppl 15):1-5
243 Marmont AM, van Lint MT, Frassoni F, Bacigalupo A: Adult respiratory distress syndrome (ARDS) after Bone Marrow Transpl in patients receiving cyclosporin A. Exp Hematol 1984 (12 Suppl 15):73-74
244 Weiner RS, Bortin MM, Gale RP et al: Interstitial pneumonitis after bone marrow transplantation: assesment of risk factors. Ann Intern Med 1986 (104):168-175
245 Zwaan FE, Lyklema A, Hermans J: Factors associated with the occurrence of interstitial pneumonitis after bone marrow transplantation. Exp Hematol 1984 (12 Suppl 15):15-16
246 Emanuel D, Cunningham I, Jules-Elysee K et al: Cytomegalovirus pneumonia after marrow transplantation successfully treated with the combination of gangiclovir and high-dose intravenous immune globulin. Ann Intern Med 1988 (109):777-782
247 Reed EC, Bowden RA, Dandliker PS et al: Treatment of cytomegalovirus pneumonia with gangiclovir and intravenous cytomegalovirus immunoglobulin in patients with bone marrow transplants. Ann Intern Med 1988 (109):783-788
248 Verdonck LF, de Gast GC, Dekker AW et al: Treatment of cytomegalovirus pneumonia after bone marrow transplantation with cytomegalovirus immunoglobulin combined with gangiclovir. Bone Marrow Transpl 1989 (4):187-189
249 Editorial: Lung disease following allogeneic marrow transplantation. Lancet 1989 (2):1368-1369
250 Roca J, Granena A, Rodriguez-Roisin R et al: Fatal airway disease in an adult with chronic graft-versus-host disease. Thorax 1983 (37):77-78
251 Holland HK, Wingard JR, Beschorner WE et al: Bronchiolitis obliterans in bone marrow transplantation and its relationship to chronic graft-versus-host disease and low serum IgG. Blood 1988 (72):621-627
252 Clark JG, Crawford SE, Madres DK, Sullivan K: Obstructive lung disease after allogeneic bone marrow transplantation. Ann Intern Med 1989 (111):368-376
253 McDonald GB, Shulman HM, Wolford JL, Spencer GD: Liver disease after human marrow transplantation. Semin Liver Dis 1987 (7):210-229
254 Farthing MJG, Clark ML, Sloane JP et al: Liver disease after bone marrow transplantation. Gut 1982 (23):465-474
255 Aach RD, Kahn RA: Post-transfusion hepatitis: current prospectives. Ann Intern Med 1980 (92):539-546
256 Beschorner WE, Pino J, Boitnott JK et al: Pathology of the liver with bone marrow transplantation: effects of busulfan, carmustine, acute graft-versus-host disease, and cytomegalovirus infection. Am J Pathol 1980 (99):369-386
257 Shulman HM, McDonald GB: Liver disease after bone marrow transplantation. In: Sale GE, Shulman HM (eds) The Pathology of Bone Marrow Transplantation. Masson, New York 1984 p 104
258 Locasciulli A, Bacigalupo A, Alberti A et al: Predictability before transplant of hepatic complications following allogeneic bone marrow transplantation. Transplantation 1989 (48):68-72
259 McDonald GB, Sharma P, Matthews DE et al: Veno-occlusive disease of the liver after bone marrow transplantation: Diagnosis, incidence and predisposing factors. Hepatology 1984 (4):116-122
260 Jones RJ, Lee KSK, Beschorner WE et al: Veno-occlusive disease of the liver following bone marrow transplantation. Transplantation 1987 (44):778-783
261 Bearman SI, Appelbaum FR, Buckner CD et al: Regimen-related toxicity in patients undergoing bone marrow transplantation. J Clin Oncol 1988 (6):1562-1566
262 Marmont AM: Allogeneic bone marrow transplantation for chronic granulocytic leukaemia: progress and controversies. Haematol 1987 (72):285-289
263 Champlin R, Golde DW: Chronic myelogenous leukemia: recent advances. Blood 1985 (65):1039-1047
264 Dreazen O, Canani E, Gale RP: Molecular biology of chronic myelogenous leukaemia. Sem Hematol 1988 (25):35-49
265 Goldman JM: Chronic myeloid leukemia: pathogenesis and management. In: Hoffbrand AV (ed) Recent Advances in Haematology. Churchill-Livingstone, Edinburgh-New York 1988 pp 131-152
266 Gale RP, Goldman JM: Rapid progress in chronic myelogenous leukemia. Leukemia 1988 (2):234-321

267 Morgan GJ, Wiedemann LM: Molecular biology of the Philadelphia positive leukaemias. Rec Progr Med 1989 (80):508-519

268 Talpaz M, Kantarjan HM, Kurzock R, Gutterman J: Therapy of chronic myelogenous leukaemia: chemotherapy and interferons. Sem Hematol 1988 (25):62-73

269 Goldman JM: Bone marrow transplantation for chronic myeloid leukaemia. Hematol Oncol 1987 (5):265-279

270 Champlin RE, Goldman JM, Gale RP: Bone marow transplantation in chronic myelogenous leukaemia. Sem Hematol 1988 (25):74-80

271 Thomas ED, Clift RA: Indications for marrow transplantation in chronic myelogenous leukaemia. Blood 1989 (73):861-864

272 Degliantoni G, Mangoni L, Rizzoli V: In vitro restoration of polyclonal hematopoiesis in a chronic myelogenous leukemia after in vitro treatment with 4-Hydroxycyclophosphamide. Blood 1985 (65):753-757

273 Bacigalupo A, Frassoni F, van Lint MT et al: Bone marrow transplantation for chronic granulocytic leukemia. Cancer 1986 (59):2307-2311

274 Baughan ASJ, Goldman JM, Worsley AM et al: Haematologic reconstruction and severity of graft-versus-host disease after bone marrow transplantation for chronic granulocytic leukaemia: influence of previous splenectomy. Br J Haematol 1984 (56):445-454

275 Gratwohl A, Goldman JM, Gluckman E, Zwaan F: Effect of splenectomy before bone marrow transplantation on survival in chronic granulocytic leukaemia. Lancet 1985 (2):1290-1291

276 Spiers ASD: Metamorphosis of chronic granulocytic leukaemia: diagnosis, classification and management. Br J Haematol 1979 (41):1-7

277 Martin PJ, Clift RA, Fisher LD et al: HLA-identical marrow transplantation during accelerated-phase chronic myelogenous leukaemia: analysis of survival and remission duration. Blood 1988 (72):1978-1984

278 Przepiorka D, Thomas ED: Prognostic significance of cytogenetic abnormalities in patients with chronic myelogenous leukaemia. Bone Marrow Transpl 1988 (3):113-119

279 Sokal JE, Baccarani M, Russo D, Tura S: Staging and prognosis in chronic myelogenous leukaemia. Sem Hematol 1988 (25):49-61

280 Prischl FC, Haas OA, Lion T et al: Duration of first remission as an indicator of long-term survival in chronic myelogenous leukaemia. Br J Haematol 1989 (71):337-342

281 Segel GB, Simon W, Lichtman MA: Variables influencing the timing of bone marrow transplantation in patients with chronic myelogenous leukaemia. Blood 1986 (68):1055

282 Thomas ED, Clift RA, Fefer A et al: Marrow transplantation for the treatment of chronic myelogenous leukaemia. Ann Intern Med 1986 (104):155-163

283 Goldman JM, Gale RP, Horowitz MM et al: Bone marrow transplantation for chronic myelogenous leukemia in chronic phase. Increased risk of relapse associated with T-cell depletion. Ann Intern Med 1988 (108):806-814

284 Schaefer-Rego K, Dudek M, Popenol D et al: CML patients in blast crisis have breakpoints localized to a specific region of the BRC. Blood 1987 (70):448-455

285 Shtalrid M, Talpaz M, Kurzrock R et al: Analysis of breakpoints within the bcr gene and their correlation with the clinical course of Philadelphia-positive chronic myelogenous leukemia. Blood 1988 (72):485-490

286 Miles KI, Mackenzie ED, Birnie GD: The site of breakpoint within the bcr is a prognostic factor in Philadelphia-positive CML. Blood 1988 (72):1237-1241

287 Dreazen O, Berman M, Gale RP: Molecular abnormalities of bcr and c-abl in chronic myelogenous leukemia associated with a long chronic phase. Blood 1988 (71):797-799

288 Birnie GD, Mills KI, Benn P: Does the site of the breakpoint on chromosome 22 influence the duration of the chronic phase in chronic myeloid leukemia? Leukemia 1989 (3):545-547

289 Butturini A, Gale RP: Oncogenes and leukemia. Leukemia 1990 (4):138-160

290 Daley CQ, Van Etten RA, Baltimore D: Induction of chronic myelogenous leukemia in mice by the P210 bcr/abl gene of Philadelphia chromosome. Science 1990 (247):824-830

291 Sanders JE, Buckner CD, Thomas ED et al: Allogeneic bone marrow transplantation for children with juvenile chronic myelogenous leukemia. Blood 1989 (71):1144-1146

292 Arthur CK, Apperley JF, Guo AP et al: Cytogenetic events after bone marrow transplantation for chronic myeloid leukaemia in chronic phase. Blood 1988 (71):1179-1186

293 Cooperative Study Group on Chromosomes in Transplanted Patients: Cytogenetic follow up of 100 patients submitted to bone marrow transplantation for Philadelphi chromosome-positive chronic myeloid leukemia. Eur J Haematol 1988 (40):50-57

294 Rosti G, Zaccaria A, Testoni N et al: Ph chromosome persistence after allogeneic BMT for PH+CML: long follow up of 9 patients. Bone Marrow Transpl 1989 (4 Suppl 2):22

295 Borgies P, Ferrant A, Delannoy A et al: Interferon alpha induced and maintained complete remission in chronic granulocytic leukemia in relapse after bone marrow transplantation. Bone Marrow Transpl 1989 (4):127-128

296 Newland AC, Jones L, Mir N et al: Alpha 2 interferon in chronic myeloid leukaemia following relapse post-allogeneic transplant. Br J Haematol 1987 (66):141-143

297 Arcese W, Mauro FR, Alimena G et al: Interferon therapy for Ph-1 positive CML patients relapsing after T-cell depleted allogeneic bone marrow transplantation. Bone Marrow Transpl 1990 (5):310-315

298 Morgan GJ, Hughes T, Janssen JWG et al: Polymerase chain reaction for detection of residual leukaemia. Lancet 1989 (1):928-929

299 Lee MS, Chang KS, Freireich EJ et al: Detection of minimal residual bcr/abl transcripts by a modified polymerase chain reaction. Blood 1988 (72):893-897
300 Dohrovic A, Trainor KJ, Morley AA: Detection of the molecular abnormality in chronic myeloid leukemia by use of polymerase chain reaction. Blood 1988 (72):2063-2065
301 Roth MS, Antin JH, Bingham EL, Ginsburg D: Detection of Philadelphia chromosome-positive cells by the polymerase chain reaction following bone marrow transplantation for chronic myelogenous leukemia. Blood 1989 (74):882-885
302 Gabert J, Thuret I, Lafage M et al: Detection of residual bcr-abl translocation by polymerase chain reaction in chronic myeloid leukaemia patients after bone marrow transplantation. Lancet 1989 (2):1125-1128
303 Bartram CR, Janssen JWG, Schwidberger M et al: Minimal residual leukaemia in chronic myeloid leukaemia patients after T-cell depleted bone marrow transplantation. Lancet 1989 (1):1260
304 Hughes TP, Economou K, Mackinnon S et al: Slow evolution of chronic myeloid leukaemia relapsing after BMT with T-cell depleted donor marrow. Br J Haematol 1989 (73):462-467
305 Hughes TP, Goldman JM: Biological importance of residual leukaemic cells after BMT for CML: does the polymerase chain reaction help? Bone Marrow Transpl 1990 (5):3-6
306 Arnold R, Bartram CR, Heinze B et al: Evaluation of remission state in chronic myeloid leukemia patients after bone marrow transplantation using cytogenetic and molecular genetic approaches. Bone Marrow Transpl 1989 (4):389-392
307 McGlave P, Beatty P, Ash R, Hows J: Therapy for chronic myelogenous leukemia with unrelated donor bone marrow transplantation: results in 102 cases. Blood 1990 (75):1728-1732
308 Ash RC, Horowitz MM, Gale RP et al: Bone marrow transplantation from related donors other than HLA-identical siblings: effects of T-cell depletion. Submitted for publication
309 Apperley JF, Jones L, Hale G et al: Bone marrow transplantation for chronic myeloid leukaemia: T-cell depletion reduces the risk of graft-versus-host disease but may increase the risk of leukaemic relapse. Bone Marrow Transpl 1986 (1):53-66
310 Arcese W, Screnci M, Mauro FR et al: Italian survey on allogeneic bone marrow transplantation for chronic myeloid leukemia. Bone Marrow Transpl 1989 (4 Suppl 2):19
311 Hale G, Cobbold S, Waldmann H (for Campath-1 users): T-cell depletion with Campath-1 in allogeneic bone marrow transplantation. Transplantation 1988 (45):753-759
312 Frassoni F, Sessarego M, Bacigalupo A et al: Competition between recipient and donor cells after bone marrow transplantation for chronic myeloid leukaemia. Br J Haematol 1988 (69):471-475
313 Lawler SP, Harris H, Millar J et al: Cytogenetic follow-up studies of recipients of T-cell depleted allogeneic bone marrow. Br J Haematol 1987 (65):143-150
314 Prentice HG, Brenner MK, Gottlieb D: T-cell depleted bone marrow transplantation in acute myeloblastic leukaemia: the way ahead. Bone Marrow Transpl 1989 (4 Suppl 1):225-228
315 Ahmed T, Arlin ZA: Bone marrow transplantation for chronic myelogenous leukemia: some thoughts about future prospects. Leukemia 1988 (2):181
316 Gale RP and Champlin R: How does bone marrow transplantation cure leukemia? Lancet 1984 (ii):28-30
317 Butturini A, Gale RP: The role of T cells in preventing relapse in chronic myelogenous leukaemia. Bone Marrow Transpl 1987 (2):351-354
318 Butturini A, Bortin MM, Seeger RC, Gale RP: Graft-versus-leukemia following bone marrow transplantation: a model of immunotherapy in man. In: Truitt RL, Gale RP, Bortin MM (eds) Cellular Immunotherapy of Cancer. Alan R Liss Inc, New York 1987 p 390
319 Truitt RL, Lefever AV, Shih CY: Graft-versus-leukemia reactions: experimental models and clinical trials. In: Gale RP and Champlin R (eds) Progress in Bone Marrow Transplantation. Alan R Liss Inc, New York 1987 pp 219-232
320 Horowitz MM, Gale RP, Sondel PM et al: Graft-versus-leukemia reactions following bone marrow transplantation in humans. Blood 1990 (75):555-562
321 Schultz FW, Vriesendorp HM and Hagenbeek A: On the quantitative role of graft-versus-host disease in decreasing the leukemia relapse rate after allogeneic bone marrow transplantation. Submitted for publication
322 Butturini A, Gale RP: Annotation. How can we cure leukaemia? Br J Haematol 1989 (72):479-485
323 Sullivan KM, Storb R, Buckner CD et al: Graft-versus-host disease as adoptive immunotherapy in patients with advanced hematologic neoplasms. New Engl J Med 1989 (320):828-834
324 Jones RJ, Vogelsang GB, Hess AD et al: Induction of graft-versus-host disease after autologous bone marrow transplantation. Lancet 1989 (1):754-757
325 Thomas ED, Buckner CD, Banaji M et al: One hundred patients with acute leukemia treated by chemotherapy, total body irradiation, and allogeneic bone marrow transplantation. Blood 1977 (49):511-533
326 Thomas ED, Buckner CD, Clift RA et al: Marrow transplantation for acute nonlymphoblastic leukemia in first remission. N Engl J Med 1979 (301):597-599
327 Bacigalupo A, van Lint MT, Frassoni F et al: Bone marrow transplantation (BMT) for acute non lymphoid leukemia (ANLL) in first remission: an update. Haematol 1989 (74):418-489
328 Santos GW: Marrow transplantation in acute nonlymphocytic leukemia. Blood 1989 (74):901-908
329 Clift RA, Buckner CD, Thomas ED et al: The treatment of acute non-lymphoblastic leukemia by allogeneic marrow transplantation. Bone Marrow Transpl 1987 (2):243-258
330 Dinsmore R, Kirckpatrick D, Flomenberg N et al: Allogeneic bone marrow transplantation for

patients with acute nonlymphocytic leukemia. Blood 1984 (62):381-388
331 Weisdorf DJ, McGlave P, Ramsay N et al: Allogeneic bone marrow transplantation for acute leukaemia: comparative outcomes for adults and children. Br J Haematol 1988 (69):351-358
332 Sanders JE, Thomas ED, Buckner CD et al: Marrow transplantation for children in first remission of acute nonlymphoblastic leukemia: an update. Blood 1985 (88):400-402
333 Feig SA, Nesbit ME, Buckley J et al: Bone marrow transplantation for acute nonlymphocytic leukemia: a report from the Children's Cancer Study Group of sixty-seven children transplanted in first remission. Bone Marrow Transpl 1987 (2):365-374
334 Siegert W, Porta F, Barrett AJ et al: Allogeneic bone marrow transplantation in children with leukemia: a report from the EBMT Working Party. Bone Marrow Transpl 1989 (4 Suppl 2):10
335 Gratwohl A, Hermans J, Barrett AJ et al: Allogeneic bone marrow transplantation for leukemia in Europe: Regional differences. Bone Marrow Transpl 1990 (in press)
336 Marmont AM, Bacigalupo A, van Lint MT, Frassoni F: Il trapianto di midollo allogenico nella terapia delle leucemie acute non-linfoidi (ANLL). Haematol 1988 (72 Suppl 1):147-158
337 Begg CB, McGlave PB, Bennet JM et al: A critical comparison of allogeneic bone marrow transplantation and conventional chemotherapy as treatment for acute nonlymphocytic leukemia. J Clin Oncol 1984 (2):369-378
338 Powles RL, Morgenstein G, Clink HM et al: The place of bone-marrow transplantation in acute myelogenous leukaemia. Lancet 1980 (1):1047-1050
339 Champlin RE, Ho WG, Gale RP et al: Treatment of acute myelogenous leukemia: a prospective controlled trial of bone marrow transplantation versus consolidation chemotherapy. Ann Intern Med 1985 (102):285-291
340 Appelbaum FR, Dahlberg S, Thomas ED: Bone marrow transplantation or chemotherapy after remission induction for adults with acute nonlymphoblastic leukemia: a prospective study. Ann Intern Med 1984 (101):581-588
341 Appelbaum FR, Fisher LD, Thomas ED and the Seattle Transplantation Team: Chemotherapy versus marrow transplantation for adults with acute nonlymphoblastic leukemia: a five-year follow up. Blood 1988 (72):179-184
342 Zittoun R, Jah V, Fiére D et al: Alternative versus repeated post-remission treatment in adult acute myelogenous leukemia: a randomized phase III (AMLG) trial of the EORTC-Leukemia Cooperative Group. Blood 1989 (73):896-906
343 Wolff SN, Herzig RH, Fay JW et al: High-dose cytarabine and daunorubicinas consolidation therapy for acute myeloid leukemia in first remission: long-term follow up and results. J Clin Oncol 1989 (7):1260-1287
344 Hermans J, Sucin S, Stijnen Th: Treatment of acute myelogenous leukemia. Allogeneic or autologous bone marrow transplantation. Eur J Cancer Clin Oncol 1989 (25):545-550
345 Marmont AM, van Lint MT, Frassoni F, Bacigalupo A: Second marrow transplants for relapsed leukaemia after allogeneic bone marrow transplantation. Bone Marrow Transpl 1988 (3 Suppl 1):332-333
346 Wright SE, Thomas ED, Buckner CD et al: Experience with second marrow transplants. Exp Hematol 1976 (4):221-226
347 Champlin RE, Ho WG, Lenarsky C et al: Successful second bone marrow transplants for acute myelogenous leukemia or acute lymphoblastic leukemia. Transplant Proc 1985 (17):496-499
348 Atkinson K, Biggs J, Concannon A et al: Second marrow transplants for recurrence of haematological malignancy. Bone Marrow Transpl 1986 (1):159-166
349 Wagner JE, Santos GW, Burus WH, Saral R: Second marrow transplantation after leukemia relapse in 11 patients. Bone Marrow Transpl 1989 (4):115-118
350 Sanders JE, Buckner CD, Clift RA et al: Second marrow transplants in patients with leukemia who relapse after allogeneic marrow transplantation. Bone Marrow Transpl 1988 (3):11-19
351 Barrett AJ, Helenglass G, Treleaven J, Gratwohl A: Second transplants in leukaemia: the EBMT experience. Bone Marrow Transpl 1989 (4 Suppl 2):11
352 Mickels SD, Mckenna RW, Arthur DC, Brunning RD: Therapy-related acute myeloid leukemia and myelodysplastic syndrome: a clinical and morphologic study of 65 cases. Blood 1983 (65):1364-1372
353 Brusamolino E, Pagnucco G, Bernasconi D: Acute leukemia occurring in a primary neoplasia (secondary leukemia). A review of biological, epidemiological and clinical aspects. Haematol 1986 (71):60-83
354 Francis GR, Hoffbrand AV: The myelodysplastic syndromes and preleukemia. In: Hoffbrand AV (ed) Recent Advances in Haematology. Churchill-Livingstone, London 1985 pp 239-267
355 Boogaerts MA: Progress in the therapy of myelodysplastic syndromes. Blut 1989 (58):265-270
356 Rowley JD, Golomb HM, Vardiman JW: Nonrandom chromosome abnormalities in acute leukemia and dysmyelopoietic syndromes in patients with previously treated malignant disease. Blood 1981 (58):759-767
357 Le Beau MM, Albain KS, Larson RA et al: Clinical and cytogenetic correlation in 63 patients with therapy-related myelodysplastic syndromes and acute nonlymphocytic leukemia: further evidence for characteristic abnormalities of chromosomes no. 5 and 7. J Clin Oncol 1986 (4):325-345
358 Coltman CA, Dahlberg S: Treatment-related leukemia. N Engl J Med 1990 (322):52-53
359 Bennett JM, Catovsky D, Daniel MD et al: Proposals for the classification of the myelodysplastic syndromes. Br J Haematol 1982 (51):189-199

360 Hamblin TJ, Oscier DG: The myelodysplastic syndrome: a practical guide. Hematol Oncol 1987 (5):19-34
361 Lichtman MA, Brennan JK: Preleukemia and oligoblastic leukemia (myelodysplastic disorders). In: Williams WJ, Beutler E, Erslev AJ, Lichtman MA (eds) Hematology. McGraw-Hill, New York-Toronto 1990 pp 175-187
362 Arnold R, Heimpel H: Allogeneic bone marrow transplantation for myelodysplastic syndromes (MDS). Bone Marrow Transpl 1989 (4 Suppl 4):101-103
363 International Bone Marrow Transplant Registry: Unpublished data
364 Appelbaum FR, Storb R, Ramberg RE et al: Allogeneic marrow transplantation in the treatment of preleukemia. Ann Intern Med 1984 (100):689-693
365 Lin Yin JA, Love EM, Hows JM et al: Bone marrow transplantation in the treatment of the myelodysplastic syndromes. Bone Marrow Transpl 1987 (Suppl 1):25
366 Appelbaum FR, Storb R, Ramberg RE et al: Treatment of preleukemic syndromes with marrow transplantation. Blood 1987 (69):92-96
367 Belanger R, Gyger M, Perreault G et al: Bone marrow transplantation for myelodysplastic syndrome. Br J Haematol 1988 (69):29-33
368 O'Donnell MR, Nademanee AP, Snyder DS et al: Bone marrow transplantation for myelodysplastic and myeloproliferative syndromes. J Clin Oncol 1987 (5):1822-1826
369 De Witte T, Zwaan F, Hermans J et al: Allogeneic bone marrow transplantation for secondary leukaemia and myelodysplastic syndrome: a survey by the Leukaemia Working Party of the European Bone Marrow Transplantation Group (EBMTG). Br J Haematol 1990 (74): 151-155
370 Tricot G, Van Hoof P, Zachee P, Vermilghen RL: Bone marrow transplantation performed as first-time treatment in two cases of secondary acute myeloid leukemia. Leukemia Res 1984 (8):93-96
371 Marmont AM, van Lint MT, Bacigalupo A et al: Bone marrow transplantation for secondary (therapy-related) acute nonlymphoblastic leukaemia: report of a case associated with adoptive beta-thalassaemia. Bone Marrow Transpl 1987 (2):91-97
372 Greaves MF, Chan LC: Is spontaneous mutation the major "cause" of childhood acute lymphoblastic leukaemia? Br J Haematol 1986 (64):1
373 Champlin R, Gale RP: Acute lymphoblastic leukemia: recent advances in biology and therapy. Blood 1989 (73):2051-2066
374 Rivera G, Mauer AM: Controversies in the management of childhood acute lymphoblastic leukemia: treatment intensification, CNS leukemia and prognostic factors. Sem Hematol 1987 (24):27-39
375 Pinkel D: Curing children of leukemia. Cancer 1987 (59):1683-1691
376 Riehm H, Feickert HJ, Schrappe M et al: Therapy results in five ALL-BFM studies since 1970. Implication of risk factors for prognosis. In: Büchner T, Schellong G, Hiddeman W, Urbaniz D, Ritter J (eds): Acute Leukemia. Springer Verlag, Berlin 1987 p 139
377 Hoelzer D, Gale RP: Acute lymphoblastic leukemia in adults: recent progress, future directions. Sem Hematol 1987 (24):27-39
378 Hoelzer D: Which factors influence the different outcome of therapy in adults and children with ALL? Bone Marrow Transpl 1989 (4 Suppl 1):98-100
379 Gale RP, Ben Bassat I: Hybrid acute leukaemia. Br J Haematol 1987 (65):261
380 Niethammer D, Dopfer R, Klingebiel T et al: Actual role and perspectives of BMT in children. Bone Marrow Transpl 1989 (4 Suppl 4):7-11
381 Sobel RE, Mick R, Royston I et al: Clinical importance of myeloid antigen expression in adult acute lymphoblastic leukemia. N Engl J Med 1987 (326):1111-1117
382 Bordigoni P, Vernant JP, Souillet G et al: Allogeneic bone marrow transplantation for children with acute lymphoblastic leukaemia in first remission. A study of the GEGMO-France. Bone Marrow Transpl 1988 (3 Suppl 1):148-149
383 McCarthy DM, Barrett AJ, McDonald D et al: Bone marrow transplantation for adults and children with poor risk ALL in first complete remission. Bone Marrow Transpl 1988 (3):315-322
384 Herzig RH, Bortin MM, Barrett AJ et al: Bone marrow transplantation in high risk acute lymphoblastic leukaemia in first and second remission. Lancet 1987 (1):786-789
385 Barrett AJ, Horowitz MM, Gale RP et al: Marrow transplantation for acute lymphoblastic leukemia: factors affecting relapse and survival. Blood 1989 (74):862-871
386 Johnson FL, Thomas ED, Clark BS et al: A comparison of marrow transplantation with chemotherapy for children with acute lymphoblastic leukemia in second or subsequent remission. N Engl J Med 1981 (305):846-851
387 Bacigalupo FL, Van Lint MT, Frassoni F et al: Allogeneic bone marrow transplantation versus chemotherapy for childhood acute lymphoblastic leukaemia in second remission. Bone Marrow Transpl 1986 (1):75-80
388 Butturini A, Rivera GK, Bortin MM, Gale RP: Which treatment for childhood acute lymphoblastic leukemia in second remission? Lancet 1987 (1):429-432
389 Rivera GK, Santana V, Mahmoud H et al: Acute lymphocytic leukemia of childhood: the problem of relapses. Bone Marrow Transpl 1989 (4 Suppl 1):80-85
390 Barrett AJ, Horowitz MM, McCarthy D et al: Bone marrow transplantation for acute lymphoblastic leukaemia in first and second remission. Bone Marrow Transpl 1989 (4 Suppl 1):247-249
391 Blume K, Schmidt GM, Chao NJ et al: Bone marrow transplantation from histocompatible sibling donors for patients with acute lymphoblastic leukemia. Bone Marrow Transpl 1989 (4 Suppl 2):18
392 International Bone Marrow Transplant Registry: Effect of methotrexate on relapse after bone

marrow transplantation for acute lymphoblastic leukaemia. Lancet 1989 (1):535-536
393 Prentice HG, Hermans J, Zwaan FE: Relapse risk in allogeneic BMT with T-cell depletion of donor marrow. Bone Marrow Transpl 1988 (3 Suppl 1):30-32
394 Ringdèn O, Backman L, Tollemar J et al: Long-term follow up of randomised trial comparing graft-versus-host disease prophylaxis using cyclosporin or methotrexate in patients with haematological malignancies. Bone Marrow Transpl 1989 (4 Suppl 2):119
395 Bacigalupo A, Van Lint MT, Frassoni F et al: A randomized trial comparing cyclosporin A 1 us 5mg/kg/day in allogeneic bone marrow transplantation. Bone Marrow Transpl 1989 (4 Suppl 2):118
396 Butturini A, Gale RP: Chemotherapy versus transplantation. II. Acute lymphoblastic leukemia. Haematol 1989 (74):337-339
397 Hoelzer D, Triel E, Loeffler H et al: Prognostic factors in a multicenter study for treatment of acute lymphoblastic leukemia in adults. Blood 1988 (71):123-131
398 Atkinson K, Barrett AJ, Gale RP et al (for the IBMTR): ALL BMT versus chemotherapy. In preparation
399 Champlin RE, Gale RP: Bone marrow transplantation for acute leukemia. Recent advances and comparison with alternative therapies. Sem Hematol 1987 (24):55-67
400 Bernasconi C, Lazzarino M, Canevari A et al: Allogeneic versus autologous bone marrow transplantation versus intensive post-remission chemotherapy in acute leukemias. Bone Marrow Transpl 1989 (4 Suppl 4):65-68
401 Gale RP, Rai KR (eds) Chronic Lymphocytic Leukemia. Recent Progress and Future Directions. Alan R Liss Inc, New York 1986
402 Binet JL, Dighiero G (eds) IV International Workshop of Chronic Lymphocytic Leukemia. Nouv Rev Franç Hématol 1988 (30):281-481
403 Rozman C, Montserrat E: Chronic lymphocytic leukaemia: when and how to treat. Blut 1989 (59):467-474
404 Michallet M, Corront B, Hollard D et al: Allogeneic bone marrow transplantation in chronic lymphocytic leukaemia: 9 cases. Bone Marrow Transpl 1989 (4 Suppl 2):12
405 Barlogie B: Management of multiple myeloma. Blut 1990 (60):1-7
406 Tura S, Cavo M, Baccarini M et al: Bone marrow transplantation in multiple myeloma. Scand J Haematol 1986 (36):176-179
407 Cavo M, Tura S, Bandini G et al: High-dose multi-agent chemoradiotherapy and allogeneic BMT for multiple myeloma (MM). Bone Marrow Transpl 1989 (4 Suppl 2):76
408 Gallamini A, Buffa E, Bacigalupo A et al: Allogeneic bone marrow transplantation in multiple myeloma. Acta Haematol 1987 (77):111-114
409 Gahrton G, Tura S, Flesch M et al: Bone marrow transplantation in multiple myeloma: report from the European Cooperative Group for Bone Marrow Transplantation. Blood 1987 (69):1262-1264
410 Gahrton G, Gratwohl A, Ernst P et al: Allogeneic bone marrow transplantation in haematological malignancies. Bone Marrow Transpl 1989 (4 Suppl 4):4-6
411 Cheever MA, Fefer A, Greenberg PD: Treatment of hairy cell leukemia with chemoradiotherapy and identical twin bone marrow transplantation. N Engl J Med 1982 (307):479-481
412 Izzi T, Polchi P, Muretto P, Lucarelly G: Syngeneic bone marrow transplant in a patient with hairy cell leukemia. Exp Hematol 1984 (12 Suppl 15)
413 Lichtman MA: Agnogenic myeloid metaplasia. In: Williams WJ, Beutler E, Erslev AJ, Lichtman M (eds) Hematology. McGraw-Hill, New York-Toronto 1990 pp 223-232
414 Wolf JL, Sprace WE, Bearman RM et al: Reversal of acute ("malignant") myelosclerosis by allogeneic bone marrow transplantation. Blood 1982 (59):191-193
415 Smith JW, Shulman HM, Thomas ED et al: Bone marrow transplantation for acute myelosclerosis. Cancer 1981 (48):2198-2203
416 McGlave PB, Brunning RD, Hurd DD, Kin TH: Reversal of severe bone marrow fibrosis and osteosclerosis following allogeneic bone marrow transplantation for chronic granulocytic leukemia. Br J Haematol 1982 (52):189-194
417 Oblon DJ, Elfenbein GJ, Braylan RC et al: The reversal of myelofibrosis associated with chronic myelogenous leukemia after allogeneic bone marrow transplantation. Exp Hematol 1983 (11):881-883
418 Vowels MR, White L, Lam-Po-Tong PRL: Bone marrow transplantation for malignant histiocytosis. Cancer 1985 (56):2786-2788
419 Ringdèn O, Ahström M, Lonnquist B: Allogeneic bone marrow transplantation in a patient with chemotherapy-resistant progressive histiocytosis X. N Engl J Med 1987 (316):733-735
420 Stoll M, Link H, Freund M et al: Allogeneic bone marrow transplantation in a case of chemotherapy resistant progressive histiocytosis X. Bone Marrow Transpl 1988 (3 Suppl 1):316
421 Troussard X, Girard A, Leporrier N et al: Treatment of disseminated malignant histiocytosis with allogeneic bone marrow transplantation. Bone Marrow Transpl 1986 (1 Suppl 1):226
422 Geller RB, Esa AH, Beschorner WE et al: Successful in vitro graft-versus-tumor effect against an Ia-bearing tumor using cyclosporine-induced syngeneic graft-versus-host disease in the rat. Blood 1989 (74):1165-1171
423 Juttner CA, To LB, Haylock DN et al: Circulating autologous stem cells collected in very early remission from acute non-lymphoblastic leukaemia produce prompt but incomplete haemopoietic reconstitution after high-dose melphalan or supralethal chemoradiotherapy. Br J Haematol 1985 (61):739-745
424 Kessinger A, Armitage JO, Landwark JD et al: Autologous peripheral hematopoiesis stem cell transplantation restores hematopoietic function following marrow ablative therapy. Blood 1988 (71):723-727

425 Williams SF, Bitran JD, Richards JM et al: Peripheral blood-derived stem cell collection for use in autologous transplantation after high dose chemotherapy: an alternative approach. Bone Marrow Transpl 1990 (5)129-133
426 Siena SG, Bregni M, Brando B et al: Circulation of CD 34+ hematopoietic stem cells in the peripheral blood of high-dose cyclophosphamide-treated patients: enhancement by intravenous recombinant human granulocyte-macrophage colony-stimulating factor. Blood 1989 (74):1905-1914
427 Molgaard HV, Spurr NK, Greaves MF: The hemopoietic stem cell antigen, CD34, is encoded by a gene located on chromosome 1. Leukemia 1989 (3):773-776
428 Vaughan WP, Civin CI, Weisenburger DD et al: Acute leukemia expressing the normal hematopoietic stem cell membrane glycoprotein CD34 (MY10). Leukemia 1988 (2):661-666
429 Gorin NC: Collection, manipulation and freezing of haemopoietic stem cells. Clin Haematol 1986 (15):19-48
430 Davis JM, Rowley SD, Braine HG et al: Clinical toxicity of cryopreserved bone marrow graft infusion. Blood 1990 (75):781-786
431 Appelbaum FR, Buckner CD: Overview of the clinical relevance of autologous bone marrow transplantation. Clin Haematol 1986 (15):1-18
432 Gale RP, Butturini A: Autotransplants in leukaemia. Lancet 1989 (2):315-317
433 Gale RP, Armitage JO, Butturini A: Editorial. Is there a role for autotransplants in acute leukaemia? Bone Marrow Transpl 1989 (4):217-219
434 Spitzer G, Verma DS, Fisher R et al: The myeloid progenitor cell - Its value in predicting hematopoietic recovery after autologous bone marrow transplantation. Blood 1980 (55):317-323
435 Andreeff M, Welte K: Hematopoietic colony-stimulating factors. Sem Oncol 1989 (16):211-229
436 Mumcuoglu M, Naparstek E, Slavin S: The use of recombinant cytokines for enhancing innumohaematopoietic reconstitution following bone marrow transplantation II. The influence of lymphokines on CFU-GM colonies from human untreated, ASTA-Z or campath-1M treated bone marrow. Bone Marrow Transpl 1990 (5):153-158
437 Gordon MY, Hibbin JR, Kearney V et al: Colony formation by primitive haemopoietic progenitor cells in cocultures of bone marrow cells and stromal cells. Br J Haematol 1985 (60):129-136
438 Rizzoli V, Mangoni L, Carella AM et al: Drug-mediated marrow purging: mafosfamide in adult acute leukaemia in remission. The experience of the Italian study group. Bone Marrow Transpl 1989 (4 Suppl 1):190-194
439 International Cooperative Study: Bone marrow autotransplantation in man. Lancet 1986 (2):960-961
440 International Autologous Bone Marrow Transplant Registry (ABMT): Autologous bone marrow transplants: different indications in Europe and North America. Lancet 1989 (2):317-318
441 Burnett AK: Editorial. Autologous bone marrow transplantation in acute leukemia. Leukemia Res 1988 (12):531-536
442 Santos GW, Yeager AM, Jones RJ: Autologous bone marrow transplantation. In: Creger WP, Coggins CH, Hancock WE (eds) Annual Review of Medicine. Ann Rev Inc, Palo Alto 1989 pp 40-99
443 Armitage J: Bone marrow transplantation in the treatment of patients with lymphoma. Blood 1989 (7):1749-1758
444 Appelbaum FR, Sullivan K, Thomas ED et al: Treatment of malignant lymphoma in 100 patients with chemoradiotherapy and marrow transplantation. Exp Hematol 1985 (13):321-324
445 Goldstone AH, Singer CRJ, Gribben JG et al: European experience of ABMT in non-Hodgkin's lymphoma and Hodgkin's disease. In: Gale RP, Champlin RD (eds): Bone Marrow Transplantation: Current Controversies. Alan R Liss Inc, New York 1989 pp 265-278
446 Gribben JG, Linch DC, Singer CRJ et al: Successful treatment of refractory Hodgkin's disease by high-dose combination chemotherapy and autologous bone marrow transplantation. Blood 1989 (73):340-344
447 Carella AM, Marmont AM: Treatment of resistant Hodgkin's lymphoma with bone marrow transplantation in Italy. In: Diehl V, Pfreundschuh M, Loeffler M (eds) New aspects in the diagnosis and treatment of Hodgkin's disease. Rec Res Cancer Res 1989 (117):239-241 Springer Verlag, Berlin-Hong Kong
448 Armitage JO, Barnett MJ, Carella AM et al: Bone marrow transplantation in the treatment of Hodgkin's lymphoma: problems, remaining challenges, and future prospects. In: Diehl V, Pfreundschuh M, Loeffler M (eds) New aspects in the diagnosis and treatment of Hodgkin's disease. Rec Res Cancer Res 1989 (117):246-253. Springer Verlag, Berlin-Hong Kong
449 Phillips T, Armitage JO, Spitzer G et al: High-dose therapy and autologous bone marrow transplantation after failure of conventional chemotherapy in adults with intermediate grade or high grade non-Hodgkin's lymphoma. N Engl J Med 1987 (316):1493-1497
450 Takvorian T, Canellos GP, Ritz J et al: Prolonged disease-free survival after autologous bone marrow transplantation in patients with non-Hodgkin's lymphoma with a poor prognosis. N Engl J Med 1987 (316):1499-1504
451 Dini G, Philip T, Hartmann R et al: Bone marrow transplantation for neuroblastoma: a review of 509 cases. Bone Marrow Transpl 1989 (4 Suppl 4):42-46
452 Hortobagyi GN: The role of high-dose chemotherapy with autologous bone marrow transplantation in the treatment of breast cancer. Bone Marrow Transpl 1988 (3):525-530
453 Frei E III, Antman K, Teicher B et al: Bone marrow transplantation for solid tumours - Prospects. J Clin Oncol 1989 (7):515-526
454 Hagenbeek A, Martens ACM: Toxicity of Asta-Z (INN Mafosfamide) to normal and leukemic stem cells: Implications for autologous bone marrow

transplantation. Invest New Drugs 1984 (2):237-244
455 Hagenbeek A, Schultz FW, Arkesteijn GJA et al: Animal models of bone marrow transplantation for acute myelocytic leukemia. In: Gale RP, Champlin RD (eds): Bone Marrow Transplantation: Current Controversies. Alan R Liss Inc, New York 1989 pp 179-183
456 Hagenbeek A, Martens ACM: On the fate of leukemic cells infused with the autologous marrow graft. In: Buchner Th, Schellong A, Urbanitz D, Hiddeman W, Ritter R (eds) Acute Leukemias. Springer Verlag, Berlin-Heidelberg. Hematology and Blood Transfustion 1989 (30):353-359
457 Brandwein JM, Callum J, Sutcliffe SB et al: Evaluation of cytoreductive therapy prior to high dose treatment with autologous bone marrow transplantation in relapsed and refractory Hodgkin's disease. Bone Marrow Transpl 1990 (5):99-103
458 Favrot MC, Philip I, Philip T et al: Bone marrow purging procedure in Burkitt lymphoma with monoclonal antibodies and complement. Quantification by a liquid cell culture monitoring system. Br J Cancer 1986 (64):161-167
459 Reynolds CP, Black AT, Woody JN: Sensitive method for detecting viable cells seeded into bone marrow. Cancer Res 1986 (46):5878-5883
460 Evinger-Hodges MJ, Spinolo JA, Spencer V et al: Detection of minimal residual disease in acute myelogenous leukemia by RNA-in situ hybridization. Bone Marrow Transpl 1989 (4 Suppl 1):13-15
461 Bregni M, Siena S, Neri A et al: Minimal residual disease in acute lymphoblastic leukemia detected by immune selection and gene rearrangement analysis. J Clin Oncol 1989 (7):338-343
462 Janossy G, Campana D, Burnett A et al: Autologous bone marrow transplantation in acute lymphoblastic leukemia. Preclinical immunologic studies. Leukemia 1988 (2):485-495
463 Favrot MC, Philip T: Bone marrow purging. In: Magrath I (ed) New Directions in Cancer Treatment. Springer Verlag, Berlin-Tokyo 1989 pp 343-357
464 Hagenbeek A, Martens ACM: Cell separation studies in autologous bone marrow transplantation for acute leukemia. In: Gale RP (ed) Recent Advances in Bone Marrow Transplantation. Alan R Liss Inc, New York 1983 pp 717-735
465 Porcellini A, Manna M, Marchetti-Rossi MT et al: Purging by dye-mediated photosensitization. Bone Marrow Transpl 1989 (4 Suppl 1):188-189
466 Sharkis SJ, Santos GW, Colvin M: Elimination of acute myelogenous leukemia cells from marrow and tumor suspension in the rat with 4-hydroxyperoxycyclophosphamide. Blood 1980 (55):521-523
467 Santos GW, Colvin OM: Pharmacological purging of bone marrow with reference to autografting. Clin Haematol 1986 (15):67-83
468 Sindermann H, Penkert M, Hilgard P: Bone marrow purging with mafosfamide. A critical survey. Blut 1989 (5):432-441
469 Deconinck E, Tamayo E, Hervé P; In vitro chemosensitivity of leukemic progenitor cells (AML-CFU) to a combination of mafosfamide-lysine (ASTA-Z 7654) and etoposide (VP16-213). Bone Marrow Transpl 1990 (5):13-18
470 Gorin NC, Douay L, Laporte JP et al: Autologous bone marrow transplantation using marrow incubated with Asta-Z 7557 in adult acute leukemia. Blood 1986 (67):1367-1376
471 Douay L: Pharmacological purging of bone marrow with drugs other than cyclophosphamide derivatives. Bone Marrow Transpl 1989 (4 Suppl 1):195
472 Hervé P, Tamayo E, Lamy B et al: Comparative studies between mafosfamide and etoposide on myeloid progenitor cells, T-cell response and clonogenic cell lines. Int J Cell Cloning 1985 (3):275-276
473 MacIntyre EA: The use of monoclonal antibodies for purging autologous bone marrow in the lymphoid malignancies. Clin Haematol 1986 (15):249-267
474 Bast RC, De Fabritiis P, Lipton J et al: Elimination of malignant clonogenic cells from human bone marrow using multiple monoclonal antibodies and complement. Cancer Res 1985 (45):499-507
475 Treleaven JG, Kemshead JT: Removal of tumor cells from bone marrow: an evaluation of the available techniques. Haematol Oncol 1985 (3):65-75
476 Kemshead JT, Gibson FM: Monoclonal antibodies and magnetic microspheres used for the depletion of tumour cells from bone marrow. Bone Marrow Transpl 1987 (suppl 2):84-88
477 Janssen WE, Johnson KE, Lee C, Cassano W: Relative efficiency of leukemic cell depletion using anti-murine-IgG1 (Fc) or anti-murine-IgG coated immunomagnetic microbeads. Bone Marrow Transpl 1990 (5):19-22
478 Krlocick KA, Uhr JW, Vitetta S: Selective killing of leukaemia cells by antibody-toxin conjugates: implications for autologous bone marrow transplantation. Nature 1982 (295):604-605
479 Filipovich AH, Vallera DA, Youle RJ et al: Ex vivo treatment of donor bone marrow with anti-T cell immunotoxins for prevention of graft-versus-host disease. Lancet 1984 (1):469-472
480 Casellas P, Canal X, Fauser AA et al: Optimal elimination of leukemic T cells from human bone marrow with T101-ricin A chain immunotoxin. Blood 1985 (65):289-295
481 Myers CD, Thorpe PE, Ross WCJ et al: An immunotoxin with therapeutic potential in T cell leukemia. Blood 1984 (63):1178-1185
482 Uckun FM, Gaijl-Peczalska KJ, Kersey JH et al: Use of a novel colony assay to evaluate the cytotoxicity of an immunotoxin containing pokeweed antiviral protein against blast progenitor cells freshly obtained from patients with common B lineage acute lymphoblastic leukemia. J Exper Med 1986 (163):347-353
483 Wagner JE, Johnson RJ, Santos GW, Shin HS: Systemic monoclonal antibody therapy for eliminating minimal residual leukemia in a rat bone marrow transplant model. Blood 1989 (73):614-618

484 Gorin NC, Aegerter P, Auvert B et al: Autologous bone marrow transplantation for acute myelocytic leukemia in remission: decreased risk of relapse associated with marrow purging by mafosfamide. Blood 1990 (75):1606-1614

485 Gorin NC, Hervé P, Aegerter P et al: Autologous BMT for acute leukaemia in remission. Br J Haematol 1986 (64):385-395

486 Zander AR, Dicke KA, Vellekoop L et al: Autografting in acute leukemia. In: Gale RP (ed) Recent Advances in Bone Marrow Transplantation. Alan R Liss Inc, New York 1983 p 659

487 Meloni G, De Fabritiis P, Papa G et al: Cryopreserved autologous bone marrow infusion following high dose chemotherapy in patients with acute myeloblastic leukemia in first relapse. Leuk Res 1985 (9):407-412

488 Stewart P, Buckner CD, Bensinger W et al: Autologous marrow transplantation in patients with acute nonlymphocytic leukemia in first remission. Exp Hematol 1985 (13):267-271

489 Burnett AK, Watkins R, Maharaj D et al: Transplantation of unpurged autologous bone marrow in acute myeloid leukaemia in first remission. Lancet 1984 (2):1068-1070

490 Carella AM, Gaozza E, Santini G et al: Autologous unpurged bone marrow transplantation for acute non-lymphoblastic leukaemia in first complete remission. Bone Marrow Transpl 1988 (3):537-541

491 Linch DC, Burnett AK: Clinical studies of ABMT in acute myeloid leukaemia. Clin Haematol 1986 (15):167-186

492 Yeager AM, Kaizer H, Santos GW et al: Autologous bone marrow transplantation in patients with acute nonlymphocytic leukemia, using ex vivo marrow treatment with 4-hydroxyperoxycyclophosphamide. N Engl J Med 1986 (315):141-147

493 Rowley SD, Jones RJ, Piantadosi S et al: Efficacy of ex vivo purging for autologous bone marrow transplantation in the treatment of acute nonlymphoblastic leukemia. Blood 1989 (74):501-506

494 Gorin NC, Aegerter P, Parlier Y: Autologous bone marrow transplantation for acute leukemia in remission: Second European survey. Exp Hematol 1985 (suppl 17):177-190

495 Meloni G, De Fabritiis P, Carella AM: Autologous bone marrow transplantation in patients with AML in first complete remission. Results of two different conditioning regimens after the same induction and consolidation therapy. Bone Marrow Transpl 1990 (5):29-32

496 Beelen DW, Quabeck K, Graeven U et al: Acute toxicity and first clinical results of intensive postinduction therapy using a modified busulfan and cyclophosphamide regimen with autologous bone marrow rescue in first remission of acute myeloid leukemia. Blood 1989 (74):1507-1516

497 Goldstone AH, Linch DC, Anderson CC et al: Double ablative chemotherapy with autologous marrow rescue in the treatment of acute leukemia. In: Minimal Disease in Acute Leukemia. Nijhoff, Boston 1984 pp 287-292

498 Mascret B, Maraninchi D, Gastant JA et al: Repeated high-dose melphalan with autologous bone marrow transplantation in acute nonlymphocytic leukemia. Blood Transf Immuno-Haematol 1985 (28):477-488

499 Beaujean F, Hartmann O, Benhamon E et al: Hemopoietic reconstitution after repeated autologous transplantation with mafosfamide-purged marrow. Bone Marrow Transpl 1989 (4):373-541

500 Lowenberg B, Verdonck LJ, Dekker AW et al: Autologous bone marrow transplantation in acute myeloid leukemia in first remission: results of a Dutch prospective study. J Clin Oncol 1990 (8):287-294

501 Kersey JH: The role of marrow transplantation in acute lymphoblastic leukemia. J Clin Oncol 1989 (7):1589-1590

502 Carella AM: Autologous bone marrow transplantation in acute lymphoblastic leukemia: biological and clinical aspects. Haematol 1990 (75):79-83

503 Gorin NC, Aegerter P, Auvert B: Autologous bone marrow transplantation (ABMT) for acute leukemia in remission: an analysis of 1322 cases. Bone Marrow Transpl 1989 (4 Suppl 2):3-5

504 Kersey JH, Weisdorf D, Nesbit ME et al: Comparison of autologous and allogenic bone marrow transplantation for treatment of high-risk refractory acute lymphoblastic leukemia. N Engl J Med 1987 (317):461-467

505 Simonsson B, Burnett AK, Prentice HG et al: Autologous BMT with monoclonal antibody purgerd marrow for high-risk acute lymphoblastic leukemia. Leukemia 1989 (9):631-636

506 Sallan SE, Niemeyer CM, Billett AL et al: Autologous bone marrow transplantation for acute lymphoblastic leukemia. J Clin Oncol 1989 (7):1594-1601

507 Dicke KA, Spitzer G: Clinical studies of autografting in acute lymphocytic leukaemia. Clin Haematol 1986 (15):85-103

508 Ramsay NKC, Kersey JH: Perspective: indications for marrow transplantation in acute lymphoblastic leukemia. Blood 1990 (75):815-818

509 Butturini A, Keating A, Goldman J, Gale RP: Autotransplants in chronic myelogenous leukaemia: strategies and results. Lancet 1990 (335):1255-1258

510 Coulombel L, Kalousek DK, Eaves CJ: Long-term culture reveals chromosomally normal hemopoietic progenitor cells in patients with Philadelphia-chromosome positive chronic myelogenous leukemia. N Engl J Med 1981 (304):700-704

511 Barnett MJ: quoted by 517

512 McGlave PB: quoted by 517

513 Buckner CD, Clift RA, Fefer A et al: Treatment of blastic transformation of chronic granulocytic leukemia by high-dose cyclophosphamide, total body irradiation and infusion of cryopreserved autologous marrrow. Exp Hematol 1974 (2):138-146

514 Goldman JM, Catovsky D, Goolden AWG et al: Buffy coat autografts for patients with chronic

granulocytic leukaemia in transformation. Blut 1981 (42):149-155
515 Haines MA, Goldman JM, Worsley AM et al: Chemotherapy and autografting for chronic granulocytic leukaemia in transformation: probable prolongation of survival for some patients. Br J Haematol 1984 (58):711-721
516 Marcus RE, Goldman JM, Worsley AM et al: Autografting in chronic granulocytic leukaemia. Clin Haematol 1986 (15):235-247
517 Goldman JM, Grosveld G, Baltimore D, Gale RP: Congress letter. Chronic myelogenous leukemia. The unfolding saga. Leukemia 1990 (4):163-167
518 Vogler WR, Winton EF, James S et al: Autologous marrow transplantation after karyotype conversion to normal in blastic phase of chronic myelocytic leukemia. Am J Med 1983 (75):1080-1085
519 Goldman JM: quoted by 517
520 Carella AM, Frassoni F, Gaozza E et al: Autografting for patients with chronic myeloid leukemia in blastic crisis: promising results achieved with intensive conventional chemotherapy, peripheral blood stem cell collection, high-dose chemoradiotherapy and reinfusion. Submitted for publication

The Impact of Cytogenetics and Molecular Genetics on Diagnosis and Treatment

Emil J Freireich

Director, Adult Leukaemia Research Programme, University of Texas M.D. Anderson Cancer Centre, Houston, Texas

Chromosomal abnormalities have long been associated with malignant transformation. For many years such aneuploidy was considered to be random and therefore an epi-phenomenon of malignancy. However, the discovery by Nowell and Hungerford that a specific cytogenetic aneuploidy was associated with a specific disease, the Philadelphia chromosome and its association with the clinical diagnosis of chronic granulocytic leukaemia, initiated a new era of the study of chromosomes in leukaemia [1]. This cytogenetic aneuploidy was called Philadelphia One, because it was expected that other non-random chromosome abnormalities would be rapidly discovered. There is no Philadelphia Two to date. In acute leukaemia, somewhere between 40 and 80% of patients were found to have aneuploidy, but, again, multiple abnormalities were discovered [2] and it was not until 1973 that an association with clinical characteristics for a specific non-random chromosome aneuploidy, the 8;21 translocation, was described [3]. It now seems clear that non-random chromosome abnormalities are associated with specific diagnoses, that is, distinctive natural histories of the disease and perhaps more important have proven to be an independent and important prognostic factor in predicting response to therapy [4,5].

Chronic Granulocytic Leukaemia (CML)

Almost a decade after Nowell and Hungerford's description of the Philadelphia chromosome and its association with chronic granulocytic leukaemia, Dr. Rowley discovered this aneuploidy represented not a loss of genetic material but a reciprocal translocation between chromosomes 9 and 22 [6]. Studies of patients who had the haematological picture of chronic granulocytic leukaemia (CML), but lacked the Philadelphia chromosome, revealed that these patients comprised approximately 15% of all CML patients, and their clinical course was characterised by a shorter overall survival, poor response to therapy, lower platelet counts, and a more rapid progression to blastic transformation [7,8]. Thus, the Philadelphia chromosome abnormality identified a more favourable subset of patients with chronic granulocytic leukaemia when treated conventionally with an alkylating agent such as myleran.

The discovery that the ABL oncogene was located on the long arm of chromosome 9 led investigators to study the ABL oncogene in patients with chronic granulocytic leukaemia, which soon resulted in the discovery that it was translocated to chromosome 22 and the gene was rearranged [9]. That is, after treatment with restriction enzymes, a new size gene was discovered in patients with CML. This led to the molecular studies which revealed that the breakpoint on chromosome 22 clustered in a small region of the gene (5.8 kb), which was characterised as the breakpoint cluster region (bcr) [10]. Thus, in patients with chronic granulocytic leukaemia who had the Philadelphia chromosome it was possible, using molecular techniques, to identify a new gene, the bcr/abl gene. This new gene can be identified by Southern blotting and the necessary probe for studying the gene is commercially available, so that this has become a generally available laboratory procedure for the diagnosis of chronic granulocytic leukaemia. When done by Southern blotting, this test can detect as few as 1% of the nucleated cells as having this unique gene. This gene is only present in the leukaemic cells of patients with chronic granulocytic leukaemia. In the patients afflicted with this diagnosis, all the other somatic cells that have been studied are normal so that this new gene indeed characterises the malignant clone. To date the gene has not been discovered in any haematologically normal individuals.

The bcr/abl gene has been found to have a unique transcript, that is, a unique RNA product which, like the DNA, exists only in patients with chronic granulocytic leukaemia and is confined to the leukaemic cells [11]. Finally, it has recently been demonstrated that there is a unique protein product of this gene which has different biochemical activity, that is, increased tyrosine kinase activity [12].

The Impact of Treatment on the Natural History of Chronic Granulocytic Leukaemia

The discovery of alkylating agent activity against chronic granulocytic leukaemia in the early 1950s had a profound effect on the natural history of this disease. Instead of complications of thrombocytosis and leukocytosis such as haemorrhage, infection, tumour formation and anaemia, alkylating agent therapy was able to control the haematological manifestations of the disease in 85% of patients. It was then realised that a high proportion of the patients, approaching 100%, transformed into a blastic pattern at which time the disease was quite refractory to treatment. Thus, although myleran therapy could control the haematological manifestations of the disease and change the biology and natural history of the disease, the overall effect was only modest increases in overall survival from diagnosis. With the discovery of the 9;22 translocation it was soon recognised that patients treated to complete haematological remission still had virtually 100% of the metaphases in their blood and bone marrow identified by the Philadelphia chromosome. Thus, it was clear that the control of the haematological manifestations was not associated with any substantial change in the cytogenetic abnormality specifically associated with the disease [13]. This created a new therapeutic target for the clinical scientist.

Efforts to intensify myleran therapy to bone marrow aplasia were largely unsuccessful in changing the proportion of Philadelphia chromosome positive cells. However, Dr. Clarkson and the group at Memorial Hospital attempted to use intensive anti-metabolite therapy that was useful for causing complete remissions in acute myeloblastic leukaemia, and they reported the recovery of normal diploid cells from the bone marrow of patients receiving such intensive treatment [14]. Unfortunately, the period of Philadelphia chromosome negativity was short and virtually all patients promptly had recurrence of the Ph chromosome positivity. Combination chemotherapy can suppress Ph-positive cells in a majority of patients, but the suppression is not sustained despite continued chemotherapy [15].

Interferon Therapy

The observation that interferon had a significant anti-proliferative effect on CML cells *in vitro* led to clinical trials of interferon for the control of chronic granulocytic leukaemia [16]. It was soon reported that interferon could induce haematological remissions in a high proportion, in excess of 80%, of patients in the benign phase of this disease. However, the important new observation was made that a significant fraction, approximately 30%, had a major reduction in the proportion of Philadelphia chromosome positive metaphases in the bone marrow with the return of diploid metaphases. Unlike the Philadelphia negative state induced by cytotoxic chemotherapy, a proportion of the patients treated with interferon had prolonged periods of Philadelphia chromosome negativity. Thus, at the very least the recurrence of diploid metaphases in the bone marrow following interferon therapy was an important prognostic factor for predicting improved survival and a prolonged interval between diagnosis and the occurrence of blast transformation. These observations greatly strengthened the hypothesis that the treatment objective for the control of CML was now shifted from haematological criteria to cytogenetic criteria for response. Thus, the absence of detectable Philadelphia chromosome positive metaphases was at least necessary if not sufficient for prolonged disease control.

The Role of Molecular Genetics in CML

As already emphasised, somewhere between 5 and 15% of patients who have the clinical picture of chronic granulocytic leukaemia lack the 9;22 translocation on cytogenetic study. The availability of molecular techniques to determine the presence of the unique bcr/abl gene has made it possible to investigate Philadelphia chromosome negative patients for the presence of this gene [17]. It was found that almost half of the Philadelphia chromosome negative patients had the bcr/abl gene. Even more important was the fact that, when the natural history of this subset of patients was examined, it was found that they had a clinical picture which was not significantly different from the ordinary patients with the Philadelphia chromosome. Thus, these patients have a masked Philadelphia chromosome translocation which is not visibly detected by the usual banding cytogenetic procedures but is easily detected by molecular techniques. It was important that these patients had a response to interferon which was identical to the patients who had the Philadelphia chromosome. This further emphasises the fact that treatment effects reveal heterogeneity in the biology of the underlying diseases.

With the availability of the molecular techniques for detecting the bcr/abl gene, it is now believed that the subset of patients who were believed to have chronic granulocytic leukaemia but were negative for both the Philadelphia chromosome and the bcr/abl gene, do not have chronic granulocytic leukaemia. After careful review in a number of centres, it has been found that these patients have various types of myeloproliferative disorders which are responsible for the notion that the Ph-negative patients have a poorer prognosis than the Ph-positive patients. Thus, it is possible to ascribe the entire clinical picture of chronic granulocytic leukaemia to the presence of this single genetic event, the bcr/abl gene. Individuals who have a clone of cells with this gene have the entire clinical spectrum of the disease, chronic granulocytic leukaemia; for individuals lacking this gene, other diagnostic categories should be seriously considered.

The Polymerase Chain Reaction in CML

Dr. Ming Lee was the first to utilise the polymerase chain reaction to amplify a gene that is tumour specific. In his initial research he studied the bcl 2 gene initially cloned by Tsuyimoto and Croce. Because the breakpoint site (mbr) was narrow (within 450 base pairs), it was technically feasible to identify primers which could be used for the polymerase chain reaction [18]. The polymerase chain reaction employs denaturation and renaturation of DNA in the presence of the appropriate chemicals necessary for copying DNA. For new genes, particularly translocations, each cycle makes two copies of the neogenes and only one copy of each of the other two normal genes. Thus, after 20 cycles one has a circumstance where the new gene is amplified a million-fold in the optimum situation, whereas the normal genes are only copied 20 times. This test has found extensive application to molecular genetics limited only by the availability of the appropriate reagents for applying to specific problems.

In the case of the bcr/abl gene, the polymerase chain reaction conducted on DNA was technically difficult to accomplish because of the variability in the bcr breakpoints. Dr. Lee and others conceived of isolating the RNA transcripts and to reverse transcribe the RNA manufacturing a cDNA *in vitro* which can then be amplified with the polymerase chain reaction [19]. The polymerase chain reaction now greatly expands the sensitivity of methods for detecting the unique bcr/abl gene. Patients with chronic granulocytic leukaemia were studied when in stable cytogenetic complete remission, that is, Philadelphia chromosome negative for more than a year as a result of interferon therapy. All of these patients to date had residual RNA transcripts of the bcr/abl detectable by the polymerase chain reaction in their peripheral blood at the time of complete remission [20]. This finding suggests that the interferon therapeutic effect on CML, while profound, is still in the palliative category and these studies predict that the majority of these patients will have recurrence of their disease either when the interferon therapy ceases to be effective or is discontinued.

In contrast to the interferon treatment effect, the use of intensive chemotherapy plus allogeneic bone marrow transplantation has resulted in between 30 and 50% prolonged survivors in CML [21,22]. Initially, it was reported that, like interferon therapy, allogeneic transplantation is associated with a high proportion of patients losing the Philadelphia chromosome aneuploidy, and the engrafted donor cells were cytogenetically diploid. The question is whether these patients have any residual CML cells. To date, a number of studies have been reported from a number of transplant centres applying the polymerase chain reaction to the problem of detecting residual disease. At this point, the final result is not in but it is clear that a significant proportion of patients fail to show RNA transcripts by the polymerase chain reaction [23,24]. This suggests that a fraction of these patients are candidates for having truly curative treatment for their disease.

In summary, for chronic granulocytic leukaemia, molecular genetics and cytogenetics have substantially altered our understanding of the biology and natural history of the disease. But, perhaps most important, we have seen an evolution in the treatment strategies for this disease based on our ability to detect the abnormal clone. We have moved from using clinical and haematological criteria to using cytogenetic criteria of the Philadelphia chromosome, and in the modern era the use of the molecular genetic techniques, particularly coupled with the polymerase chain reaction, has created a unique and important target for continuing therapeutic research with the goal of eradicating the disease.

Acute Myeloblastic Leukaemia

Between 40 and 80% of patients with acute myeloblastic leukaemia have cytogenetic aneuploidy [25]. Patients who achieve complete haematological remission virtually always show a return to the normal diploid pattern with disappearance of this cytogenetic aneuploidy. Although 20 to 50% of patients with acute myeloblastic leukaemia who achieve complete haematological remission remain disease free for prolonged periods of time and may be cured, the majority of patients have recurrence of their leukaemia. It has been regularly observed that the cytogenetic aneuploidy which was characteristic of the patients own disease at diagnosis is almost invariably present in the recurrent leukaemia. At the present time, the cytogenetic studies have approximately the same degree of sensitivity for the detection of residual leukaemic cells as ordinary haematological criteria. Recently, we have studied bone marrows in patients in remission who had cytogenetically defined clinical syndromes and we have found a small fraction, approximately 1/4, who had one or more aneuploid metaphases in their remission marrow; all of these patients had recurrence of disease. For many of these patients, morphological examination of the bone marrow at the time of the cytogenetic study did not reveal any suspicious evidence of leukaemic cell persistence and this suggested that cytogenetics may also be useful, as it is in CML, as a method for detecting residual leukaemia and as a guide to further treatment. In patients who had diploid cytogenetics, approximately half of the patients did have recurrence of the disease, thus, although achieving a diploid cytogenetic status is necessary for achieving prolonged disease-free survival, with the present state of sensitivity it is not sufficient since approximately half of the patients will nonetheless have recurrence of their disease [26].

Non-Random Chromosome Abnormalities in Acute Myeloblastic Leukaemia

In the early 1970s a number of researchers reported specific cytogenetic patterns in AML patients. One of the first to show prognostic significance was the 8;21 translocation which was found to have a favourable impact on response to therapy [27]. The recognition that the patients with promyelocytic leukaemia or the FAB M-3 type had a 15;17 translocation, also was important from a prognostic point of view because not only were these patients younger but they had a major haemorrhagic diathesis associated with disseminated intravascular coagulation [28]. Finally, the description of an elevated number of eosinophilic leukaemic cells associated with a myelomonocytic morphology of the FAB M-4 class was found to be strongly associated with an inversion 16-chromosome aneuploidy and the association of central nervous system chloroma with this cytogenetic pattern was also recognised [29]. Elderly patients who had a history of an antecedent haematologic disturbance or extensive treatment for another malignancy were patients who frequently presented with deletions of the long arm of chromosomes 5 or 7, while another subset of patients who demonstrated a trisomy of chromosome 8 were also found to be in the unfavourable prognostic group.

It was soon recognised that at least for these specific cytogenetic aneuploidies there was a unique and highly specific clinical syndrome, and it was subsequently reported that recognition of the cytogenetic aneuploidy was not only an independent variable predicting for both response and survival, but proved to be extremely important in predicting the natural history of the treated disease [5].

From 1975 to the present at the University of Texas M.D. Anderson Cancer Centre, we have had the good fortune to have the support of Dr. Trujillo, the Head of our Division of Laboratory Medicine, such that all of our patients with acute myeloblastic leukaemia who were referred without having received prior therapy had a banded cytogenetic study conducted. During that period of time we were able to study 725 patients (Table 1).

Table 1. 1975-1987 Cytogenetic Study Group (AML)

	No. Pts.	% CR
Aneuploid Study Group	266 (.37)	58
Others	459 (.63)	62
Total	725	60

Of these patients, 266 or 37% had a non-random chromosome abnormality associated with a definite impact on the natural history of their disease. The remaining patients were predominantly diploid by conventional cytogenetic study, however, there were a number of patients who had other less frequently observed non-random chromosome aneuploidies and a number of miscellaneous abnormalities that are not clearly associated with clinical syndromes. Over this period of time, 60% of the patients achieved a complete remission as a result of combination chemotherapy and on average the frequency of response was not different between the aneuploid study group of patients who are going to be discussed in detail and the remaining patients.

This study focuses on six specific cytogenetic aneuploidies; three of these are favourable as related to frequency of response, duration of response and overall survival, and three are distinctly unfavourable (Table 2).

Table 2. Cytogenetics on response rate (AML)

	No. Pts.	% CR
INV 16	40	92.5
t8;21	43	93
t15;17	40	57.5
Favourable	**123**	**81**
tri 8	55	45
-5,-7	79	29
ph'	9	56
Unfavourable	**143**	**37**

Approximately half of the patients could be grouped into a favourable category and these patients had an overall frequency of remission of 81%, which is significantly better than the 60% average for the group as a whole, while the three unfavourable categories, i.e., trisomy of chromosome 8, deletions of the long arm of chromosomes 5 or 7, and the Philadelphia-like chromosome aneuploidy,

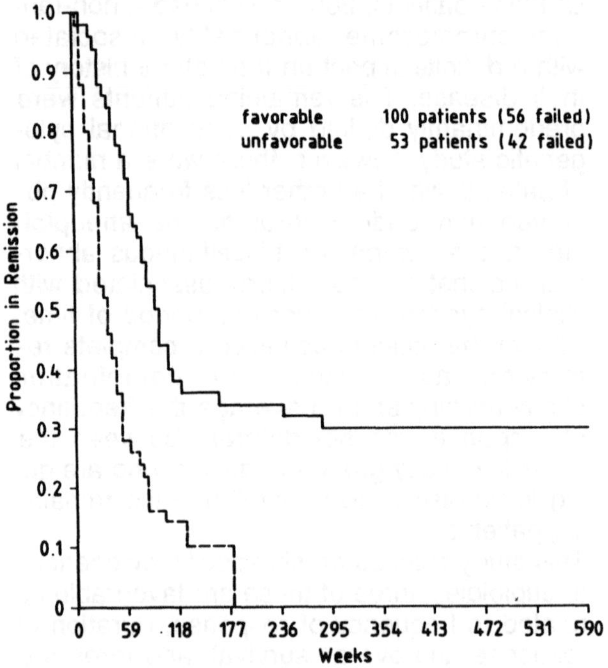

Fig. 1. Patients with acute myeloblastic leukaemia in the cytogenetic study groups. All patients achieving complete remission are considered for duration of first remission dated from onset of remission. Favourable patients have inv 16, t8;21 or t15;17. Unfavourable patients have -5q, -7q, tri 8 or ph1.

had an overall response rate which was less than half of the favourable group. Ignoring all other prognostic variables which were previously known to be important, such as age and extent of disease, knowledge of the cytogenetic aneuploidy alone predicts for more than 100% increase in the frequency of achieving complete remission.

It has been realised that patients who fail to achieve complete haematological remission have a short median survival which can be measured in months. After studying over 200 consecutive such patients in our institution, we have no patient who has survived without achieving complete haematological remission for more than two years. Therefore, all of the patients who have prolonged survivorship beyond two years and all of those who are candidates for being cured of their disease achieve a complete haematological remission.

If we consider the impact of the cytogenetic pattern on the duration of remission for those who achieve complete remission (Fig. 1), we find that patients in the unfavourable categories who achieve remission almost invariably relapse with a median duration of remission measured in months, being substantially less than a year, and virtually no patients survive relapse free beyond two years. In contrast, in the favourable cytogenetic group, between 30 and 40% have prolonged disease-free survivorship. When compared to the entire group of patients who are found to have prolonged survivorship, they are represented in the prolonged survivorship group more than twice as often as the average patient [30]. Thus, the appreciation of the cytogenetic aneuploidy is a powerful predictor both for the frequency of response and for the quality or the duration of that response.

The two variables may be considered simultaneously by projecting the time to treatment failure for each of the five major cytogenetic categories under study (Fig. 2). In this projection, the proportion of patients who are in complete remission at each time interval is measured. Therefore, this is disease-free survivorship on the initial treatment. Patients who fail to achieve remission have no duration of remission and therefore the ordinate is reduced at time zero. This figure dramatically shows the enormous impact that cytogenetics alone, without considering any other biological feature of the patient or of his disease, has on the overall duration of complete remission. The patients in the inv 16 and 8;21 groups have far and away the best overall survival. The patients with the 15;17 translocation are

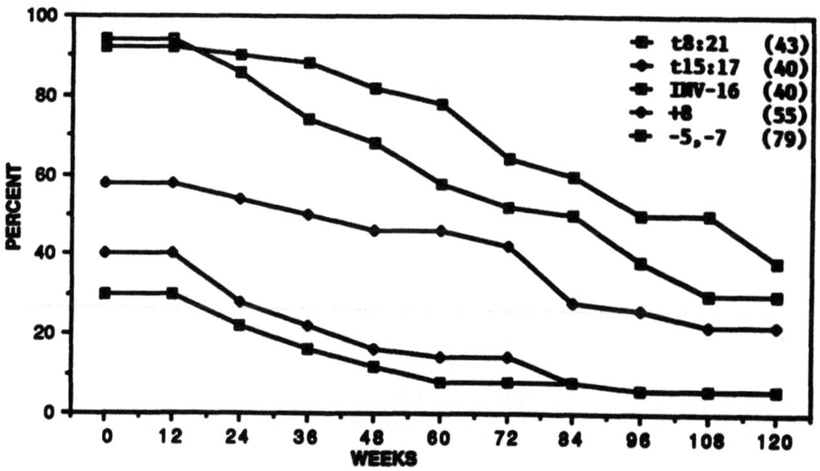

Fig. 2. Time to treatment failure for initial therapy for the first 120 weeks

intermediate because they have a high mortality during remission induction as a result of our inability to effectively control their haemorrhagic diathesis. But the patients who achieve remission have the best proportion of prolonged survivorship so that the slope of their time to treatment failure is the shallowest of the three favourable groups. These three contrast sharply with the unfavourable cytogenetic types, the trisomy 8 and the -5, -7, where the fraction of time that all patients are free of disease is dramatically lower.

The impact of the cytogenetics on prognosis is better demonstrated by considering the area under the time to treatment failure curve for the first two years of the patient's life after his diagnosis. Stated positively, this shows for all of the patients studied the average fraction of the two years immediately after diagnosis that the patient spends free of the disease (Fig. 3). This measurement provides in a single bar graph an impressive portrayal of the profound impact that cytogenetics alone has on the natural history of the treated disease. I need to emphasise, again, that in the absence of treatment the impact of these aneuploidies was relatively minor since the prognosis for all groups was extremely poor. It is the treatment effect which reveals the enormous heterogeneity in the diseases we previously thought were acute myeloblastic leukaemia because there is this dramatic difference in response to treatment. The most favourable group, the inv 16 patients, on average spend almost 75% of the first two years post diagnosis free of disease. In contrast, patients with deletions of chromosomes 5 and 7 have the inverse situation with only 15% of the time free of disease.

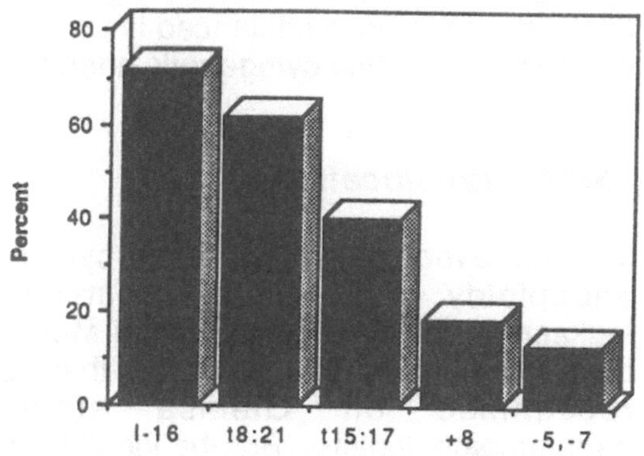

	I-16	t8:21	t15:17	+8	-5,-7
# Patients	40	43	40	55	79
# Failed	22	26	31	49	74

Fig. 3. Area under the time to treatment failure curves expressed as a percent of the first 120 weeks in complete remission

Specific Cytogenetic Categories of AML

Inversion 16 Disease

The recognition of the association of eosinophilia in the bone marrow with the inv 16 chromosome aneuploidy has defined an important new clinical syndrome, because this disease is one of the most sensitive to all the known active anti-leukaemic drugs for the treatment of acute myeloblastic leukaemia. The patients virtually all have a FAB classification M-4 myelomonocytic acute leukaemia.

The Giemsa-stained bone marrow has a classical appearance because the increased eosinophilic granules are distinctly abnormal both to the light and electron microscope and most haematopathologists can recognise this clinical syndrome morphologically with a high degree of accuracy. The cytogenetic aneuploidy confirms the diagnosis.

Recognising this clinical syndrome is extremely important because of the high probability of ending up disease-free after effective and appropriately intensive therapy. On average the patients are younger than the median, and with full dose therapy essentially all patients respond with a rapid anti-leukaemic effect. Failure is confined to patients who die of pre-existing complications or of infection or haemorrhage that occurs during the remission induction process. Chemotherapy resistance is rarely observed. When these patients were treated with maintenance chemotherapy, we observed that a significant proportion showed the development of intracerebral chloromatous tumours, which in several patients occurred while the marrow was still in remission. This disease was different from the usual diffuse subarachnoid leukaemic infiltration that is found with lymphoid neoplasms. It was observed, however, that patients who had this central nervous system disease retained their sensitivity to chemotherapy, and whatever pharmacological sanctuary was provided by the intracerebral location could be overcome with high-dose ara-C chemotherapy, that is, treatment given at doses of three grams per meter every 12 hours for at least six doses. Treatment with high-dose ara-C resulted in regression of these intracerebral deposits.

Therefore, it is important that for patients with this disease, intensive high-dose early intensification therapy is a mandatory part of the treatment of these patients in remission. Unfortunately, despite effective induction, early intensification, and a variety of maintenance type schedules, the majority of patients with inv 16 disease at least to date have had recurrence of their leukaemia. We have recently observed, after studying 20 patients in complete remission, seven who had persistent abnormalities in chromosome 16. All of the patients with these persistent abnormalities predicted for recurrent disease. The median time to recurrence from the abnormal chromosome study in remission was over 50 weeks and therefore it suggests that cytogenetic aneuploidy may provide an important parameter of residual disease and may help to identify patients in remission who are in need of additional treatment in order to be converted to the cured fraction.

Translocation Between Chromosomes 8 and 21

This abnormality is associated with a FAB classification M-2 type morphology, with granules in the cytoplasm and Auer rods. At least to date these patients cannot be regularly recognised or separated from the other FAB M-2 type patients using ordinary light microscopy. The importance of this particular cytogenetic aneuploidy is that, like inv 16 disease, the frequency of response is extremely high and resistance to chemotherapy is rare. Like inv 16 disease, although the median duration of remission is significantly longer and a high proportion of these patients remain in the cured category, there are still a major fraction of the patients who have recurrence of their leukaemia. It is important to recognise this group of patients because for both chemotherapy treatments during remission and for bone marrow transplantation offered to AML patients in first remission, a high proportion of patients with this leukaemic disorder are identified in the cured fraction of patients, therefore, the decision as to what appropriate treatment should be given to patients in remission is influenced importantly by the presence of this cytogenetic aneuploidy.

15;17 Translocation

Virtually every patient with this cytogenetic aneuploidy has acute promyelocytic leukaemia, the FAB classification M-3. Most have the classical promyelocytes that can be recognised on Giemsa stain by haematopathologists. But the identification of the cytogenetic aneuploidy has helped clarify an important subset of these patients who have a microgranular form of promyelocyte that was previously difficult to identify as acute progranulocytic leukaemia. While there have been reports of patients who morphologically have acute promyelocytic leukaemia but do not have the 15;17 translocation, and although there are rare individuals with the chromosome aneuploidy that cannot be recognised as acute promyelocytic leukaemia, the association is so strong that, like chronic granulocytic leukaemia, it is reasonable to propose that the cytogenetic aneuploidy is a sufficient diagnostic criterion for making the diagnosis of acute promyelocytic leukaemia. As already emphasised, these patients have a high mortality, somewhere between 25 and 40% during remission induction, and the major cause of this mortality is a haemorrhagic diathesis. The granules of the leukaemic cells have a high order of procoagulant activity and a consumptive type coagulopathy is associated with major catastrophic haemorrhage. Many efforts to control the haemorrhagic diathesis using extensive replacement of consumed procoagulants, plasmapheresis to deplete fibrin split products, and the use of heparin to interfere with the coagulopathy, have all been used with varying degrees of success. Nonetheless, these patients constitute a group of patients who require extraordinarily intensive and aggressive therapy to achieve remission with our currently available therapeutic methods. The efforts, regardless of cost and time, that are devoted to it are certainly justified because, as already emphasised, once these patients achieve a haematological remission they have the highest fraction of cured patients who remain prolonged disease-free survivors.

Unfavourable Cytogenetic Categories

The patients who have a partial or complete deletion of chromosomes 5 and 7 are undoubtedly the poorest prognosis group. A high proportion of these patients have had an antecedent haematological disturbance, usually some form of myelodysplastic syndrome. Virtually all patients who have secondary leukaemias, that is, leukaemias secondary to another primary malignancy such as multiple myeloma, Hodgkin's disease, breast cancer, etc., end up in this cytogenetically aneuploid group. We have studied a patient who had a FAB M-2 type of acute myeloblastic leukaemia who remained disease and treatment free for 15 years and who presented after being cured of his original acute myeloblastic leukaemia with a -5 cytogenetically aneuploid leukaemia which responded transiently to therapy but subsequently resulted in his demise. For this group of patients recognition that they are in this unfavourable category allows the clinical scientist and the physician to recognise that currently available therapy is ineffective and largely palliative. If there are innovative treatments for which the clinical experience would justify treating a previously untreated patient, then it would be reasonable to offer innovative treatments to this class of patients because the benefit they derive from conventional treatment is minor.

Patients with the trisomy 8 are slightly more responsive to chemotherapy but are readily grouped with this poor prognosis group of patients. However, an occasional trisomy 8 patient has a favourable duration of remission and it might be considered more favourably for treatment, particularly if the patients are young and the host prognostic factors are favourable for tolerating chemotherapy. The small subset of Philadelphia chromosome positive AML patients are a challenge. At the present time, it is not clear whether all of these patients have the classical Philadelphia chromosome defect of CML at the molecular level. It is clear that some do and it is conceivable that these patients have a myeloblastic transformation of a chronic granulocytic leukaemia which was not detected during the benign phase. Certainly the presence of a 9;22 translocation in this small group of patients with AML is generally associated with an unfavourable response to therapy and it allows them to be grouped with the poor prognosis patients.

Diploid and Other Patients

For the 63% of patients who have either diploid cytogenetics, that is, no abnormality detectable with banded cytogenetics, or patients who have other aneuploidies that occur less frequently, all of the characteristics discussed above that are typical of the syndromes with specific cytogenetic aneuploidy are intermediate between the favourable and unfavourable groups. The frequency of response for this entire group of patients was 62%, (Table 1), which is not different from the frequency of response for the combined study group. However, the cytogenetic study group is clearly divisible into a favourable and unfavourable group. Likewise, for relapse-free survival or duration of complete remission, this diploid and other group of patients is intermediate, having approximately one-half of the long-term survivor rate of the favourable cytogenetic group and having a median survival which is halfway between the favourable and unfavourable cytogenetic groups. These findings suggest strongly that the remaining patients with acute myeloblastic leukaemia are made up of different prognostic groupings which have an average prognosis that is identical to the entire group. It suggests that this group, although it appears homogenous, is also heterogenous with regard to its fundamental biology. One important observation is the realisation that patients with chronic granulocytic leukaemia who lack the Philadelphia chromosome aneuploidy, that is, the 9;22 translocation, when examined by banded cytogenetics in a significant fraction, are positive when studied for rearrangement of the bcr/abl. This indicates that it is possible to have major cytogenetic aneuploidy which is "masked", that is, the translocation occurs in such a way that it cannot be visualised by the morphological techniques of cytogenetic analysis. It is possible that this miscellaneous remaining group of AML patients may contain masked translocations that are not visualised with current techniques.

There is already clear evidence of heterogeneity in this group based on findings of cell surface phenotype with monoclonal antibodies.

Molecular Genetics of Acute Myeloblastic Leukaemia

Patients with acute promyelocytic leukaemia of the FAB class M-3 that have the 15;17 translocation show a substantial over-expression of the protein myeloperoxidase. This enzyme is extremely useful in classifying cells as being of the myeloid origin. Dr. Chang therefore cloned the myeloperoxidase gene and was able to localise it to chromosome 17 [31]. The in-situ hybridisation studies revealed that the myeloperoxidase gene localised to the q22-24 region of the gene which is very close to the breakpoint on chromosome 17 in the 15;17 translocation. However, studies of patients with promyelocytic leukaemia failed to show a rearrangement in the gene. Further analysis revealed that the gene is translocated from chromosome 17 to chromosome 15 in patients with acute promyelocytic leukaemia, and therefore it is clearly distal to the breakpoint on chromosome 17 [32]. It is believed that the translocation is at least in part responsible for the over-expression of this gene in the patients with the 15;17 translocation. Many investigators are pursuing the actual unique gene at the 15;17 breakpoint and one strategy is to either walk or jump along the chromosome from the myeloperoxidase gene to the putative neogene at the breakpoint on chromosome 15.

For the other reciprocal translocations, the inversion 16 and the 8;21 translocation, the genes located at the breakpoints have not yet been identified. However, many laboratories are pursuing this goal. It is clear from analogy with the chronic granulocytic leukaemia situation that this is an important research objective since identification of these unique genes will allow for novel therapeutic strategies using these genes as a target for therapy and as a marker for minimal residual disease. At the same time, identification of these genes offers the potential for a better understanding of the mechanism of leukogenesis and should provide leads for new approaches to therapeutic interventions.

For the unfavourable cytogenetic categories it has been found that a number of important stimulators of myeloid colony growth are localised to the long arm of chromosome 5 in the area that is usually deleted in patients who have a partial or a complete deletion of the long arm of chromosome 5 [33]. The discovery of both oncogenes and their counterpart anti-oncogenes has provided potential insight into the mechanism of these deletions in terms of tumorigenesis. In the best established cases, the loss of genetic heterozygosity which results from the deletion of a portion of a chromosome or a specific gene allows an oncogene, that is, a specific gene, to be overexpressed and contribute importantly to carcinogenesis. This has been demonstrated for retinoblastoma and for a number of other common malignancies including colon cancer [34,35]. It is possible that replacement of the gene products might have a major effect on the natural history of these diseases, another important lead which is being actively pursued in a number of centres.

Myelodysplastic Syndromes

The FAB classification separates patients with dysplastic bone marrows into acute myeloblastic leukaemia or into the preleukaemic myelodysplastic syndromes, based on the percentage of blasts in the differential count of the bone marrow. It was initially reported by Nowell that patients who were cytogenetically aneuploid had an unfavourable prognosis as it relates to progression to acute leukaemia and to shortened survival [36]. A high proportion of patients with these preleukaemic conditions have cytogenetically similar types of abnormalities to the unfavourable patients with acute myeloblastic leukaemia. Specifically, they frequently show deletions of the long arm of chromosomes 5 or 7 or a trisomy of chromosome 8. When patients with these unfavourable cytogenetic aneuploidies are compared to the other patients with the myelodysplastic syndromes, they are found to have an unfavourable natural history as it relates to survival.

It has been observed that the survival of patients with myelodysplastic syndromes and unfavourable cytogenetic aneuploidy, that is, blast differentials of between 5 and 30%, are similar, if not identical, to the natural history of patients with the same cytogenetic aneuploidies who have more than 30% blasts and are classified as acute myeloblastic leukaemia. We have proposed that the cytogenetic pattern of the leukaemic disorder is more important than the percentage of blasts in the differential [37]. Although there have not been studies to date where patients have received the identical treatments, it is entirely possible that the cytogenetic aneuploidy will be of more prognostic importance in this subgroup of patients as it is in acute myeloblastic leukaemia patients.

Ras Gene Mutations

It was initially reported by Liu and Bishop that RAS gene point mutations were associated with conversion from benign phase to blast crisis in chronic granulocytic leukaemia and with progression to acute leukaemia in patients with myelodysplastic syndromes [38]. This work has been confirmed but the frequency of RAS gene mutations is quite low [39]. However, it has been observed that mutations of the RAS gene occur quite frequently in patients with chronic myelomonocytic leukaemia. This observation is extremely interesting since these patients usually have a prolonged benign phase and therefore it is unlikely that this predicts for malignant transformation. Moreover, patients with FAB M-4 or M-5 myelomonocytic and monocytic acute leukaemia also show a high frequency of RAS mutations [40]. While the significance of the point mutations is not clear, it is possible that they may be useful in detecting minimal residual disease in patients who have such abnormalities.

Acute Lymphoblastic Leukaemia

As with acute myeloblastic leukaemia, a majority of patients with acute lymphoblastic leukaemia also have cytogenetic aneuploidy [41]. Patients who have hyperploid phenotypes are the most favourable. These patients have the highest likelihood of having the common form of childhood acute lymphoblastic leukaemia and have the highest cured fraction and the best overall prognosis. Particularly striking is the observation of the Philadelphia chromosome aneuploidy in patients who appear to have acute lymphoblastic leukaemia. A small fraction of these patients prove to have the translocation 9;22, which, at the molecular genetic level, is identical to that observed in chronic granulocytic leukaemia, that is, a breakpoint within the breakpoint cluster region. These patients are at least conceptually candidates for having a lymphoid blast transformation of chronic granulocytic leukaemia with an unrecognised benign phase. However, the majority of ALL patients who have the Philadelphia chromosome have the breakpoint on chromosome 22 outside of the breakpoint cluster region. Thus, although these patients cytogenetically have a 9;22 translocation at the molecular genetic level, they have a unique breakpoint, and these patients have a unique biology [42]. Specifically patients with the Philadelphia chromosome have an exceptionally poor prognosis with a low frequency of complete remission and a very infrequent prolonged disease-free survivorship.

Recently it has been reported that, using molecular genetic techniques, there are in ALL patients like CML patients individuals who have a masked 9;22 translocation. Again, it has been reported that the masked translocations are associated with the same poor prognosis as the cytogenetically determinable cytogenetic aneuploidy. It has been estimated that, if one includes all ALL patients who have the molecular genetic evidence of the 9;22 translocation, this may constitute as many as 25% of adults with ALL, and this may account for the striking difference between adults and children in terms of lower response to treatment and a lower cured fraction. Recently it has been possible to use the pcr to detect minimal disease in ALL patients by detecting monoclonal B and T cell genes in complete remission patients [43].

Conclusions

The techniques of cytogenetics and molecular genetics have revealed enormous heterogeneity in the leukaemic disorders. This heterogeneity is of fundamental importance to our understanding of the biology of these diseases since the abnormalities are specific for the tumour. The interaction of treatment effects with the natural history of the disease accentuates the enormous heterogeneity of these diseases. The responses to treatment are quite unique and specific for those cytogenetic and molecular genetic subtypes that have been clearly identified. Thus, it is clear that cytogenetic and molecular genetic studies are an essential component of the staging and diagnosis of patients with leukaemia. Moreover, it is now clear that this knowledge can influence the choice of therapy for specific subsets of patients. Both the choice of drug and the strategy employed can be fundamentally effected by the nature of the underlying malignancy. The observation that patients in haematological remission may have either cytogenetic or molecular genetic evidence of residual disease opens a whole new field of therapeutic research for the clinical scientist. The clinical and biological significance of these abnormalities in remission remain to be defined. Yet it is clear that the targets for therapy have moved from morphology to cytogenetics, and to molecular genetic techniques. Even more important than the prognostic importance of these abnormalities is the potential for new approaches to the diagnosis, prevention and treatment of the leukaemias. We are now in an era where the long sought for specific difference between the tumour cell and the normal host cell has been identified. The potential for therapeutic agents which either correct deficiencies or antagonise and overcome stimulatory effects is a new area of tumour biology and therapeutic research.

REFERENCES

1 Nowell PC and Hungerford DA: A minute chromosome in human chronic granulocytic leukemia. JNCI 1960 (25):85-109

2 Sandberg AA, Takagi N, Sofuni T and Crosswhite LH: Chromosomes and causation of human cancer and leukemia-V. Karyotypic aspects of acute leukemia. Cancer 1968 (22):1268-1282

3 Rowley JD: Identification of a translocation with quinacrine fluorescence in a patient with acute leukemia. Ann Genet (Paris) 1973 (16):109

4 Bloomfield CD and de la Chapelle A: Chromosome abnormalities in acute nonlymphocytic leukemia: Clinical and biological significance. Semin Oncol 1987 (14):372-382

5 Keating MJ, Cork A, Broach Y, Smith T, Walters RS, McCredie KB, Trujillo J and Freireich EJ: Toward a clinically relevant cytogenetic classification of acute myelogenous leukemia. Leukemia Res 1987 11(2):119-133

6 Rowley JD: A new consistent chromosomal abnormality in chronic myelogenous leukaemia identified by quinacrine fluorescence and Giemsa staining [Letter]. Nature 1973 (243):290-293

7 Kantarjian HM, Keating MJ, Walters RS, McCredie KB, Smith TL, Talpaz M, Beran M, Cork A, Trujillo JM and Freireich EJ: Clinical and prognostic features of Philadelphia chromosome-negative chronic myelogenous leukemia. Cancer 1986 (58):2023-2030

8 Whang-Peng J, Canellos GP, Carbone PP and Tjio JH: Clinical implications of cytogenetic variants in chronic myelocytic leukemia (CML). Blood 1968 (32/5):755-766

9 de Klein A, Geurts van Kessel A, Grosveld G, Bartram CR, Hagemeijer A, Bootsma D, Spurr NK, Heisterkamp N, Groffen J and Stephenson JR: A cellular oncogene is translocated to the Philadelphia chromosome in chronic myelocytic leukaemia. Nature 1982 (300):765-767

10 Groffen J, Stephenson JR, Heisterkamp N, de Klein A, Bartram CR and Grosveld G: Philadelphia chromosomal breakpoints are clustered within a limited region, bcr, on chromosome 22. Cell 1984 (36):93-99

11 Canaani E, Gale RP, Steinder-Saltz D, Berrebi A, Aghai E and Januszewicz E: Altered transcription of an oncogene in chronic myeloid leukaemia. Lancet 1984 (i):593-595

12 Konopka JB, Watanabe SM, Singer JW, Collins SJ and Witte ON: Cell lines and clinical isolates derived from Ph^1-positive chronic myelogenous leukemia patients express c-abl proteins with a common structural alteration. Proc Nat Acad Sci USA 1985 (82):1810-1814

13 Kantarjian HM, Talpaz M and Gutterman JU: Chronic myelogenous leukemia-past, present, and future. Hematol Pathol 1988 (2/2):91-120

14 Cunningham I, Gee T, Dowling M, Chaganti R, Bailey R, Hopfan S, Bowden L, Turnbull A, Knapper W and Clarkson B: Results of treatment of Ph^1 + chronic myelogenous leukemia with an intensive treatment regimen (L-5 protocol). Blood 1979 (53):375-396

15 Kantarjian HM, Vellekoop K, McCredie KB, Keating MJ, Hester J, Smith T, Barlogie B, Trujillo J and Freireich EJ: Intensive combination chemotherapy (ROAP) and splenectomy in the management of chronic myelogenous leukemia. J Clin Oncol 1985 (3):192-200

16 Talpaz M, McCredie K, Mavligit GM and Gutterman JU: Leukocyte interferon-induced myeloid cytoreduction in chronic myelogenous leukemia. Blood 1983 (62):689-692

17 Kantarjian HM, Shtalrid M, Kurzrock R, Blick M, Dalton WT, LeMaistre A, Stass SA, McCredie KB, Gutterman J, Freireich EJ and Talpaz M: Significance and correlations of molecular analysis results in patients with Philadelphia chromosome-negative chronic myelogenous leukemia and chronic myelomonocytic leukemia. Am J Med 1988 (85):639-643

18 Lee M-S, Chang K-S, Cabanillas F, Freireich EJ, Trujillo JM and Stass SA: Detection of minimal residual cells carrying the t(14;18) by DNA sequence amplification. Science 1987 (237):175-178

19 Lee M-S, Chang K-S, Freireich EJ, Kantarjian HM, Talpaz M, Trujillo JM and and Stass SA: Detection of minimal residual bcr/abl transcripts by a modified polymerase chain reaction. Blood 1988 72(3):893-897

20 Lee M-S, LeMaistre A, Kantarjian HM, Talpaz M, Freireich EJ, Trujillo JM and Stass SA: Detection of two alternative bcr/abl mRNA junctions and minimal residual disease in Philadelphia chromosome positive chronic myelogenous leukemia by polymerase chain reaction. Blood 1989 (73/8):2165-2170

21 Thomas ED, Clift RA, Fefer A, Appelbaum FR, Beatty P, Bensinger WI, Buckner CD, Cheever MA, Deeg J, Doney K, Flournoy N, Greenberg P, Hansen JA, Martin P, McGuffin R, Ramberg R, Sanders JE, Singer J, Stewart P, Storb R, Sullivan K, Weiden PL and Witherspoon R: Marrow transplantation for the treatment of chronic myelogenous leukemia. Ann Intern Med 1986 (104):155-163

22 McGlave P, Arthur D, Haake R, Hurd D, Miller W, Vercellotti G, Weisdorf D, Kim T, Ramsay N and Kersey J: Therapy of chronic myelogenous leukemia with allogeneic bone marrow transplantation. J Clin Oncol 1987 (5):1033-1040

23 Roth MS, Antin JH, Bingham EL and Ginsburg D: Detection of Philadelphia chromosome-positive cells by the polymerase chain reaction following bone marrow transplant for chronic myelogenous leukemia. Blood 1989 74(2):882-885

24 Ely P and Miller W: Patterns of detection of bcr/abl mRNA following bone marrow transplantation for chronic myelogenous leukemia. Clin Res 1989 (37/2):544A

25 Sandberg AA: Cytogenetic data and prognosis in acute leukemia. In Therapy of Acute Leukemias, Mandelli F (ed), Proceedings of International Symposium, Rome, Lombardo Editore, 1977 pp 186-192

26 Freireich EJ, Cork MA, Stass SA, Bahrych S, McCredie KB, Keating MJ, Estey EH, Kantarjian HM and Trujillo JM: Cytogenetics for detection of

minimal residual disease in acute myeloblastic leukemia (AML). Blood 1988 72(5) 708a

27 Trujillo JM, Cork A, Ahearn MJ, Youness EL and McCredie KB: Hematologic and cytologic characterization of 8/21 translocation acute granulocytic leukemia. Blood 1979 53(4):695-706

28 Rowley JD, Golomb HM and Dougherty C: 15/17 translocation, a consistent chromosomal change in acute promyelocytic leukemia. Lancet 1977 (i):549

29 Holmes R, Keating MJ, Cork A, Broach Y, Trujillo JM, Dalton WT, McCredie KB and Freireich EJ: A unique pattern of central nervous system leukemia in acute myelomonocytic leukemia associated with inv (16) (p13q22). Blood 1985 (65/5):1071-1078

30 Kantarjian HM, Keating MJ, Walters RS, McCredie KB and Freireich EJ: The characteristics and outcome of patients with late relapse acute myelogenous leukemia. J Clin Oncol 1988 (6/2):232-238

31 Chang KS, Schroeder W, Siciliano MJ, Thompson LH, McCredie KB, Beran M, Freireich EJ, Liang JC, Trujillo JM and Stass SA: The localization of the human myeloperoxidase gene is in close proximity to the translocation breakpoint in acute promyelocytic leukemia. Leukemia 1987 1(5):458-462

32 Liang JC, Chang K-S, Schroeder WT, Freireich EJ, Stass SA and Trujillo JM: The myeloperoxidase gene is translocated from chromosome 17 to 15 in a patient with acute promyelocytic leukemia. Cancer Genet Cytogenet 1988 (30):103-107

33 Le Beau MM, Lemons RS, Espinosa III R, Larson RA, Arai N and Rowley JD: Interleukin-4 and interleukin-5 map to human chromosome 5 in a region encoding growth factors and receptors and are deleted in myeloid leukemias with a del(5q). Blood 1989 73(3):647-650

34 Knudson Jr AG: Hereditary cancer, oncogenes, and antioncogenes. Cancer Res 1985 (45)1437-1443

35 Friend SH, Dryja TP and Weinberg RA: Oncogenes and tumor-suppressing genes. N Engl J Med 1988 (318):618-622

36 Nowell PC, Besa EC, Stelmach T and Finan J: Chromosome studies in preleukemic states. V. Prognostic significance of single versus multiple abnormalities. Cancer 1986 (58):2571-2575

37 Estey EH, Keating MJ, Dixon DO, Trujillo JM, McCredie KB and Freireich EJ: Karyotype is prognostically more important than the FAB system's distinction between myelodysplastic syndrome and acute myelogenous leukemia. Hematologic Pat. 1987 (1/4):203-208

38 Liu R, Hjelle B, Morgan R, Hecht F and Bishop JM: Mutations of the Kirsten-RAS proto-oncogene in human preleukemia. Nature 1987 (330):186-188

39 LeMaistre A, Lee MS, Talpaz M, Kantarjian HM, Freireich EJ, Deisseroth AB, Trujillo JM and Stass SA: RAS oncogene mutations are rare late stage events in chronic myelogenous leukemia. Blood 1989 (73/4):889-891

40 Bos JL: RAS oncogenes in human cancer: A review. Cancer Res 1989 (49):4682-4689

41 Bloomfield CD, Goldman AI, Alimena G, Berger R, Borgstrom GH, Brandt L, Catovsky D, de la Chapelle A, Dewald GW, Garson OM, Garwicz S, Golomb HM, Hossfeld DK, Lawler SD, Mitelman F, Nilsson P, Pierre RU, Philip P, Prigogina E, Rowley JD, Sakurai M, Sandberg AA, Secker Walker LM, Tricot G, Van Den Berghe H, Van Orshoven A, Vuopio P and Whang-Peng J: Chromosomal abnormalities identify high-risk and low-risk patients with acute lymphoblastic leukemia. Blood 1986 (67):415-420

42 Hooberman AL, Rubin CM, Barton KP and Westbrook CA: Detection of the Philadelphia chromosome in acute lymphoblastic leukemia by pulsed-field gel electrophoresis. Blood 1989 (74/3):1101-1107

43 Yamada M, Hudson S, Tournay O, Bittenbender S, Shane SS, Lange B, Tsujimoto Y, Caton AJ and Rovera G: Detection of minimal disease in hematopoietic malignancies of the B-cell lineage by using third-complementarity-determining region (CDR-III)-specific probes. Proc Natl Acad Sci USA 1989 (86):5123-5127

Recent Advances in Chemotherapy for Certain Leukaemias

Peter H. Wiernik

Albert Einstein Cancer Center, Montefiore Medical Center, 111 East 210th Street, New York, NY 10467, U.S.A.

Major advances in the chemotherapy of some leukaemias have recently been achieved. Although new combinations of established agents have contributed to these advances, the discovery of new agents with major antileukaemic activity has been primarily responsible for recently reported improved treatment results.

Acute Myeloid Leukaemia

Therapy for acute myeloid leukaemia (AML) has been considerably improved recently as a result of the development of new, promising agents, including some with unique presumed mechanisms of action.

Mitoxantrone

Mitoxantrone (dihydroxyanthracenedione), an anthraquinone, has significant activity against AML. This activity was noted in early phase I trials [1] and subsequently confirmed in phase II trials in relapsed patients [2,3]. Mitoxantrone, 10 mg/m^2, given daily for 3 days as a brief intravenous infusion together with a continuous 7-day infusion of cytarabine at the standard rate of 100 mg/m^2 day, yielded a 65.5% complete response rate in 32 patients in first relapse of AML and a 23% complete response rate in 13 patients who were refractory to initial therapy with an anthracycline and cytarabine [4].

More recently, mitoxantrone, 12 mg/m^2, and daunorubicin, 45 mg/m^2, each given daily for 3 days in conjunction with the standard cytarabine infusion described above, were compared in a randomised multicentre trial of previously untreated adult patients with AML and a median age of 60 years [5]. Mitoxantrone plus cytarabine (M+A) was given to 98 evaluable patients and 102 received daunorubicin plus cytarabine (D+A). Post-remission therapy consisted of 2 consolidation courses of cytarabine for 5 days with either mitoxantrone or daunorubicin administered for 2 days during each course. Complete remission was obtained in 63% of patients who received M+A and 53% of patients treated with D+A. The difference was not significant. However, 89% of complete responders required only 1 course of M+A, whereas only 68% of complete responders to D+A achieved remission with a single treatment course. There was no significant difference in response duration or survival of all treated patients or of responding patients, and there were no significant differences in frequency or severity of toxicities between the two regimens. The study suggests that M+A may be better treatment than D+A for previously untreated patients with AML since response rate and treatment time necessary for response favour M+A, especially in patients less than 60 years of age.

A combination of mitoxantrone, 12 mg/m^2/day, and etoposide, 100 mg/m^2/day, both given for 5 days, yielded a 44% complete response rate in 34 patients with AML in first relapse, with a median duration of complete response of 5.3 months [6]. The regimen was much less effective in patients who were refractory to initial induction therapy. Although the regimen is active, it is difficult to compare these results with results of other treatments since the distribution of prognostic factors among the patients studied has not yet been published.

Idarubicin

Idarubicin (4-demethoxydaunorubicin) is a synthesised analogue of daunorubicin that lacks the methoxyl group in position 4 of the aglycone of the parent compound. The new analogue is significantly more active against certain mouse leukaemias than daunorubicin [7]. Phase I studies in leukaemia patients employing a 3-day schedule recommend a dose of 8-12 mg/m^2/day [8-10], and the significant antileukaemic activity observed was subsequently confirmed in phase II trials of pediatric and adult patients with AML and acute lymphocytic leukaemia [10,11]. In 8 phase II trials of intravenous idarubicin in which 132 relapsed or refractory pediatric and adult ALL and AML patients were included [11], an overall complete response rate of 47% was obtained. When 150 previously untreated patients with AML or ALL were treated with idarubicin and cytarabine on various schedules with or without other drugs, a complete response rate of 81% was observed.

Several trials of cytarabine plus idarubicin (I+A) compared with cytarabine plus daunorubicin (D+A) in previously untreated patients with AML have now been completed in the United States. Those studies utilised a daily x 3 schedule of idarubicin with an intravenous dose of 12-13 mg/m^2. Two studies [12,13] employed the standard dose of cytarabine and one utilised cytarabine for 5 days at a dose of 200 mg/m^2/day [14]. All studies utilised the 3-day schedule of daunorubicin, 45 mg/m^2 [12,13] or 50 mg/m^2 daily [14]. In all 3 randomised studies, the complete response rate is higher with I+A than with D+A and in one of the studies [14], the difference is significant (I+A=80%, D+A=58%, p=0.03). The median duration of remission in the Memorial study was greater in the I+A group (p=0.07) and survival was significantly better in the I+A group than in the D+A group (p=0.01). In the multicentre study [12], which is the largest, the median duration of complete remission was significantly longer with I+A compared to D+A (285 vs. 256 days, p=0.021), as was the median duration of survival of all treated patients (393 vs. 281 days, p=0.04). In that study, 78% of patients randomised to I+A and 65% of patients randomised to D+A achieved complete remission with one induction course (p=0.10). There was no major difference in toxicity between the groups treated with I+A and D+A in any of the studies [12-14]. These data suggest that I+A is more effective remission induction therapy for adults with AML than is D+A.

Carboplatinum

Although cisplatin has no useful role in the treatment of acute leukaemia, a recent study suggests that carboplatinum may have significant antileukaemic activity [15].

Carboplatinum was given as a 5-day continuous infusion at the rate of 155 mg/m^2/day initially, and doses were escalated in some patients. Six complete and 2 partial responses (28.5% overall response rate) were achieved in 28 patients with relapsed leukaemia. Extramedullary toxicity was minimal. The Eastern Cooperative Oncology Group is currently exploring the activity of carboplatinum in acute leukaemia as a result of this interesting study.

Etoposide

The Australian Leukaemia Study Group [16] studied the effect of adding etoposide to D+A for induction therapy of AML. A standard 7-day infusion of cytarabine was used together with daunorubicin at a dose of 50 mg/m^2/day for 3 days. Patients were randomised to have or not have etoposide, 75 mg/m^2 daily for 7 days added to the regimen. There was no difference in the remission induction rate between the two regimens in 264 patients. However, remission duration was significantly better with the 3 drugs. Furthermore, in patients less than 55 years old, the 3-drug regimen resulted in a significantly better overall survival for all treated patients, compared with the 2-drug regimen. Further study of the 3-drug regimen is clearly warranted.

Trans-Retinoic Acid

Chinese investigators [17] reported a remarkable 100% complete remission rate in 24 patients with acute promyelocytic leukaemia (APL) with all-trans retinoic acid. Eight patients were resistant to or relapsed from prior chemotherapy and 16 others were previously untreated. All patients achieved a complete remission without developing bone marrow hypoplasia. Eight patients relapsed after 2-5 months and the others were in remission from 1+ to 11+ months at the time of their report. Toxicity was minimal and no patients experienced a clinically evident haemorrhagic diathesis.

Those results have been confirmed and extended by Degos et al. [18]. They treated 20 patients with APL with oral trans-retinoic acid, 45 mg/m^2 daily for 3 months. Sixteen patients were relapsed, 2 were primarily resistant, and 2 were previously untreated. Complete responses were observed in 14 patients (64%) after 30-90 days of treatment. Toxicity was identical to that described by the Chinese investigators [17]. Virtually all clinical responders demonstrated differentiation induction in *in vitro* studies of their leukaemia cells. These data are exciting because they suggest that leukaemic cell differentiation sufficient enough to produce complete remission may be reproducibly obtained in the clinic without significant cytotoxicity. This agent is currently under investigation in the United States.

Additional Agents of Interest

Two new anthracyclines have shown sufficient activity against AML to merit further study. Esorubicin (4'-deoxydoxorubicin) differs from the parent compound, doxorubicin, in that the amino-sugar moiety of the former has been modified at the 4'-position by replacing the hydroxyl radical with 2 hydrogens. As a result, the new agent is more lipophilic than its parent and drug uptake by certain tumour cells is enhanced. Preclinical studies suggest that esorubicin is a more potent antileukaemic agent and less cardiotoxic than doxorubicin. In a phase I-II trial which included 14 evaluable patients with relapsed or refractory AML, a 28.5% partial response rate was obtained with esorubicin [19]. Two partial responders were refractory to prior therapy with other anthracyclines, and the other two responders were in second relapse. The pharmacokinetics of the new agent were similar to those of doxorubicin in that study. This agent deserves evaluation in less advanced patients in a phase III study. The recommended dose for further study as a single agent is 16 mg/m^2 daily for 5 days [19].

Menogaril is a semi-synthetic derivative of the antitumour antibiotic, nogalamycin. Nogalamycin analogues differ structurally from the other anthracyclines due to the attachment of the sugar moiety to the D rather than the A ring. Menogaril, unlike other anthracyclines, forms only a weak bond to DNA and does not inhibit DNA or RNA polymerases. The mechanism of action of menogaril is unknown, but is presumably different from traditional anthracyclines [20]. This drug was also less cardiotoxic and more active against animal leukaemias than standard anthracyclines. In a phase I-II study by Dutcher et al. [21], a response rate similar to that of esorubicin was observed in a similar population of patients. However, complete responses were documented with menogaril. The agent will undergo a confirmatory phase II study shortly in the Eastern Cooperative Oncology Group (ECOG) at a dose of 100 mg/m^2 daily for 5 days.

Perhaps even more interesting is the significant antileukaemic activity noted for taxol in a phase I trial [22]. Taxol is a unique antimicrotubule agent that has shown significant activity against previously treated ovarian cancer [23] and melanoma [24]. The non-haematologic toxicity of this natural product is relatively mild and it is therefore highly suitable for further study in leukaemia. The ECOG will soon conduct a phase II trial of this agent in AML also.

Hairy Cell Leukaemia

The results of the first major interinstitutional study of interferon in hairy cell leukaemia (HCL) have recently been updated [25] after a median follow-up of 36 months. Seven complete and 152 partial responses were obtained in 195 patients after treatment with alpha-2b interferon, 2 million units/m^2 given thrice weekly. Fourteen of 25 patients with little or no response have expired, whereas only 3 patients who achieved a partial response or better have died.

Durrleman et al. [26] reviewed 60 HCL patients treated with 2'-deoxycoformycin (DCF) after failure of alpha interferon. A complete response was obtained in 22 (37%) and partial responses were observed in an equal number. Responses were, as expected, durable. This report confirmed the previous observations of Spiers et al. [27] that DCF was more productive of complete remissions in HCL than was alpha interferon. However, in a small study reported by Wiernik et al. [28], beta-ser interferon, 90 million units thrice weekly, yielded a complete response rate in HCL comparable to that of DCF. In that study, 7 complete and 3 partial responses were obtained in 12 patients. Most of the patients had had a splenectomy or chemotherapy prior to entry into the study. The responses have been durable, ranging from 26+ to 40+ months.

Many recent studies have continued the investigation of the role of DCF in HCL after failure of interferon. Haberman et al. [29] found that the sequential use of alpha-2a interferon and DCF reduced the early infectious complication rate below that observed in some studies of DCF alone and yielded response rates comparable to those obtained with DCF. Others have found that alternating treatment with leucocyte A interferon and DCF leads to a lower complete response rate than that obtained with DCF treatment alone [30]. Chun et al. [31] reported that only one of 31 alpha interferon failures had progressive disease when subsequently treated with DCF, and that 13 of the patients obtained a complete or partial response. Dutcher et al. [32] reported 3 patients who failed alpha or beta interferon who, when treated with DCF, obtained complete responses of 11+ to 30+ months' duration, and Holland et al. [33] have confirmed the high response rate and durable remissions achieved with DCF in patients who are intolerant or resistant to alpha interferon. It seems clear from these studies that DCF is superior to alpha interferon for the treatment of HCL. The relative merits of beta-ser interferon and of sequential therapy with interferon followed by DCF requires further study.

Piro et al. [34] studied 2-chlorodeoxyadenosine (CDA) in 12 patients with HCL and produced results at least comparable to those obtained with DCF, but with less treatment. CDA was administered as a 7-day continuous infusion at a dose of 0.1 mg/kg/day and not repeated. Eleven complete responses were obtained. None of the patients has relapsed after a median duration of response of 15.5 months (maximum observation, 3.8 years). No serious toxicity of CDA was observed. This study strongly suggests that CDA is the most effective and least toxic therapy for HCL described to date. Confirmatory studies will be of major interest.

Chronic Lymphocytic Leukaemia

Chronic lymphocytic leukaemia (CLL) has also yielded to a significant degree to several new agents. CDA was first studied in this disease, and the early report of Piro et al. [35] has recently been updated. They treated 30 evaluable, previously treated B-CLL patients with advanced and progressive disease with CDA, 0.05-0.015 mg/kg/day given as a continuous 7-day intravenous infusion. Unlike HCL patients, however, the CLL patients were retreated monthly for a median of 3 courses. Sixteen major responses were obtained, of which 2 were complete and 14 were partial. The median duration of the responses was 4 months. Four of 6 patients with Coombs-positive haemolytic anaemia had resolution of haemolysis. Less impressive results were reported by others in T-CLL [36]. On the whole, it would appear that CDA is less active in CLL than in HCL. On the other hand, CLL patients treated to date have had more advanced disease for significantly longer time than HCL patients studied. The study of CDA in previously untreated patients will be of major interest.

DCF, another major new drug for HCL, has also been studied in B-CLL [37,38] and found to be active. More than three-quarters of the 29 patients studied by Ho et al. [37] were in Rai stage 4 and heavily pretreated, and 7 achieved a partial response with a median duration of 6.5 months. These results may be comparable to those obtained with CDA by others.

Fludarabine, a fluorinated adenosine analogue, has been extensively studied in CLL after Keating et al. [39] reported its major activity. Recent reports suggest that overall response rates of 40-50% with complete response rates of 10-15% are routinely obtained in B-CLL [40,41]. More importantly, true complete responses identified by immunophenotype and molecular studies are obtained in some CLL patients with fludarabine [41]. Complete response rates may be lower in heavily previously treated patients with advanced disease who are treated with less than usual dose intensity [32].

Conclusion

The steady erosion of resistance to curability that has characterised the last 35 years of clinical research in AML continues, largely due to the development of new drugs with greater antileukaemic activity and therapeutic index than their predecessors. During the same period, there has been little, if any, real progress in the treatment of HCL and CLL until recently. Several new agents with major activity against these chronic leukaemias have now been described, and they promise to change the natural history of these deadly illnesses.

REFERENCES

1 Van Echo DA, Whitacre MY, Aisner J, Wiernik PH: A phase I trial of dihydroxyanthracenedione. Cancer Treat Rep 1981 (65):831-834

2 Prentice HG, Robbins G, Ma DD, Ho AD: Sequential studies on the role of mitoxantrone in the treatment of acute leukaemia. Cancer Treat Rev 1983 (10 Suppl B):57-63

3 Arlin ZA, Silver R, Cassileth P: Phase I-II trials of mitoxantrone in acute leukemia. Cancer Treat Rep 1985 (69):61-64

4 Paciucci PA, Dutcher JP, Cuttner J et al: Mitoxantrone and Ara-C in previously treated patients with acute myelogenous leukemia. Leukemia 1987 (1):565-567

5 Arlin Z, Case DC Jr, Moore J et al: Randomized multicenter trial of cytosine arabinoside with mitoxantrone or daunorubicin in previously untreated adult patients with acute nonlymphocytic leukemia (ANLL). Leukemia 1990 (4):177-183

6 Rowe JM, Mazza JJ, Hines JD et al: Mitoxantrone (MITOX) and etoposide (VP-16-213) in patients with relapsed and refractory acute non-lymphocytic leukemia (ANLL). Proc Am Soc Clin Oncol 1990 (9):209

7 Casazza AM, Pratesi G, Giuliani F et al: Antileukemic activity of 4-demethoxydaunorubicin in mice. Tumori 1980 (66):549-564

8 Hayat M, Huterloup P, Parmentier C: Phase I trial of idarubicin (4-demethoxydaunorubicin) in adult acute leukemia. Invest New Drugs 1984 (2):375-378

9 Sessa C, Tschopp L, Lopp M, Cavalli F: Phase I trials of 4-demethoxydaunorubicin in acute leukemia. Invest New Drugs 1985 (3):357-361

10 Daghestani AN, Arlin ZA, Leyland-Jones B et al: Phase I-II clinical and pharmacology study of 4-demethoxydaunorubicin (idarubicin) in adult patients with acute leukemia. Cancer Res 1985 (45):1408-1410

11 Carella AM, Berman E, Maraone MP, Ganzina T: Idarubicin in the treatment of acute leukemias: An overview of preclinical and clinical studies. Haematologica 1990 (75):1-11

12 Wiernik PH, Case DC Jr, Periman PO et al: A multicenter trial of cytarabine plus idarubicin or daunorubicin as induction therapy for adult nonlymphocytic leukemia. Semin Oncol 1989 (16 Suppl 2):25-29

13 Vogler WR, Velez-Garcia E, Omura G et al: A phase three trial comparing daunorubicin or idarubicin combined with cytosine arabinoside in acute myelogenous leukemia. Semin Oncol 1989 (16 Suppl 2):21-24

14 Berman E, Raymond V, Gee T et al: Idarubicin in acute leukemia: Results of studies at Memorial Sloan-Kettering Cancer Center. Semin Oncol 1989 (16 Suppl 2):30-34

15 Myers FJ, Welborn J, Lewis JP, Flynn N: Infusion carboplatin treatment of relapsed and refractory acute leukemia: Evidence of efficacy with minimal extramedullary toxicity at intermediate doses. J Clin Oncol 1989 (7):173-178

16 Bishop JF, Lowenthal RM, Jochua D et al: Etoposide in acute nonlymphocytic leukemia. Blood 1990 (75):27-32

17 Meng-er H, Yu-Chen Y, Shu-song C et al: Use of all-trans retinoic acid in the treatment of acute promyelocytic leukemia. Blood 1988 (72):567-572

18 Degos L, Chomienne C, Ballerini P et al: All-trans retinoic acid: A novel differentiation therapy for acute promyelocytic leukemia. Proc Am Soc Clin Oncol 1990 (9):207

19 Dutcher JP, Riggs CE, Strauman JJ et al: A phase I-II trial of 4'-deoxydoxorubicin (esorubicin) in refractory or relapsed acute leukemia. Clin Pharmacol Ther 1989 (45):424-428

20 McGovern JP, Nelson KG, Lassus M et al: Menogaril: A new anthracycline agent entering clinical trials. Invest New Drugs 1984 (2):359-367

21 Dutcher JP, Wiernik PH: unpublished data

22 Rowinsky EK, Burke PJ, Karp JE et al: Phase I and pharmacodynamic study of taxol in refractory acute leukemias. Cancer Res 1989 (49):4640-4647

23 McGuire WP, Rowinsky EK, Rosenshein NB et al: Taxol: A unique antineoplastic agent with significant activity in advanced ovarian epithelial neoplasms. Ann Intern Med 1989 (111):273-279

24 Wiernik PH, Schwartz EL, Einzig A et al: Phase I trial of taxol given as a 24-hour infusion every 21 days: responses observed in metastatic melanoma. J Clin Oncol 1987 (5):1232-1239

25 Golumb H, Fefer A, Golde D et al: Update of a multi-institutional study of 195 patients (PTS) with hairy cell leukemia (HCL) treated with interferon alfa-2b (IFN). Proc Am Soc Clin Oncol 1990 (9):215

26 Durrleman S, Grem JL, Cheson BD: 2'-deoxycoformycin after failure of alpha-interferon in hairy cell leukemia. Eur J Haematol 1989 (43):297-302

27 Spiers ASD, Moore D, Cassileth PA et al: Remissions in hairy cell leukemia with pentostatin (2'-deoxycoformycin). N Engl J Med 1987 (316):8825-8830

28 Wiernik PH, Schwartz B, Dutcher JP et al: Successful treatment of hairy cell leukemia with B-ser interferon. Am J Hematol 1990 (33):244-248

29 Habermann T, Vangeneugden T, Cassileth P et al: A phase II trial for the evaluation of recombinant alpha-2a interferon (Roferon-A) followed by 2'-deoxycoformycin (pentostatin) (dCF) in the therapy of hairy cell leukemia in previously splenectomized patients. Proc Am Soc Clin Oncol 1990 (9):211

30 Martin A, Nerenstone S, Urba WJ et al: Treatment of hairy cell leukemia with alternating cycles of pentostatin and recombinant leukocyte A interferon: Results of a phase II study. J Clin Oncol 1990 (8):721-730

31 Chun HG, Grem J, Vena A et al: Treatment of active hairy cell leukemia (HCL) refractory or intolerant to alpha interferon (IFN-A) with pentostatin under the group C protocol. Proc Am Soc Clin Oncol 1990 (9):214

32 Dutcher JP, Salva K, Wiernik PH: Successful treatment of hairy cell leukemia with 2'-deoxycoformycin after failure of interferons alpha or beta. Am J Clin Oncol 1990 (in press)

33 Holland DR, Connors JM, Gascoyne RD: Superior quality and duration of response to deoxycoformycin in hairy cell leukemia patients previously exposed to alpha-interferon. Proc Am Soc Clin Oncol 1990 (9):202
34 Piro LD, Carrera CJ, Garson DA, Beutler E: Lasting remissions in hairy-cell leukemia induced by a single infusion of 2-chlorodeoxyadenosine. N Engl J Med 1990 (322):1117-1121
35 Saven A, Carrera CJ, Garson DA et al: Phase II trial update of 2-chloroadenosine treatment of advanced chronic lymphocytic leukemia. Proc Am Soc Clin Oncol 1990 (9):212
36 Estey E, Freireich E, Koller C et al: Treatment of advanced, refractory T-cell CLL with 2-chlorodeoxyadenosine (2CdA). Proc Am Assoc Cancer Res 1990 (31):191
37 Ho AD, Thaler J, Stryckmans P et al: Pentostatin in resistant chronic lymphocytic leukemia - A phase II trial of the European Organization for Research and Treatment of Cancer. Proc Am Soc Clin Oncol 1990 (9):206
38 Dillman RO, Mick R, McIntyre OR: Pentostatin in chronic lymphocytic leukemia: A phase II trial of Cancer and Leukemia Group B. J Clin Oncol 1989 (7):433-438
39 Keating MJ, Kantarjian H, Talpaz M et al: Fludarabine: A new agent with major activity against chronic lymphocytic leukemia. Blood 1989 (74):19-25
40 Reich SD, Tessman DK: Analysis of two studies of fludarabine, a drug active against chronic lymphocytic leukemia (CLL), using the new NCI guidelines for response. Proc Am Soc Clin Oncol 1990 (9):214
41 Robertson L, Huh Y, Horsch-Ginsberg C et al: Immunophenotypic assessment of response in chronic lymphocytic leukemia after fludarabine (FLU). Proc Am Soc Clin Oncol 1990 (9):205
42 Puccio C, Mittelman A, Lichtman S et al: Phase II study of fludarabine phosphate (FAMP) in chronic lymphocytic leukemia (CLL). Proc Am Soc Clin Oncol 1990 (9):206

MIX
Papier aus verantwortungsvollen Quellen
Paper from responsible sources
FSC® C105338

If you have any concerns about our products, you can contact us on
ProductSafety@springernature.com

In case Publisher is established outside the EU, the EU authorized representative is:
Springer Nature Customer Service Center GmbH
Europaplatz 3, 69115 Heidelberg, Germany

Printed by Libri Plureos GmbH
in Hamburg, Germany